Forensic Odontology

Sam Evans
To Emma, Jacob, Zach, Eli and Mabel

Romina Carabott
To Lee

Forensic Odontology: An Essential Guide

Edited by

Catherine Adams
UKDVI & Powys Teaching Health Board, UK

Romina Carabott
expertFORENSICS Ltd, Cardiff, UK

Sam Evans
School of Dentistry, Cardiff University, UK

WILEY Blackwell

Registered office: John Wiley & Sons, Ltd, The Atrium, Southern Gate, Chichester, West Sussex, PO19 8SQ, UK

Editorial offices: 9600 Garsington Road, Oxford, OX4 2DQ, UK
The Atrium, Southern Gate, Chichester, West Sussex, PO19 8SQ, UK
111 River Street, Hoboken, NJ 07030-5774, USA

For details of our global editorial offices, for customer services and for information about how to apply for permission to reuse the copyright material in this book please see our website at www.wiley.com/wiley-blackwell.

Library of Congress Cataloging-in-Publication Data

Forensic odontology (Adams)
Forensic odontology : an essential guide / [edited by] Catherine Adams, Romina Carabott, and Sam Evans.
p. ; cm.
Includes bibliographical references and index.
ISBN 978-1-119-96145-1 (cloth)
I. Adams, Catherine, 1960- editor of compilation. II. Carabott, Romina, editor of compilation. III. Evans, Sam, 1976- editor of compilation. IV. Title.
[DNLM: 1. Forensic Dentistry–methods. W 705]
RA1062
614′.18–dc23

2013024348

A catalogue record for this book is available from the British Library.

Wiley also publishes its books in a variety of electronic formats. Some content that appears in print may not be available in electronic books.

Typeset in 10/12pt Times-Roman by Laserwords Private Limited, Chennai, India.

1 2014

Contents

List of contributors **xi**

Acknowledgements **xiii**

1 Brief introduction to forensic odontology **1**
Romina Carabott

1.1 Introduction 1
1.2 Forensic odontology in the 21st century 3
1.3 Training and experience 4
1.4 How to use this book 6
1.5 References 6

2 Development of the dentition **9**
Alastair J. Sloan

2.1 Early tooth development 9
2.2 Later tooth development 13
2.3 Dentinogenesis 14
2.4 Tooth root formation 16
2.5 Epithelial/mesenchymal interactions in tooth development 17
2.6 Amelogenesis 19
2.7 Biomineralisation of enamel 20
2.8 Further reading 21

3 Acting as an expert witness **23**
Jason Tucker

3.1 Introduction 23
3.2 The nature of expert evidence 23
3.2.1 What is evidence? 23
3.2.2 What is expert evidence? 24
3.2.3 Who can act as an expert witness? 25
3.2.4 The expert witness's role in court proceedings 25
3.3 The rules of court 26
3.3.1 Why is expert evidence governed by rules of court? 26
3.3.2 Which rules apply? 26
3.3.3 Key differences between the procedural regimes 27

3.4 The expert's duties 28
3.4.1 The Ikarian Reefer 28
3.4.2 The overriding duty 29
3.4.3 The particular duties 29
3.5 Report writing 30
3.5.1 The content of an expert's report 31
3.5.2 Drafting your reports: Some suggestions 32
3.5.3 The required declarations 34
3.6 Giving evidence at court 36
3.6.1 The process of giving evidence 37
3.6.2 Questioning 38
3.6.3 Addressing the court 40
3.7 Ancillary topics 41
3.7.1 Written questions to experts 41
3.7.2 Experts' meetings and 'hot tubbing' 42
3.7.3 Obtaining directions from the court 43
3.7.4 Acting as a single joint expert 43
3.7.5 Getting feedback on your work 44
3.7.6 Keeping up to date 44
3.8 Things to avoid 45
3.8.1 Being sued for negligence 45
3.8.2 Being reported for misconduct 46
3.8.3 Wasted-costs orders 47
3.8.4 Contempt and perjury 47
3.9 A final thought 47
3.10 References 48

4 Mortuary practice **49**
Alison Anderson

4.1 Definitions of a mortuary 49
4.1.1 Permanent mortuary 49
4.1.2 Emergency mortuary 49
4.2 The Human Tissue Act and the Human Tissue Authority 50
4.3 Legal requirements for licence issue 51
4.3.1 Designated individuals 52
4.3.2 Licence holders 52
4.4 Mortuary facilities 52
4.4.1 Mortuary layout 52
4.4.2 Mortuary equipment 54
4.5 The Anatomical Pathology Technologist 54
4.5.1 Training and qualifications of APTs 55
4.5.2 Responsibilities of APTs 55
4.6 The odontologist in the mortuary: Specialist resection techniques 56
4.7 Health and safety in the mortuary 57
4.7.1 Safe working practices 58
4.7.2 Hygiene 59
4.7.3 Personal protective equipment (PPE) 60
4.7.4 Cleaning and decontamination 60
4.7.5 Waste disposal 61
4.7.6 Immunisation 62
4.8 References 62

5 Dental human identification 65
Romina Carabott

5.1 Introduction 65
5.1.1 Why is human identification necessary? 65
5.1.2 Why comparative dental analysis? 66
5.1.3 What if there is no presumptive identification? 67
5.1.4 When does the forensic dentist 'come on the scene'? 68
5.2 Comparative dental identification 70
5.2.1 Post-mortem examination 70
5.2.2 Incinerated remains 77
5.2.3 Ante-mortem data collection 78
5.2.4 Reconciliation: The comparative process 80
5.2.5 Problems with comparative dental identification 85
5.3 Radiography in dental identification 87
5.3.1 Post-mortem radiography 89
5.3.2 Ante-mortem radiographs 91
5.3.3 Computed tomography 93
5.4 Dental appliances in identification 93
5.4.1 Dental models (casts) 94
5.4.2 Palatal rugae 95
5.4.3 Removable appliances 96
5.4.4 Denture marking 97
5.4.5 Bleaching trays 99
5.4.6 Fixed prostheses 99
5.5 Dental profiling 100
5.5.1 Gender 101
5.5.2 Ethnicity 101
5.5.3 Age assessment 102
5.5.4 Habits 102
5.5.5 Developmental tooth anomalies 103
5.5.6 Fluorosis 103
5.5.7 Tetracycline staining 105
5.5.8 Isotope and trace element analysis 105
5.5.9 Dental restorations 106
5.5.10 Facial reconstruction 106
5.5.11 Craniofacial superimposition 107
5.6 Teeth as a source of DNA 107
5.7 Conclusion 110
5.8 References 110

6 Disaster victim identification 117
Catherine Adams

6.1 Introduction 117
6.2 Disaster management 118
6.3 DVI planning 119
6.4 DVI and the dentist 120
6.5 The dental DVI team structure 121
6.6 Documentation 122
6.7 Retrieval of dental records 125
6.8 Post-mortem dental examination 127
6.9 Ante-mortem dental records 129

6.10 Dental reconciliation 130
6.11 Equipment for the dental DVI team 132
6.12 Maintaining dental team morale 135
6.13 References 135

7 Dental age assessment **137**
Sakher AlQahtani

7.1 The importance of knowing age 137
7.2 The chronological age 138
7.3 The dental age 139
7.4 Dentition as an age indicator 140
7.4.1 Dental development 140
7.4.2 Dental age assessment 140
7.4.3 Techniques using dental development 141
7.4.4 Accuracy of dental age estimation techniques 141
7.4.5 Schemas of dental development 145
7.5 Age estimation methods in children and young adults 146
7.5.1 Essentials 146
7.5.2 Neonatal issues 148
7.5.3 Infants from birth to 2 years 149
7.5.4 Children and adolescents from 2 to 18 years 150
7.5.5 Adults aged 18 years and above 151
7.6 Age assessment after tooth development 151
7.6.1 Pulp ratio 152
7.6.2 Other markers 152
7.6.3 Biomarkers 153
7.7 Writing a dental age report 153
7.8 Final comments 155
7.9 References 155

8 Bite marks – I **167**
Douglas R. Sheasby

8.1 Introduction 167
8.2 Bite mark components 167
8.2.1 Dentition and mouth parts 167
8.2.2 Skin 169
8.2.3 Episode of contact 171
8.3 Nature of the injury 172
8.4 Bite mark incidence 174
8.5 Principles of bite mark analysis 174
8.5.1 Distortion 174
8.5.2 Uniqueness of the human dentition 179
8.5.3 Representation of uniqueness 180
8.5.4 Interpretation of representation of uniqueness 182
8.6 Bite mark evidence recording 184
8.6.1 Initial examination of the alleged/suspected bite mark 184
8.6.2 Photography of the bite mark 185
8.6.3 Dental examination of the suspect biter 187

8.7 Bite mark analysis techniques 188
8.7.1 Biological comparison 188
8.7.2 Physical comparison 191
8.7.3 Principles of physical comparison 192
8.7.4 Feature-based analysis 194
8.7.5 Superimposition-based analysis 200
8.8 Feature-based analysis conclusions 200
8.8.1 Exclusion of the suspect 201
8.8.2 Limited conclusion 201
8.8.3 Inclusion of the suspect 201
8.9 Feature-based analysis report 202
8.10 Limitations of bite mark analysis 204
8.11 References 207

9 Bite marks – II **211**
Roland Kouble

9.1 Guidelines for bite mark analysis 211
9.2 Collection of evidence 211
9.3 Assessment of the suspected bite mark injury 212
9.4 Examination of the dentition of the suspected biter/biters 214
9.5 Bite mark comparisons 214
9.5.1 Feature-based analysis 214
9.5.2 Comparison with overlays and dental casts 214
9.5.3 Conclusion 217
9.5.4 Open and closed populations 218
9.6 Bite mark reports and presentation of evidence to a court 220
9.7 References 221

10 Forensic photography and imaging **223**
Sam Evans

10.1 Introduction 223
10.2 The photography of bite marks 223
10.3 Relevant equipment 226
10.4 Digital image file formats 231
10.5 Guidance for preparation of equipment for forensic photography 234
10.6 Photographing a bite mark 235
10.6.1 Minimising image distortion 235
10.6.2 Can distortion be corrected? 239
10.6.3 Magnification ratios: a tool for consistency 240
10.6.4 Sequence of images when photographing a bite mark 240
10.7 Photographing dentition 241
10.7.1 Equipment 243
10.7.2 Sequence of images for the dentition 243
10.8 Image downloading and storage 247
10.8.1 Guidance on downloading and image workflow 249
10.8.2 Storage of images 249
10.9 Imaging modalities 250
10.9.1 Reflected ultraviolet and near-infrared 250
10.9.2 Cross-polarised imaging 253

10.10 Three-dimensional technology 256
10.10.1 Triangulation laser scanners (active) 256
10.10.2 Hand-held laser scanners (active) 258
10.10.3 Structured light scanners (active) 258
10.10.4 Stereophotogrammetry (passive or active) 260
10.10.5 Other 3-dimensional devices 262
10.10.6 3D versus 2D 263
10.11 Image enhancement and processing 264
10.11.1 Examples of enhancement 264
10.11.2 Published guidelines 269
10.11.3 Case law 271
10.11.4 Comment 273
10.12 References 273

11 Role of the forensic odontologist in the protection of vulnerable people 277
Barbara Chadwick and Catherine Adams

11.1 Introduction 277
11.2 Bite marks and vulnerable people 278
11.3 Dental neglect in childhood 279
11.3.1 Introduction 279
11.3.2 Defining dental neglect 279
11.3.3 When is decay neglect? 281
11.3.4 Parental response to dental disease 284
11.3.5 Identifying neglect in dental practice 284
11.3.6 Responding to neglect in dental practice 286
11.4 Legislative framework for child protection in the UK 287
11.5 Protection of the vulnerable adult 288
11.5.1 The dentist and the vulnerable adult 288
11.5.2 Confidentiality 288
11.5.3 The Mental Capacity Act 2005 289
11.6 Record keeping 290
11.7 Summary chart 292
11.8 Further reading 294
11.9 References 294

Index 297

List of contributors

Catherine Adams
Consultant in Forensic Odontology, UKDVI & Powys Teaching Health Board, UK

Sakher AlQahtani
Paediatric and Forensic Dentist, Assistant Professor, King Saud University, Riyadh, Saudi Arabia

Alison Anderson
Senior Anatomical Pathology Technologist, NHS Greater Glasgow and Clyde Mortuaries, UK

Romina Carabott
Consultant and Senior Lecturer in Forensic Odontology, Director of expertFORENSICS Ltd, Cardiff, UK

Barbara Chadwick
Professor of Paediatric Dentistry, School of Dentistry, College of Biomedical and Life Sciences, Cardiff University, UK

Sam Evans
Chief Clinical and Forensic Photographer, School of Dentistry, Cardiff University, UK

Roland Kouble
Dental Surgeon and Forensic Odontologist, Sheffield, UK

Douglas R. Sheasby
Honorary Senior Clinical Lecturer in Forensic Odontology, University of Glasgow, UK

Alastair J. Sloan
Professor of Bone Biology and Tissue Engineering, School of Dentistry, Cardiff University, UK

Jason Tucker
Lecturer, Teaching and Scholarship, Solicitor, Centre for Professional Legal Studies, Law School, Cardiff University, UK

Acknowledgements

The editors would, first and foremost, like to thank all the contributors to this book. Their hard work and dedication have been instrumental in the completion of this joint effort.

Furthermore, without the tireless support from the editing team at Wiley this project would have ground to a halt long ago. Fiona, Nicky and Celia, we give you our thanks.

The editors would also like to thank all the colleagues who have supported us in this endeavour, with a special mention for the team at the Dental Illustration Unit, Cardiff University.

Lastly, the editors would like to give personal thanks to our loved ones who have supplied the endless patience and understanding we needed to finish this project.

1

Brief introduction to forensic odontology

Romina Carabott
expertFORENSICS Ltd, Cardiff, UK

1.1 Introduction

According to Keiser Neilsen (1970; cited in Cameron and Sims, 1974), forensic odontology is:

> that branch of dentistry which – in the interests of justice – deals with the proper handling and examination of dental evidence and with the proper evaluation and presentation of dental findings.

Forensic odontology, or dentistry, has been around for a long time: the identification of Lollia Paulina from her 'distinctive' teeth being as early as AD49, and the first use of bite mark evidence in court in a case of grave robbing in 1814.

The recent attention of the media on forensic 'specialities' featured in various fictional television series has seen an increased interest in this already fascinating subject. This heightened interest, however, has not always been for the right reasons. The use of dental identification in mass fatalities as the more efficient means of identification of severely decomposed bodies has attracted particular attention in natural disasters such as the Boxing Day tsunami in Thailand (2004), the Black Saturday bushfires in Australia (2009) and the Christchurch earthquake in New Zealand (2011). On the other hand, The Innocence Project (see references) has highlighted the 'abuse' and 'misuse' of bite mark analysis as reliable evidence in court; see also Bowers (2006), Pretty and Sweet (2010), Bush (2011) and Metcalfe *et al.* (2011).

To those involved in bite mark analysis research, this 'attack' on the validity of this identification science may not have come as a complete surprise (Clement and Blackwell, 2010; Pretty and Sweet, 2010). Bite mark evidence may be perceived by some in the investigative arena, who are not familiar with this area of forensic odontology, as a science akin to fingerprint analysis or DNA analysis. This is not the case, as was clearly highlighted in the report of the National Academy of Sciences

Forensic Odontology: An Essential Guide, First Edition.
Edited by Catherine Adams, Romina Carabott and Sam Evans.

(NAS) entitled *Strengthening Forensic Science in the United States: A Path Forward* (2009):

> there also are important variations among the disciplines relying on expert interpretation. For example, there are more established protocols and available research for fingerprint analysis than for the analysis of bite marks. (p. 87)
>
> Much forensic evidence – including, for example, bitemarks and forearm and tool mark identifications – is introduced in criminal trials without any meaningful scientific validation, determination of error rates, or reliability testing to explain the limits of the discipline. (p. 107)

The potential for bite mark evidence to be as useful as other forensic science disciplines may exist, but to date the very nature of the evidence renders sound and rigorous scientific research extremely difficult. Numerous publications have highlighted the lack of sound empirical evidence backing the two basic postulates of bite mark evidence and the paucity of rigorous research surrounding this discipline (Bowers, 2006; Pretty and Sweet, 2010; Bush, 2011). This is not to say that sound research has not been conducted over the years, but merely that more of such high-level research needs to come through. Until such a time when 'the barriers to such encompassing and rigorous research to support bite mark evidence' (Pretty, 2006) can be overcome, bite mark analysis needs to be applied to forensic case work with extreme caution.

A forensic odontologist's expertise in bite mark analysis lies in his/her ability to recognise the limitations of bite mark analysis for each individual case (Pretty, 2006). If such caution is applied, the credibility of bite mark analysis will not be irrevocable damage in the long term despite the wrongful convictions documented to date. With the progress of technology in leaps and bounds and 'the willingness to utilise' (Clement and Blackwell, 2010) such technology and science, there will still be a place for bite mark analysis in the investigators' arsenal.

Dental identification has attracted less media attention than bite mark analysis: the methodology is well understood and accepted, and its efficiency, cost-effectiveness and success have been witnessed on numerous occasions (Schuller-Götzburg and Suchanek, 2007; Bush and Miller, 2011; Hinchcliffe, 2011; Tengrove 2011); but that does not mean that it doesn't have challenges to contend with. Improvements in oral care – with an associated reduction of restorations available for comparison – highlight the importance of dental radiography which allows unique anatomical features to assist in establishing a dental identification. Chemical, biological, radiological and nuclear (CBRN) threats call for safe means of collecting dental evidence at the scene, such as cone-beam CT technology. Educating the members of the dental team in the advantages of dental identifications, ideally as early as undergraduate level, is required so as to continue to address the age-old problem of poor ante-mortem dental records which has always hindered the dental identification process. The advent of dental record keeping software addresses part of the problem but has been known to create other minor issues that must be kept in mind.

Mobilisation of individuals from areas of conflict into Europe has increased the requirement for a means to reliably assess the age of a living individual. Discussions are on-going, particularly in the UK, as to the reliability of dental age estimation of young adults and the ethical implications associated with exposing an individual to radiation for these purposes. In the author's view, the expertise of a forensic odontologist is not reflected in how well he/she mastered the age estimation techniques, but in his/her awareness of the limitations of these methods. Arguably, more important is the skill of explaining clearly to a judge and jury those same limitations and how they may apply to the particular case at hand. Interpreting the results and the statistical background of the methodology used in a way that is clear to the uninitiated is probably the main challenge; more so when various statistical approaches have been applied and then superseded over the years.

1.2 Forensic odontology in the 21st century

Forensic odontology has seen very few major developments over the last 20 years. Changes were mainly related to the assimilation of IT developments into this area of expertise. A very clear example is the improvement in bite mark analysis, previously relying on manual overlay production, while today it is often done with the aid of software such as Adobe Photoshop®.

Research and development in forensic odontology is hampered by two main problems:

1. Ethical issues make adequate research in bite mark analysis, child protection cases and age assessment difficult to conduct.
2. Securing funding for such research and development is notoriously difficult as most funding tends to be directed towards traditional medical and dental specialities (Pretty, 2006).

Despite these difficulties over the last few years, through the dedication of those interested in this area and postgraduate student research, the application of forensic odontology is slowly acquiring a more robust backing from rigorous scientific research (Sheets *et al.*, 2012, 2013; Bush *et al.*, 2011). The application of medical devices, software and improved technology to address difficulties in forensic dentistry is seen as a move in the right direction.

The following are some examples of recent and current research:

- *Portable X-ray units*, developed largely with the veterinary services in mind, were brought to the attention of the international forensic dental community by the New Zealand DVI (Disaster Victim Identification) team during identification of the victims of the Boxing Day tsunami in Thailand. One of these units is now on the essential equipment list of the UK DVI team and, coupled with digital x-ray software, it eliminates the need for removing jaws for radiographic examination (both in isolated identifications as well as in mass fatality scenarios), when the only purpose for such removal of jaws is radiographic examination with traditional dental radiographic equipment.

- *Mobile multi-slice computed tomography* (MSCT) has been part of various research programmes into the application of virtual autopsies in multiple fatality scenarios where CBRN contamination is known or suspected. Concomitant current studies are also assessing whether a similar principle could be applied to dental identification in such scenarios. Cone-beam CT (CBCT) technology provides superior quality dental detail to MSCT and, if applicable, may have the potential to provide post-mortem dental information without the need for direct examination of contaminated bodies.
- *Three-dimensional imaging* for patterned injuries (bite marks) is being researched in various facilities around the world. If developed adequately it could not only eliminate the photographic distortion that affects bite mark analysis but could also increase the versatility of analytical methods and the presentation of evidence in court (Evans *et al.*, 2010; Blackwell *et al.*, 2007; Thali *et al.*, 2003).
- *Computer-generated skin/human body modelling* could resolve the ethical issues with bite mark analysis, providing a means of studying the effects of force, friction, movement, time and tooth features in relation to the reaction of living human tissue, skin being such a notoriously poor impression material (Stam *et al.*, 2010, 2012; Whittle *et al.*, 2008).

However, without the investment by academic departments, funding bodies and research councils, the advance of forensic dentistry will continue to be at a very slow rate.

1.3 Training and experience

There is to date no universally accepted pathway for training to become a forensic odontologist other than the requirement of obtaining a degree in dental surgery and being registered with the national regulatory body to practice dentistry. Different countries have different courses or training pathways, so if someone is interested in getting involved in the analysis of forensic dental evidence he/she should refer to the national organisation for forensic odontology. Table 1.1 lists some of these associations with their respective website (where available). This is not a comprehensive list: new associations/groups will continue to be set up as the knowledge and awareness of the subject spreads.

The International Organisation of Forensic Odonto-Stomatology (IOFOS; www.iofos.eu) aims to liaise between forensic odontology societies on a global basis and should be an early port of call if someone is unable to identify a national association for forensic odontology in their own country.

The national associations will be able to provide advice on the accepted pathway by which a dentist may gain experience as a forensic odontologist/dentist and practise within the legal framework of the country in question following recommended guidelines of good practice. Joining these associations also allows the interested dentist to learn more about the day-to-day experience of being a forensic dentist from those who have been practising for some years. It may come as a surprise to some, how unglamorous the reality is in comparison to the life of forensic specialists portrayed in the various crime dramas aired on the media.

Table 1.1 Forensic odontology/dentistry organisations

American Board of Forensic Odontology	www.abfo.org
American Society of Forensic Odontology	www.asfo.org
Australian Society of Forensic Odontology	www.ausfo.com.au
Austrian Society of Forensic Medicine (ÖGGM)	www.oeggm.com
British Association for Forensic Odontology	www.bafo.org.uk
Canadian Society of Forensic Science	www.csfs.ca
Croatian Association of Forensic Stomatologists	
Danish Society of Forensic Odontology (Dansk RetsOdontologisk Forening)	www.retsodont.dk
Finnish Association of Forensic Odontology	www.apollonia.fi
Flemish Association of Dental Experts	
French Association of Dental Identification (Association Francaise d'Identification Odontologique)	www.adf.asso.fr
German Academy of Forensic Odontostomatology (Arbeitskreis für Forensische Odonto-Stomatologie)	www.akfos.com
Icelandic Society of Forensic Odontology	
Indian Association of Forensic Odontology	www.theiafo.org
International Association for Forensic Odonto-Stomatology	www.iofos.eu
Israel National Police Volunteer Dentists Unit	
Italy – Forensic Odontology Project (ProOF – Progetto Odontologia Forense)	www.proofweb.eu
Netherlands (Forensisch Medisch Genootschap)	www.forgen.nl
New Zealand Society of Forensic Odontology	www.nzsfo.org.nz
Norwegian Society of Forensic Odontology	
Polish Society of Forensic Odontology	www.ptos.pl
South African Society for Forensic Odonto-Stomatology	
Switzerland (Forensische Zahnärtze der Schweiz)	www.sso.ch

A handful of structured postgraduate degrees exist and have for some time been the entry point for those who express an interest in training in this field. Few as they are, these courses (ranging from Diploma to Masters levels) are becoming even rarer as some of them become victims to lack of funding.

It is the author's and editors' view that, while a structured postgraduate course is an excellent start, it is important for those who qualify to then spend some time shadowing an experienced forensic dentist in the field, ideally on a mentoring scheme. No course, no matter how in-depth and how practical it is, can recreate a case in the field, particularly when it comes to bite mark analysis. The latter requires experience not only in handling and collecting the evidence but also in the analysis itself, due to the variety of scenarios and circumstances that makes each case unique.

As an example, the British Association for Forensic Odontology (BAFO; www.bafo.org.uk) has now established a mentoring scheme whereby dentists who have qualified from a postgraduate degree in forensic odontology and who wish to practise in the field are assigned a mentor in their geographical area. The mentor is someone with some years of experience in the field and, together with the mentee, he/she puts together a personal development plan. This plan will include a period of observation by the mentee and eventually a period of being under observation during actual cases until both mentor and mentee feel confident that the mentee can practise independently.

The above applies to the practice of forensic odontology in the UK. Different recommendations/pathways will apply in other countries.

1.4 How to use this book

The intention of this book is, in the first instance, to act as an introduction to forensic odontology for the general dental practitioner who has an interest in forensic dentistry and is contemplating practising in the field. It can also be utilised as a companion and reference during practice.

Most chapters will outline accepted and recommended practices and refer to particular methodologies. Where different schools of thought exist, they will be outlined objectively. The reader is advised to use the book as a starting point rather than the one and only source of information, as well as a reference to guidelines of good practice.

It is beyond the scope of the book to cover in full detail areas such as basic dental science, the law as it pertains to practising as an expert witness, mortuary practice, and protection of the vulnerable person. Dedicated specialist texts are available that expand on these subjects.

As noted previously, the editors believe that a book or a series of lectures alone, no matter how comprehensive, are not sufficient to qualify a person to become a forensic odontologist. Such media will provide the information, but the true acquisition of knowledge in the field comes with practical mock scenarios and observation/practice on real cases under the mentorship of experienced practitioners.

The contributors to this book are all experts in their respective fields and understand the needs of the forensic odontologist and how the respective fields interact in practice.

Most of the chapters can stand alone so that the book doesn't have to be read sequentially. However, the ordering of the chapters follows what the editors believe is the correct approach to building up one's knowledge of forensic odontology.

We hope you can enjoy discovering forensic odontology and that this book will encourage you to research more about this field. We welcome any feedback or comments.

1.5 References

Blackwell S. A., Taylor R. V., Gordon I., Ogleby C. L., Tanijiri T., Yoshino M., Donald M. R. and Clement J. G. (2007) 3-D imaging and quantitative comparison of human dentitions and simulated bite marks, *International Journal of Legal Medicine* **121**: 9–17.

Bowers C. M. (2006) Problem-based analysis of bitemark misidentifications: the role of DNA, *Forensic Science International* **159S**: S104–S109. ScienceDirect [Online]. Available at: www.sciencedirect.com (accessed 20 March 2013).

Bush M. A. (2011) Forensic dentistry and bitemark analysis: sound science or junk science?, *Journal of the American Dental Association* **142**(9): 997–999. Highwire Press

American Dental Association [Online]. Available at: http://jada.ada.org (accessed 20 March 2013).

Bush M. A., Bush P. J. and Sheets H. D. (2011) A study of multiple bitemarks inflicted in human skin by a single dentition using geometric morphometric analysis, *Forensic Science International* **211**(1–3): 1–8. ScienceDirect [Online]. Available at: www.sciencedirect.com (accessed 25 March 2013).

Bush M. and Miller R. (2011) The crash of Colgan Air flight 3407: advanced techniques in victim identification, *Journal of the American Dental Association* **142**(12): 1352–1356. Highwire Press American Dental Association [Online]. Available at: http://jada.ada.org (accessed 10 September 2012).

Cameron J. M. and Sims B. G. (1974) *Forensic Dentistry*. Edinburgh:Churchill Livingstone.

Clement J. G. and Blackwell S. A. (2010) Is current bite mark analysis a misnomer?, *Forensic Science International* **201**: 33–37. ScienceDirect [Online]. Available at: www.sciencedirect.com (accessed 20 March 2013).

Evans S., Jones C. and Plassmann P. (2010) 3D imaging in forensic odontology, *Journal of Visual Communication in Medicine* **33**(2): 63–68.

Hinchliffe J. (2011) Forensic odontology. Part 2: Major disasters, *British Dental Journal* **210**(6): 269–274.

Metcalfe R. D., Lee G., Gould L. A. and Stickels J. (2011) Bite this! The role of bite mark analyses in wrongful convictions, *Southwest Journal of Criminal Justice* **7**(1): 47–64. [Online]. Available at: www.forensic-dentistry.info/wp/wp-content/uploads/2011/07/Metcalf-et-al.1.pdf (accessed 25 March 2013). National Academy of Science (2009) Strengthening Forensic Science in the United States: A Path Forward. [Online]. Available at: www.nap.edu/catalog/12589.html (accessed 20 March 2013).

Pretty I. A. (2006) The barriers to achieving an evidence base for bitemark analysis. *Forensic Science International* **159**(suppl 1): S110–S120 (review).

Pretty I. A. and Sweet D. (2010) A paradigm shift in the analysis of bitemarks, *Forensic Science International* **201**: 38–44. ScienceDirect [Online]. Available at: www.sciencedirect.com (accessed 20 March 2013).

Schuller-Götzburg P. and Suchanek J. (2007) Forensic odontologists successfully identify tsunami victims in Phuket, Thailand, *Forensic Science International* **171**(2–3): 204-207. ScienceDirect [Online]. Available at: www.sciencedirect.com (accessed 20 March 2013).

Sheets H. D., Bush P. J. and Bush M. A. (2012) Bitemarks: distortion and covariation of the maxillary and mandibular dentition as impressed in human skin, *Forensic Science International* **223**(1–3): 202–207. ScienceDirect [Online]. Available at: www.sciencedirect.com (accessed 25 March 2013).

Sheets H. D., Bush P. J. and Bush M. A. (2013) Patterns of variation and match rates of the anterior biting dentition: characteristics of a database of 3D-scanned dentitions, *Journal of Forensic Sciences* **58**(1): 60–68. Swetswise [Online]. Available at: www.swetswise.com (accessed 25 March 2013).

Stam B., van Gemert M., van Leeuwen T. and Aalders M. (2010) 3D finite compartment modelling of formation and healing of bruises may identify methods for age determination of bruises, *Medical and Biological Engineering and Computing* **48**(9): 911–921.

Stam B., Gemert M., Leeuwen T. and Aalders M. (2012) How the blood pool properties at onset affect the temporal behaviour of simulated bruises, *Medical and Biological Engineering and Computing* **50**(2): 165–171.

Tengrove H. (2011) Operation earthquake 2011: Christchurch earthquake disaster victim identification, *Journal of Forensic Odontostomatology* **29**(2): 1–7. Journal of Forensic Odontostomatology Online [Online]. Available at: www.iofos.eu/JFOSOnline2.html (accessed 20 March 2013).

Thali M. J., Braun M., Markwalder Th. H., Brüschweiler W., Zollinger U., Malik Naseem J., Yen K. and Dirnhofer R. (2003) Bite mark documentation and analysis: the forensic 3D/CAD supported photogrammetry approach, *Forensic Science International* **135**: 115–121. The Innocence Project (undated: accessed 6 June 2013): http://innocenceproject.org/Content/Cases_Where_DNA_Revealed_that_Bite_Mark_Analysis_Led_to_Wrongful_Arrests_and_Convictions.php

Whittle K., Kieser J., Ichim I., Swain M., Waddell N., Livingstone V. and Taylor M. (2008) The biomechanical modelling of non-ballistic skin wounding: blunt-force injury *Forensic Science, Medicine, and Pathology* **4**(1): 33–39.

2

Development of the dentition

Alastair J. Sloan
School of Dentistry, Cardiff University, UK

The process of tooth development – or odontogenesis – is a complex series of reciprocal cellular interactions, by which teeth form from epithelial and mesenchymal cells in the stomatodeum. Enamel, dentine, cementum and the periodontium must all develop during appropriate stages of embryonic development. Primary teeth begin to form between the sixth and eighth weeks of intrauterine (i.u.) life, and permanent teeth begin to form in the twentieth week. If teeth do not start to develop around those times, it is likely that they will not develop at all and be missing.

2.1 Early tooth development

The stomatodeum is lined by a primitive epithelium which is two or three cells in thickness. Beneath this is embryonic connective tissue, the ectomesenchyme (Figure 2.1). The first sign of tooth development within the stomatodeum is a thickening of the epithelium and this thickening is called the *primary epithelial band*. It forms at around 6 weeks of i.u. life and indicates the position of the future dental arches. The primary epithelial band rapidly divides into two structures, the *dental lamina* and the *vestibular lamina*. The latter ultimately gives rise to the *vestibule/sulcus* while the former gives rise the to the *tooth germs*. At 6 weeks there is no vestibule/sulcus between cheek and tooth-bearing area. The vestibule forms from proliferation of vestibular lamina into the ectomesenchyme. The vestibular lamina cells rapidly enlarge, then degenerate leaving a cleft which becomes the vestibule.

The dental lamina is the structure that gives rise to the tooth germs, and proliferation of the dental lamina at 6–7 weeks i.u. determines the positions of future deciduous teeth with a series of 20 epithelial ingrowths into ectomesenchyme (10 in each development jaw). This first incursion of the epithelial dental lamina into the mesenchyme leads to a bud of cells at the distal aspect of the dental lamina and is called the *bud stage* of tooth development (Figure 2.2). Each bud is separated from the ectomesenchyme by a basement membrane. There is little change in shape or function of the epithelial cells at this time. The supporting ectomesenchymal cells congregate around the bud, forming a cluster of cells which are closely packed beneath and around the epithelial bud, which is the initiation of the condensation of the ectomesenchyme. The remaining ectomesenchymal cells are arranged with less regular order.

Forensic Odontology: An Essential Guide, First Edition.
Edited by Catherine Adams, Romina Carabott and Sam Evans.

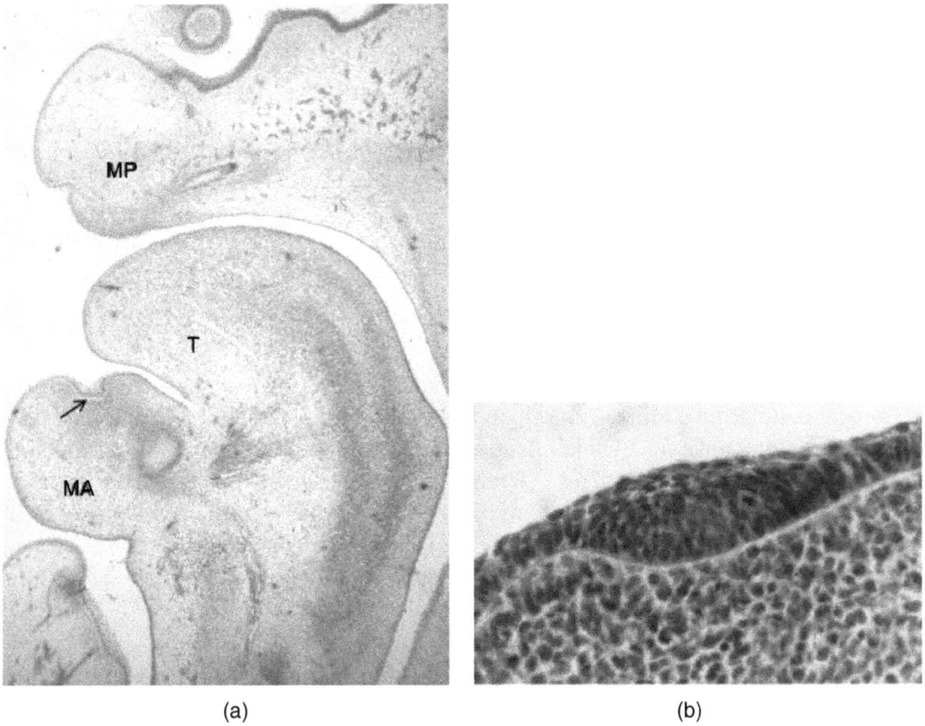

Figure 2.1 (a) Stomatodeum with primary epithelial band (arrow). MP, maxillary process; T, tongue; MA, mandibular arch. (b) Primary epithelial band at high magnification

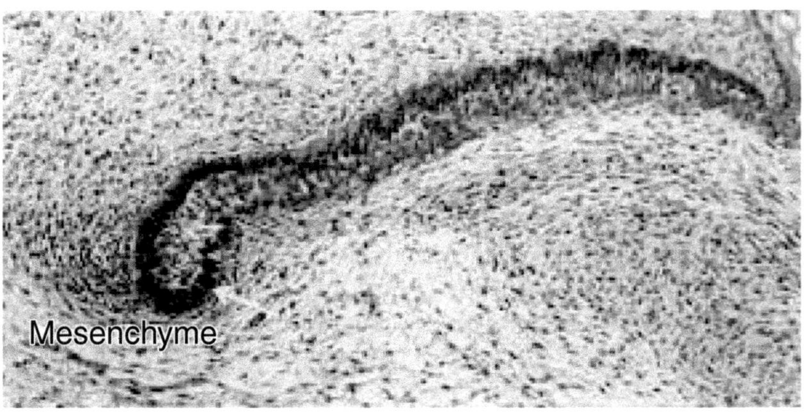

Figure 2.2 Bud stage of tooth development (arrow). The bud is formed from the invading epithelium and condensation of the surrounding ectomesenchymal cells

As tooth development progresses, two key processes become essential to development. The first is *morpho-differentiation*, which is the determination of the shape of the crown of the tooth through the shape of the amelodentinal junction of the forming tooth. The second process is *histo-differentiation*, where cells of the developing tooth differentiate (specialise) into morphologically and functionally distinct groups of cells responsible for secretion of various dental tissues. Control and regulation of this differentiation is through specific and reciprocal cellular interactions between the epithelial/mesenchymal compartments.

As the epithelial bud continues to proliferate into the ectomesenchyme, the first signs of an arrangement of cells in the tooth bud appear in the *cap stage*. A small group of ectomesenchymal cells stops producing extracellular substances and do not separate from each other, which results in an aggregation or condensation of these cells immediately adjacent to the epithelial bud. This is the developing *dental papilla*. At this point, the tooth bud grows around the ectomesenchymal aggregation, taking on the appearance of a cap, and becomes the enamel (or dental) organ. A condensation of ectomesenchymal cells called the *dental follicle* surrounds the enamel organ and limits the dental papilla (Figure 2.3). The enamel organ is responsible for the synthesis and

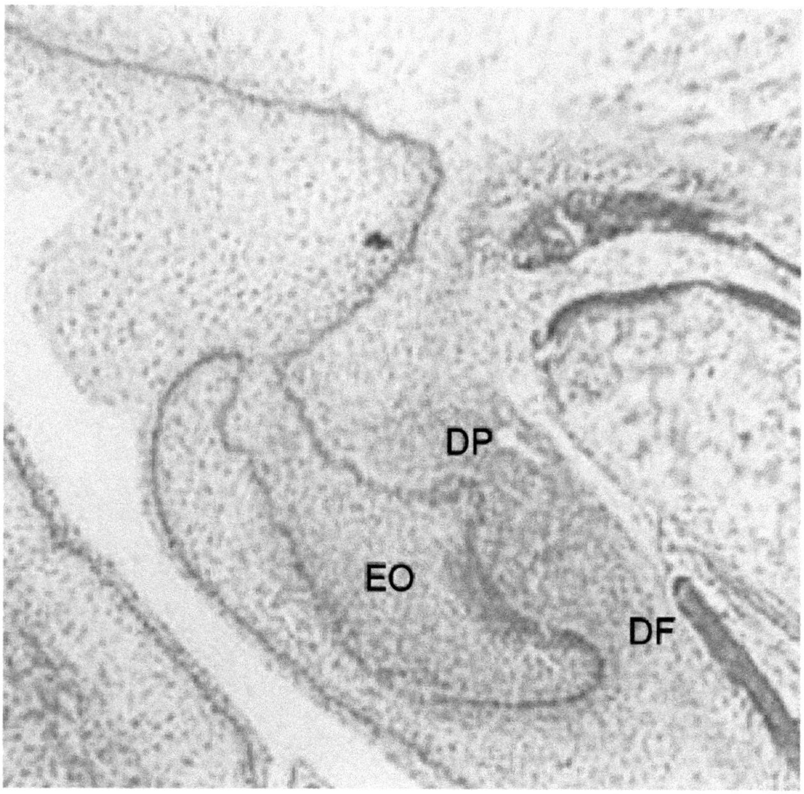

Figure 2.3 Cap stage of tooth development where the three components of the tooth germ can be observed. EO, enamel organ; DP, dental papillae; DF, dental follicle

secretion of enamel, the dental papilla will lead to the formation of the dentine and pulp, and the dental follicle will produce the supporting structures of a tooth. This explains why enamel is epithelial in origin whereas dentine, pulp and periodontal tissues are mesenchymally derived.

As tooth development proceeds there is a distinct histo- and morpho-differentation of the enamel organ as it prepares for secretory function, along with an increase in size of the tooth germ. This change signifies the transition to the *early bell stage*. The enamel organ takes on a bell shape during this stage with continued cell proliferation, and histo-differentiation of four distinct cell layers within the enamel organ can be observed (Figure 2.4).

A single layer of cubiodal cells at the periphery of the enamel organ limit its size and are known as the *outer enamel epithelium*. Conversely, the single cell layer adjacent to the dental papilla is known as *inner enamel epithelium* and it is these cells that will differentiate into ameloblasts and give rise to enamel synthesis and secretion. Where these cells of the inner and outer enamel epithelium meet is termed the *cervical loop*. The majority of the cells that are situated between the outer and inner

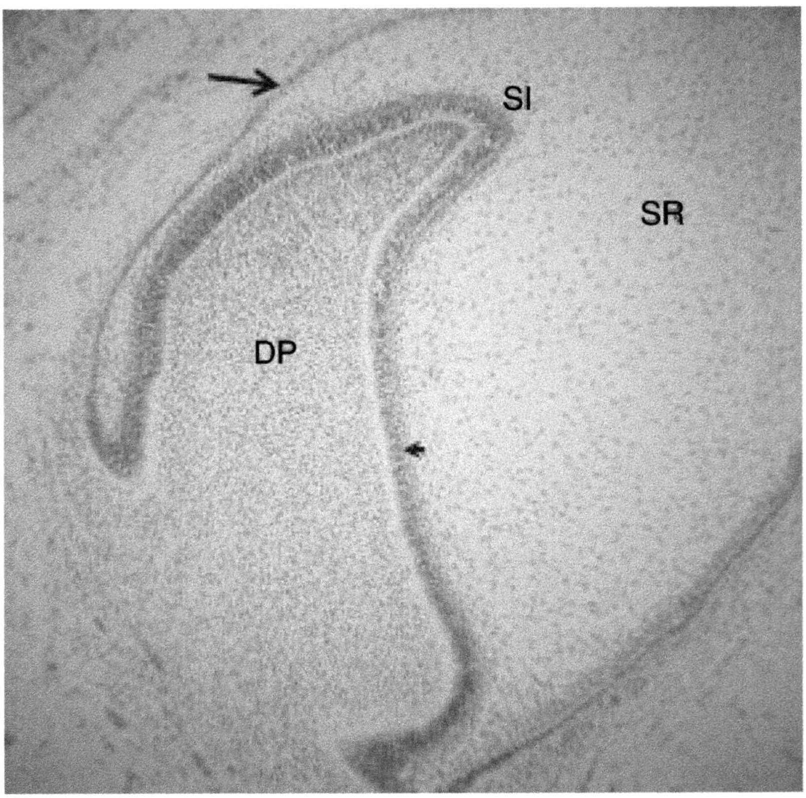

Figure 2.4 Bell stage of tooth development where the four cell layers of the enamel organ can be observed. SR, stellate reticulum; SI, stratum intermedium; arrow, outer enamel epithelium; arrowhead, inner enamel epithelium

enamel epithelium are termed the *stellate reticulum*. These cells secrete hydrophilic glycosaminoglycans which increase the extracellular space and the cells interconnect through desmosomes giving them a stellate or star-shaped appearance. A layer two or three cells thick lying next to the inner enamel epithelium, and having a flattened shape, is termed the *stratum intermedium*. In summary, the layers of the enamel organ in order of innermost to outermost consist of inner enamel epithelium, stratum intermedium, stellate reticulum and outer enamel epithelium.

During this stage of development, as it progresses from cap stage to early bell stage, a localised thickening of cells at the inner enamel epithelium around the cusp tip appears. This is known as the *enamel knot* and is a signalling centre of the tooth that provides positional information for tooth morphogenesis and regulates the growth of tooth cusps. The enamel knot produces a range of molecular signals from all the major growth factor families, including fibroblast growth factors (FGF), bone morphogenetic proteins (BMP), Hedgehog (Hh) and Wnt signals. These molecular signals direct the growth of the surrounding epithelium and mesenchyme and have putative roles in signalling and regulation of crown development. The enamel knot is transitory and the primary enamel knot is removed by apoptosis. Later, secondary enamel knots may appear that regulate the formation of the future cusps of the teeth.

2.2 Later tooth development

As tooth development progresses from the early bell stage to a *late bell stage* of development, epithelial/mesenchymal interactions signal further histo-differentiation of the four cell layers of the enamel organ in preparation for amelogenesis. Cell appearance in the enamel organ is directly related to function. The cells of the outer enamel epithelium are cuboidal with a high nuclear:cytoplasm ratio. These cells have a non-secretory protective role and will eventually become part of the dentogingival junction. The stellate reticulum cells sit in a substantial jelly-like extracellular matrix which protects the interior of a tooth germ. The cells of the inner enamel epithelium have a low columnar appearance with a central nucleus and few organelles. These cells are at a preparatory stage of becoming secretory, the ameloblast.

The inner enamel epithelial cells are separated from the ectomesenchymal dental papillae by the *dental basement membrane*. This structure mediates interactions between the epithelial and mesenchymal compartments of the tooth germ during development and odontoblast differentiation prior to dentine secretion. At this time, the dental papillae contains undifferentiated ectomesenchymal cells with relatively small amounts of extracellular matrix (apart from a few fine collagen fibrils) and these cells are not yet specialised for secretory function.

The late bell stage is also known as the *crown stage* of tooth development and further cellular changes occur at this time. In all prior stages of tooth development, all of the inner enamel epithelium cells were proliferating to contribute to the increase of the overall size of the tooth germ. However, during the crown stage, cell proliferation stops at the location corresponding to the sites of the future cusps of the teeth. At the same time, the inner enamel epithelial cells change in shape from cuboidal to short columnar cells with nuclei polarised to the end of the cell away from the basement membrane.

The adjacent layer of cells on the periphery of the dental papilla increases in size, the cells become columnar and their nuclei polarise away from the basement membrane as they differentiate into odontoblasts. These changes to the inner enamel epithelium and the differentiation of odontoblasts begin at the site of the future cusp tips and the odontoblasts secrete an organic collagen-rich matrix called *pre-dentine*, towards the basement membrane. As the odontoblasts secrete pre-dentine, they retreat and migrate toward the centre of the dental papilla. Cytoplasmic extensions are left behind as the odontoblasts move inward, creating a unique, tubular microscopic appearance of dentine as pre-dentine is secreted around these extensions.

After dentine formation begins, the dental basement membrane breaks down and the short columnar cells of the inner enamel epithelium come into contact with the pre-dentine, terminally differentiate into ameloblasts and begin to secrete an organic-rich matrix against the dentine. This matrix is partially mineralised and will mature to become the enamel. Whereas dentine formation proceeds in a pulpal direction, enamel formation moves outwards, adding new material to the outer surface of the developing tooth.

During this stage of tooth development, the tooth germ loses attachment to oral epithelium as it becomes encased in bone of developing jaws. The dental lamina begins to disintegrate into discrete islands of cells known as the Glands of Serres. Most of these degenerate but some remain quiescent in jaw bone; if stimulated later in life they may form odontogenic cysts known as 'odontogenic keratocysts'. The vascular supply enters dental papilla during the cap stage of development and increases during the bell stage during hard tissue formation. The vasculature enters the dental papilla around sites of future root formation. The pioneer nerve fibres approach the developing tooth germ during the bud/cap stage but do not penetrate dental papilla until dentine formation begins.

Formation of the permanent dentition arises from a proliferation and extension of the dental lamina. The permanent incisor, canine and premolar germs arise from proliferation on the lingual aspect of the dental lamina next to their deciduous predecessors. The permanent molars have no deciduous predecessors and develop from backward extension of the dental lamina which gives off epithelial ingrowths giving rise to the first, second and third permanent molars.

2.3 Dentinogenesis

The secretion of dentine matrix begins at 17–18 weeks i.u., corresponding to the late bell stage (crown stage) of tooth development. Odontoblast differentiation begins at the future cusp tip, spreading apically down a gradient of differentiation down the cuspal slopes. Dentine formation, or secretion of a dentine matrix, starts immediately following odontoblast differentiation. Odontoblast differentiation can be characterised by a distinct change in cell phenotype and morphology. The ectomesenchymal cells of dental papilla have a high nucleus to cytoplasm ratio, little rough endoplasmic reticulum and few mitochondria, so they have a low synthetic/secretory activity. As these cells differentiate into odontoblasts, they become cells with a low nuclear to cytoplasm ratio and have increased rough endoplasmic reticulum, golgi and mitochondria and develop a high synthetic/secretory capacity.

The cells of the inner enamel epithelium are critical to the formation of dentine and odontoblast differentiation through molecular signalling. The basement mediates presentation of these molecules, which include the growth factors *fibroblast growth factor* and *bone morphogenetic protein*. As odontoblasts differentiate and secrete pre-dentine, the basement membrane breaks down and the cells of the inner enamel epithelium become exposed to pre-dentine which signals ameloblast differentiation. As well as receiving the chemical/molecular signals, the dental papilla cells must also be competent to respond to that signal for differentiation to occur. Competency is achieved by the cells undergoing the requisite number of cell cycles; and after the final cell division and cell alignment at the periphery of the dental papilla, the cell nearest the inner enamel epithelium receives these molecular signals from the enamel organ and differentiates into an odontoblast (Figure 2.5). The other daughter cell remains undifferentiated and exists within the developed pulp as a sub-odontoblast in the cell-rich layer. Odontoblasts are post-mitotic and they undergo no further cell division. Once differentiated, they begin to secrete pre-dentine which is an unmineralised dentine matrix.

The first formed dentine is termed *mantle dentine* and is approximately 0.15 mm thick. This matrix is synthesised and secreted from both newly differentiated odontoblasts and existing dental papilla cells (the rest of the dentine matrix is secreted from odontoblasts alone). Mineralisation of this mantle dentine is via matrix vesicles.

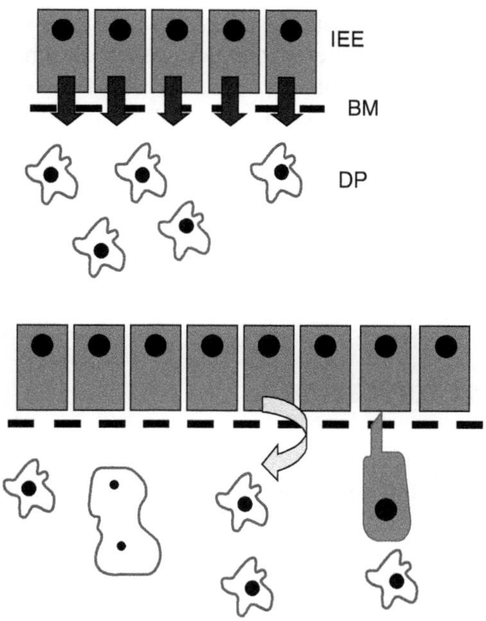

Figure 2.5 Odontoblast differentiation is controlled by reciprocal epithelium/mesenchymal interactions mediated by the dental basement membrane. Signals are passed between the inner enamel epithelium (IEE) to the cells at the periphery of the dental papillae (DP) though the basement membrane (BM). After one final cell division, the daughter cell nearest the basement membrane receives the signal which mediates differentiation into an odontoblast cell, while the other daughter cell remains undifferentiated

After mantle dentine formation, odontoblasts continue to secrete pre-dentine which mineralises to dentine, and this, secreted throughout the remainder of tooth development, is termed *primary dentine*. The odontoblasts always secrete a layer of pre-dentine which mineralises to dentine and as they secrete pre-dentine, the cells retreat pulpally. As the cells retreat, they leave a single cytoplasmic process within the matrix which allows the odontoblast to communicate with the deeper layers of matrix. This process also creates the tubular structure of dentine which runs throughout the tissue. These tubules follow an S-shaped course in coronal dentine, but a straighter course in radicular dentine.

There are two levels of matrix secretion from the odontoblast and it is this which contributes to the unique structure of dentine. The main secretion of structural components (collagen, proteoglycans) into pre-dentine comes from the cell body of the odontoblast. The pre-dentine matrix is secreted around and between the extending odontoblast process and this leads to formation of tubules within the matrix, with each tubule containing an odontoblast process. This creates the tubular structure of dentine and this dentine matrix secreted from the odontoblast cell body is termed *intertubular dentine*. A second level of secretion of a dentine matrix, rich in tissue-specific matrix components at the mineralisation front, is within each dentinal tubule. This is termed *intratubular or peritubular dentine* and is found immediately surrounding the inside of the dentinal tubule. It is highly mineralised with little collagen. It is thought that secretion of peritubular dentine is from the odontoblast process.

Dentine forms rhythmically during development, with the odontoblast alternating between periods of pre-dentine secretion and quiescence. As a result, incremental lines can be observed and these correspond to a daily rate of secretion of pre-dentine of 4 m per day. At the boundary between these daily increments, minute changes in collagen fibre orientation can be noted. In addition to these daily incremental lines, a 5-day pattern of secretion can be observed and these incremental lines run at 90 degrees to the dentinal tubules and highlight the normal rhythmic and linear pattern of dentine secretion. These incremental lines are known as the Lines of Von Ebner and are approximately 20 m apart.

2.4 Tooth root formation

Roots are incomplete at eruption and root development is completed approximately 12 months post eruption for deciduous teeth and 2–3 years post eruption for the permanent dentition.

The root is formed primarily of dentine but is lined with cementum. For root formation to begin, epithelial tissue is required to map out the shape of the tooth and initiate and mediate root odontoblast differentiation and subsequent dentine secretion. The epithelium responsible for this is known as Hertwig's Epithelial Root Sheath (HERS) and is formed from a downward growth of the cervical loop. The HERS is bilaminar, consisting of cells from both the inner and outer enamel epithelium, and it grows as a collar enclosing the future root. The inner cells of the HERS do not differentiate into ameloblasts, but they are responsible for inducing cells on the periphery of the dental papilla, adjacent to the HERS to differentiate into odontoblasts for root dentine secretion. As in the crown, a gradient of root odontoblast differentiation and root dentine secretion can be observed from crown to root apex. The HERS fragments once root dentine secretion begins and exposes the root surface to the ectomesenchymal cells of the dental follicle. This stimulates follicular cells adjacent to the root dentine to differentiation into cementoblasts which are responsible for cementogenesis and secretion of cementum. The HERS fragments lie adjacent to the root as cell clusters and are generally quiescent and functionless. These clusters are known as the Cell Rests of Malassez and, although quiescent, can be stimulated to proliferate during periods of inflammation (e.g. pulpitis) and give rise to dental (radicular) cysts.

Two types of cementum are formed: *cellular* and *acellular*. As cementoblasts differentiate from the follicular cells they begin to secrete collagen fibrils and non-collagenous proteins (e.g. bone sialoprotien, osteocalcin) along and at right-angles to the root surface before migrating away from the developing root. As the cementoblasts migrate, more collagen is deposited. This is acellular cementum and is the first formed cementum. The matrix secreted by the cementoblasts subsequently mineralises. During mineralisation the cementoblasts move away from the cementum, and the collagen fibres left along the surface of the root eventually join the forming periodontal ligament fibres. Cellular cementum is formed once the majority of the tooth development is complete and once the tooth is present in the occlusion. Cellular cementum is formed around the collagen fibre bundles and the cementoblasts become entrapped within the matrix they produce. These cells trapped within the cementum are termed *cementocytes*.

The origin of cementoblasts is thought to be different for acellular and cellular cementum. Current thinking is that cementoblasts responsible for acellular cementum arise from the ectomesenchymal cells of the dental follicle adjacent to the developing root dentine, whereas cementoblasts responsible for the synthesis and secretion of cellular cementum migrate from the adjacent area of bone. Interestingly, cellular cementum is not commonly found in single-rooted teeth; however, in premolars and molars it is found only in the part of the root closest to the apex and in interradicular areas between multiple roots.

It is also thought that the inner cells of the HERS have a very brief secretory phase prior to it fragmenting. This results in the secretion of a thin hyaline layer of tissue containing enamel-like proteins. It is most prominent in the apical area of molars and premolars and less obvious in incisors and deciduous teeth.

Differential proliferation of the HERS in multi-rooted teeth causes the division of the root into two or three roots, as local proliferation causes invaginations of the HERS. Ingrowth of the rooth sheath towards the end of root development is responsible for apical closure of the root.

2.5 Epithelial/mesenchymal interactions in tooth development

Sequential and reciprocal signalling between the epithelial (enamel organ) and mesenchymal (dental papilla) compartments of the tooth germ regulates the formation of the complex shape of individual teeth. Signalling molecules of different families mediate cell communication during tooth development. The majority of these belong to the transforming growth factor beta (TGFβ), fibroblast growth factor (FGF), Hedgehog and Wnt families. These signals generally regulate interactions between the enamel organ and dental papilla, but they may also mediate cell-to-cell communication within each tissue compartment. The genes regulated by these different signals include transcription factors and those encoding for cell surface receptors (on cells in either the enamel organ or dental papilla) that regulate the competence of those cells to respond to the next signals. They also regulate the ability of the cells to respond to new signals that act reciprocally, which maintains communication between the enamel organ and dental papilla.

The appearance of transient signalling centres in the enamel organ during tooth development is crucial to maintaining these epithelial/mesenchymal interactions and thus allowing tooth development to proceed. The first of these centres appears during the bud stage and then again when the enamel knot(s) appear. They may express many different signalling molecules, including sonic hedgehog (Shh), BMPs, FGFs and Wnts, and regulate coronal development and the initiation of the secondary enamel knot(s) at the sites of the folding of the inner enamel epithelium leading to cusp formation.

One of the first signalling events in tooth development addresses the question of how a tooth knows to become a tooth. Tissue recombination studies have shown that the jaw epithelium controls events which commit the neural crest cells of the ectomesenchyme to become teeth and the BMPs and FGFs regulate this process. It is the epithelium which induces cell competence in the mesenchyme to drive subsequent tooth development. Further tissue recombination studies using a mix of dental epithelium or dental mesenchyme and skin epithelium or skin mesenchyme confirmed this, as combining dental epithelium with skin mesenchyme gave rise to a skin-like tissue, whereas recombining skin epithelium with dental mesenchyme led to progression of dental tissue. The growth factors BMPs and FGFs induce the expression of several transcription factors in the developing dental papilla, many of which are essential for tooth development to progress. These include the transcription factors Msx1 and Pax9.

The first epithelial signals induce in the mesenchyme the expression of reciprocal signal molecules (FGF and BMP4), which act back on the epithelium regulating the formation of the primary epithelial band. Further signals then regulate formation of the bud stage and condensation of the ectomesenchymal cells. These cells of the ectomesenchyme maintain the expression of transcription factors (e.g. Msx1) which had been earlier induced by signalling from the jaw epithelium, and this upregulates the expression of new genes (such as the transcription factor Runx2 and the signalling molecule FGF3), which then regulates progression from the bud to cap stage. At the same time, BMP4 expression in the ectomesenchyme is required for the formation of the enamel knot. The enamel knot cells express many signalling molecules and these influence both epithelial and ectomesenchymal cells. Reciprocal interactions between the mesenchyme and epithelium maintain the enamel knot and mediate the formation of the four cell layers within the developing enamel organ. SHH is another important signalling molecule as its secretion from the enamel knot influences growth of the cervical loops. It also regulates crown patterning (crown shape) by initiating formation of the secondary enamel knots which determine the sites where the inner enamel epithelium folds (due to differential cell proliferation) and cusp development starts.

To understand how we get teeth of different shapes in the correct position in the dental arch (patterning of the dentition), two theories have been proposed:

- The *field model* proposes that local factors responsible for tooth shape reside in the ectomesenchyme in specific regions or fields and tell the ectomesenchyme to form a tooth of a specific shape.
- A second theory, the *clone theory*, proposes that clones of ectomesenchymal cells are already programmed by the epithelium to become a specific tooth with a specific shape.

Evidence exists to support both theories and it is likely that both may influence tooth development. The Odontogenic Homebox Code (field theory) is based on observing restricted expression of certain homeobox genes (known to be important in tooth development) in early developing ectomesenchyme. It has been observed that expression of Msx1 and Msx2 is restricted to areas of ectomesenchyme corresponding to regions where incisor teeth will eventually develop but not regions where multi-cuspid teeth will develop. Conversely, expression of the genes Dlx-1 and Dlx-2 have been observed in ectomesenchyme corresponding to regions where multi-cuspid teeth, but not single-cusped teeth, form. These areas of expression are broad and overlap, but they may provide the positional information for development of teeth of specific shape in the correct position in the dental arch.

2.6 Amelogenesis

Amelogenesis begins with secretion of a partially mineralised enamel matrix by terminally differentiated ameloblasts until a full thickness of tissue is achieved. This provides an organic scaffold for subsequent mineralisation. This is the secretory phase of amelogenesis. Following this, maturation of secreted enamel matrix is achieved beginning from the amelodentinal junction (ADJ) and proceeding outwards. During this phase there is considerable resorption of the majority of the organic matrix, which is replaced by crystal growth.

The secretory stage begins immediately after dentinogenesis at future cusp tips and following ameloblast differentiation. Ameloblasts secrete an organic enamel matrix which is almost instantly partially mineralised. This first formed enamel matrix is composed of organic, protein matrix (20% by volume), inorganic hydroxyapatite (16% by volume) and water (64% by volume). The organic matrix is comprised of two families of enamel protiens, the *amelogenins* and the *non-amelogenins*. The amelogenins are small, soluble hydrophobic proteins and have a significant role in the regulation of enamel prism orientation, enamel mineralisation and crystal growth. The non-amelogenins are a mixture of proteins including *enamelin*, *tuftelin* and *ameloblastin*. Enamelin is a larger, acidic protein encoded by the ENAM gene. Mutations in this gene can give rise to the autosomal dominant amelogenesis imperfecta, suggesting a role for the protein in amelogenesis. Tuftelin is an acidic glycoprotein which has been suggested to have a role in enamel mineralisation, as has ameloblastin.

The inorganic phase of this initial enamel matrix consists of small crystals of hydroxyapatite (HAp) and further crystal growth is observed during the maturation phase of amelogenesis. As a full thickness of enamel is secreted by the late secretory stage, changes become apparent in the first formed enamel next to the ADJ. This consists of proteolysis of the amelogenins with concurrent increase in crystal growth and an increase in mineralisation. During the maturation stage there continues to be a selective loss of protein (amelogenin) through proteolysis and resorption, loss of water and further growth of mineral crystals.

The ameloblast differentiates from inner enamel epithelium as the first pre-dentine is secreted. A number of changes to the cell are observed as it terminally differentiates, including an increase in cell length, increase in synthetic organelles, polarisation of the nuclei to the basal third of the cell, and the development of a short, stubby process at the secretory pole of the cell. This process is termed *Tome's Process* and is responsible for the formation of the structural unit of the enamel – the enamel prism or enamel rod. The first formed enamel, however, is structureless and is called *aprismatic enamel.* This is because the distinct Tome's Process has not yet developed, so amorphous secretion from the cell body of the ameloblast is observed. Enamel structure is based on numerous enamel prisms/rods and each is made by one ameloblast and consists of many Hap crystals. These prisms are perpendicular to the ADJ and define the course of the ameloblast as it moves towards the future enamel surface, secreting enamel matrix as it does so.

Once the Tome's Process develops, two sites of secretion exist. One is the proximal end of the process/cell body and gives rise to inter-rod or *interprismatic enamel.* The second site of secretion is the distal end of the process and is responsible for the formation of the enamel rods or *prismatic enamel.* One ameloblast (Tome's Process) gives rise to one enamel prism, but interprismatic enamel is formed from adjacent cells. Both interprismatic and prismatic enamel have the same biochemical composition but differ in the orientation of Hap crystals. Aprismatic enamel has a more random orientation of crystals at the ADJ. This dual level of secretion from the ameloblast gives enamel its characteristic structure, which at the light microscopic level is a fish-scale/keyhole appearance. The Tome's Process is always short and remains on the formative surface of the enamel matrix; it is not embedded in the matrix, as the odontoblast process is in the dentinal tubules. Thus, enamel is not permeable like dentine.

2.7 Biomineralisation of enamel

Enamel mineralisation occurs in a tissue-specific microenvironment. The size, morphology and stability of the formed crystals are determined by the degree of supersaturation of calcium and phosphate in the fluid phase. This is greatly influenced by the presence of a large number of regulators, which are the *matrix proteins.*

Calcium reaches the matrix through the enamel organ by intercellular and transcellular pathways. Active transport systems using carrier proteins in cell membranes may be involved, and calcium may also flow through concentration gradients from blood plasma to enamel matrix. The first formed aprismatic enamel is poorly organised with random crystal sizes and morphology. Initial crystals grow by fusion of nucleation sites, but once a prismatic structure takes shape, growth is by increased length, not width, and controlled by the amelogenin protein which forms nanospheres.

The amelogenin nanospheres control Hap crystal growth by acting as spacers between the crystals, providing space for new crystal deposition and inhibiting crystal fusion. There is good correlation between the size of the nanospheres and spacing of the enamel crystallites, suggesting that the width of the nanospheres controls the final thickness of the enamel crystals. In the maturation phase of amelogenesis, the matrix proteins have a reduced role as most organic material has been degraded through proteolysis and been removed. Matrix proteins are removed long before crystal growth ends, and they may accumulate in the extracellular space around the ameloblasts where they may inhibit cell activity and so control or limit the thickness of enamel deposition.

During enamel maturation the Tome's Process is lost, so a thin layer of structureless aprismatic enamel is found on the tooth surface. The ameloblast cell surface membrane next to the enamel modulates between a ruffled and smooth surface corresponding to proteolytic degradation and removal of the amelogenin nanospheres and influx of mineral ions. There is a reduction in cell height, loss of synthetic organelles within the cell, and an increase in surface area with the presence of the ruffled border. Further regressive changes are observed as the cell enters a protective stage.

At this point, once enamel formation is complete, the enamel organ regresses to a thin layer of cuboidal cells known as the *reduced enamel epithelium*, which fuses with the oral epithelium as the tooth erupts into the oral cavity.

2.8 Further reading

Bei M. (2009) Molecular genetics of tooth development, *Current Opinion in Genetic Development* **19**(5): 504–510.

Caton J. and Tucker A. S. (2009) Current knowledge of tooth development: patterning and mineralization of the murine dentition. *Journal of Anatomy* **214**(4): 502–515.

Smith A. J. and Lesot H. (2001) Induction and regulation of crown dentinogenesis: embryonic events as a template for dental tissue repair? *Critical Reviews in Oral Biology and Medicine* **12**(5): 425–437.

Thesleff I. and Mikkola M. (2002) The role of growth factors in tooth development. *International Review of Cytology* **217**: 93–135.

Townsend G., Harris E. F., Lesot H., Clauss F. and Brook A. (2009) Morphogenetic fields within the human dentition: a new clinically relevant synthesis of an old concept. *Archives of Oral Biology* **54**(Suppl. 1): S34–S44.

Wang Y., Li L., Zheng Y., Yuan G., Yang G., He F. and Chen Y. (2012) BMP activity is required for tooth development from the lamina to the bud stage. *Journal of Dental Research* **91**: 690–695.

3

Acting as an expert witness

Jason Tucker
Centre for Professional Legal Studies, Law School, Cardiff University, UK

3.1 Introduction

The law recognises that the court is frequently without the requisite knowledge to form judgments on complex technical questions without assistance. Where the court requires such assistance, the parties involved in the litigation will usually be permitted to obtain evidence from an expert witness. Essentially, the expert witness's function is to assist the court in its decision making.

The expert witness, therefore, has a very important role in the court process. As a result, the work of expert witnesses is governed by a series of court rules, with which both experts and those instructing them must comply. The purpose of this chapter is to explore the duties and obligations that experts owe to the court so that, when you are instructed to act as an expert witness, you will be able to undertake the role with confidence.

3.2 The nature of expert evidence

3.2.1 What is evidence?

In simple terms, evidence is the information that the parties put before the court to assist the court in determining whether a *fact in issue* occurred or not. A fact in issue is a disputed fact about which the court must make a decision.

Legal rules of evidence exist to ensure that the court has the relevant information available to it, so that court decision making is safe and reliable. Evidence will be *relevant* if it helps to prove or disprove a fact in issue. The general rule is that all relevant evidence is admissible in court unless it is excluded by a particular rule of evidence (e.g. because it is inadmissible hearsay). Any dispute regarding whether evidence is admissible will be determined by the court.

Forensic Odontology: An Essential Guide, First Edition.
Edited by Catherine Adams, Romina Carabott and Sam Evans.

Evidence falls into three main categories:

- oral testimony
- documentary evidence
- real evidence.

Oral testimony

Evidence about the facts in dispute is given by witnesses of fact. A witness must state facts only, which means that the witness may only give evidence of what he/she saw, heard and did. The rules of evidence prevent witnesses of fact from giving opinion evidence (except in the limited sense of opinions intended to convey relevant facts, such as an indication that a vehicle was travelling quickly). The reason for this is that the court is not interested in the opinions of witnesses, as it is for the court to draw the appropriate conclusions from the facts provided by the witnesses. Unless all the parties involved in the litigation agree their evidence, witnesses are usually required to attend court to give oral testimony.

Documentary evidence

In many cases, documents relevant to the issues in the litigation will be made available to the court for consideration. As well as paper records (e.g. correspondence), documentary evidence also includes various types of electronically recorded material, such as audio-visual recordings and data held on computers.

Real evidence

Occasionally, as well as oral and documentary evidence, physical objects will be produced for inspection by the court. These physical objects are known as real evidence, and an example would be a weapon used in an assault.

3.2.2 What is expert evidence?

Most witnesses involved in court proceedings give evidence of fact (matters about which they have direct knowledge). While expert witnesses may give evidence of fact, they are also permitted to give opinion evidence, provided the opinion is within their sphere of expertise. For example, a forensic scientist examining a crime scene for fingerprints may provide information about the circumstances in which any fingerprints were obtained (evidence of fact), but will also be permitted to explain whether the fingerprints match those of the defendant (opinion evidence). Therefore, expert witnesses represent an exception to the normal position limiting witnesses to only giving evidence of facts within their knowledge.

Additionally, under the *hearsay rules*, witnesses of fact are usually prevented from referring to things said or written by other people outside court. However, expert witnesses are permitted to rely on the words, thoughts and views of others, and can base their opinions on the published and unpublished material of others (including books, journals and research papers), as well as drawing on their own training and experience. Expert evidence is, therefore, an exception to the general rules relating to hearsay evidence.

Expert evidence in given in two ways, via written report and oral evidence. Both report writing and giving evidence at court are key skills, and guidance regarding these aspects of acting as an expert witness is given later in this chapter.

3.2.3 Who can act as an expert witness?

An expert witness is someone who makes his/her knowledge and experience available to help the court to understand the issues in the case, and thereby reach a sound and just decision. Therefore, an expert witness must be an expert in their field and must comply with the duties and obligations that expert witnesses owe to the court. The nature of the expert's duties to the court are discussed in detail later in this chapter.

In *RP v Nottingham City Council and the Official Solicitor (Mental Capacity of Parent)* [2008] EWCA Civ 462, it was noted that the court will receive expert evidence only where the expert has the requisite expertise to advise the court on the particular point in question. Although the onus is on the court to ensure that the expert selected is able to provide the advice sought, an expert witness will usually be required to provide a curriculum vitae setting out his/her qualifications and experience.

3.2.4 The expert witness's role in court proceedings

Expert evidence is required when the court needs assistance in resolving a key issue that is outside the court's skill and experience. However, expert evidence is likely to be only one aspect of the evidence available to the court. We do not have a system of 'trial by expert', and the court's decision is based on the totality of the evidence. Therefore, it is possible for a court to prefer the evidence of lay witnesses to that of an expert. Essentially, while an expert advises it is the court that decides.

In *R v Bonython* (1984) 38 S.A.S.R. 45, the South Australia Supreme Court noted that, where there is a dispute about whether expert evidence should be admitted, consideration should be given to:

1. whether a person (i.e. juror) without the qualification or experience of the expert would be able to form a sound judgment on the issue(s) before the court;
2. whether the subject matter of the opinion forms part of a body of knowledge or experience which is sufficiently organised or recognised to be accepted as a reliable body of knowledge or experience;

3. whether the expert has a special acquaintance with this such that their opinion would assist the court;
4. whether the expert has sufficient knowledge (through study or experience) of the subject to make their opinion on the issue(s) of assistance to the court.

While being an expert witness means you have increased responsibilities to the court, you are entitled to be paid for your work, whereas other witnesses are generally not paid.

3.3 The rules of court

3.3.1 Why is expert evidence governed by rules of court?

In his review of civil litigation in England and Wales, Lord Woolf found serious fault with the system of expert evidence, pointing out the central tension that exists between the expert's dual roles as a paid agent of one of the parties and as an independent witness giving assistance to the court (Woolf, 1996). He identified the danger that experts were being transformed into 'additional advocates of the parties' – a position which he noted already, to an extent, existed in the United States, and which should not be emulated in the courts in England and Wales. Lord Woolf was also concerned that experts were often used in cases where expert evidence was not really needed at all. Inappropriate use of experts led to increased costs and delay, and arose because the parties generally had complete control over the scope and presentation of their case. Lord Woolf argued for a series of reforms, including court control over the use of expert evidence, the wider use of the single joint expert, and new rules emphasising that the expert's primary duty is to the court rather than to the instructing party.

Lord Justice Auld noted similar issues relating to expert evidence in his subsequent review of the domestic criminal courts (Auld, 2001).

The recommendations from these reviews were the main drivers for the introduction of the procedural rules that now govern the use of expert witnesses in the courts of England and Wales.

3.3.2 Which rules apply?

The rules of court that govern the use of expert evidence vary depending on the nature of the litigation in which the expert is instructed. An expert instructed in court proceedings is going to be involved in either criminal, civil or family proceedings.

Criminal proceedings usually involve an individual being prosecuted by the state for the commission of an offence, such as murder or theft. Civil proceedings normally involve one individual bringing a claim against another individual for breaching an obligation, such as failing to fulfil a contract or committing a negligent act. Family proceedings are a form of civil proceedings, which usually involve the breakdown of a family relationship, such as a divorce or a dispute regarding the arrangements for the care of children.

Table 3.1 Rules of court: a summary

Nature of proceedings	Applicable procedural regime
Criminal	Part 33 Criminal Procedure Rules*
Civil	Part 35 Civil Procedure Rules, and Practice Direction 35 – Experts and Assessors
	Protocol for the Instruction of Experts to give Evidence in Civil Claims (2005)
	Practice Direction – Pre-action Conduct
Family	Part 25 Family Procedure Rules, and Practice Directions 25A–25F

*Expert witnesses instructed by the Crown Prosecution Service will also be required to comply with *Disclosure: Experts' Evidence, Case Management and Unused Material* (May 2010)

The three main categories of court proceedings are each governed by their own procedural rules. As the provisions of each set of rules are different, it is essential that expert witnesses understand which rules apply to the proceedings in which they have been instructed. Table 3.1 summarises the rules that apply to the different types of proceedings, and the rules are available to download from the Ministry of Justice website (www.justice.gov.uk).

3.3.3 Key differences between the procedural regimes

The three procedural regimes are each designed to address similar concerns relating to expert evidence, such as ensuring that the expert's focus is providing objective assistance to the court. However, there are some significant differences between the regimes. In particular, the rules relating to the instruction of expert witnesses and the disclosure of expert evidence differ depending on whether the expert is instructed in a criminal, civil or family case.

In criminal and civil proceedings, the parties are generally free to instruct any expert witness of their choice. However, in family proceedings the position is different. Where the proceedings relate to a child, Rule 25.4(2)(a) of the Family Procedure Rules 2010 provides that no party may instruct an expert without the court's permission. Furthermore, Rule 25.4(2)(b) provides that 'a child may not be medically or psychiatrically examined or otherwise assessed for the purposes of the provision of expert evidence in the proceedings' without the court's permission. Therefore, an expert cannot be instructed in family proceedings relating to a child without the permission of the court having first been obtained, and disclosure of information and documents without permission may amount to contempt of court. In practice, the need to have the court's permission to disclose information or documents to an expert, or to have the child examined or assessed, means that in children proceedings the court strictly controls the number, fields of expertise and identity of the experts who may be instructed to provide evidence. It is essential that any expert witness instructed in proceedings relating to a child checks that the requisite permission has been granted by the court.

The position relating to disclosure of expert evidence also differs depending on the nature of the proceedings. Generally, litigation privilege applies to expert evidence.

This means that the parties will usually be able to choose whether they wish to disclose/rely on any expert evidence which they have commissioned. In practice, this means that if a party obtains expert evidence that is unfavourable, it does not have to be disclosed to the other party or to the court. The principal exceptions to this position are expert evidence commissioned by the prosecution in criminal proceedings and expert evidence commissioned in family proceedings relating to children.

In criminal proceedings, the prosecution is under a duty to disclose any evidence that either undermines the prosecution's case or which may assist the defence. Therefore, if the prosecution commissions expert evidence, which proves to be unfavourable, that evidence has to be made available to the defence.

In family proceedings relating to children, litigation privilege does not apply. This means that the party who commissioned the expert evidence cannot refuse to disclose it to the other parties and to the court, even if it is adverse to their position. The rationale for this is that, in cases involving children, the court's paramount consideration is the welfare of the child, and thus the court needs to have access to all the available evidence in order to make the decision that accords with the child's best interests.

3.4 The expert's duties

3.4.1 The Ikarian Reefer

The Ikarian Reefer was a commercial shipping case, during which the judge, Creswell J, gave guidance on the duties and responsibilities of expert witnesses; see *National Justice Compania Naviera SA v Prudential Assurance Co. Ltd* [1993] 2 Lloyds' Rep 68. The principles set out by Creswell J have received universal approval and are, therefore, equally applicable in criminal and family proceedings. Creswell J noted that the duties and responsibilities of expert witnesses included the following:

1. Expert evidence presented to the court should be – and should be seen to be – the independent product of the expert uninfluenced as to form or content by the exigencies of litigation.
2. An expert witness should provide independent assistance to the court by way of objective unbiased opinion in relation to matters within his/her expertise. An expert witness should never assume the role of advocate.
3. An expert witness should state the facts or assumptions on which his/her opinion is based. An expert witness should not omit to consider material facts that detract from his/her concluded opinion.
4. An expert witness should make it clear when a particular question or issue falls outside his/her expertise.
5. If an expert's opinion is not properly researched because he/she considers that insufficient data is available, then this must be stated with an indication that the opinion is no more than a provisional one.

6. If, after exchange of reports, an expert witness changes his/her view on a material matter, such change of view should be communicated to the other side without delay and, when appropriate, to the court.
7. Where expert evidence refers to photographs, plans, calculations, survey reports or other similar documents, these must be provided to the opposite party at the same time as the exchange of reports.

The procedural rules of court governing expert evidence expand on these core principles, and emphasise both the expert's overriding duty to the court and the particular duties owed by expert witnesses.

3.4.2 The overriding duty

An expert witness owes an overriding duty to the court, which takes precedence over any obligation to the person from whom the expert has received instructions or by whom the expert is paid. Therefore, it is not the expert's role to promote the point of view of the party instructing them or to engage in the role of advocate for one of the parties. The expert's principal duty is to provide objective, unbiased evidence on matters within their expertise.

Without the objectivity required by the overriding objective, an expert ceases to be independent and simply becomes a 'hired gun' on behalf of the client. If that happens, the expert's testimony will be found wanting and discounted, if not entirely disregarded. For example, in the civil litigation case *Pearce v Ove Arup* [2001] EWHC 455 (Ch), the claimant's expert architect was held not to have been objective. He failed to consider all the relevant facts and documents, and was so irrational and biased that he had failed to meet his duty to the court to be objective. Instead, he had come to argue the case and any point which supported it, however flimsy. The judge noted that the expert bore a heavy responsibility for the case ever coming to trial at all. As a result, his evidence was rejected and the judge reported him to his professional body. The same principles apply equally to expert witnesses in criminal and family proceedings.

3.4.3 The particular duties

The particular duties with which an expert witness must comply are set out most fully under Family Procedure Rules 2010, Practice Direction 25B (The duties of an expert, the expert's report, and arrangements for an expert to attend court – paragraph 4.1), which notes that an expert shall have regard to the following duties:

1. to assist the court in accordance with the overriding duty;
2. to provide advice to the court that conforms to the best practice of the expert's profession;

3. to answer questions about which the expert is required to give an opinion (in children proceedings, those questions will be set out in the order of the court giving permission for an expert to be instructed, a child to be examined or otherwise assessed or expert evidence to be put before the court);
4. to provide an opinion that is independent of the party or parties instructing the expert;
5. to confine the opinion to matters material to the issues in the case and in relation only to questions that are within the expert's expertise (skill and experience);
6. where a question has been put which falls outside the expert's expertise, to state this at the earliest opportunity and to volunteer an opinion as to whether another expert is required to bring expertise not possessed by those already involved or, in the rare case, as to whether a second opinion is required on a key issue and, if possible, what questions should be asked of the second expert;
7. in expressing an opinion, to take into consideration all of the material facts including any relevant factors arising from ethnic, cultural, religious or linguistic contexts at the time the opinion is expressed;
8. to inform those instructing the expert without delay of any change in the opinion and of the reason for the change.

While neither the Criminal Procedure Rules nor the Civil Procedure Rules particularise the expert's duties to the same degree, you would be well advised to comply with the provisions of Practice Direction 25B regardless of whether you are undertaking criminal, civil or family work.

3.5 Report writing

Report writing is probably the key skill for expert witnesses, as a well-written, clearly argued report may obviate the need for the expert to attend court and give oral evidence. While the rules of court prescribe the matters that should be included in an expert's report, they do not provide a template. Some clear, common-sense advice regarding how to structure an expert's report is provided by Sir Nicholas Wall, former President of the High Court's Family Division (Wall, 2007, para. 17.5), who notes that:

> The court looks above all for clarity in presentation and in the conclusions reached. The court is concerned with:
>
> 1. the issues it asked you to address;
> 2. the material you have considered;
> 3. the conclusions you have reached; and
> 4. your reasons for reaching those conclusions.

Therefore, the basic structure for any expert's report should make clear: what the expert has been asked to do, what investigations the expert has undertaken, what conclusions the expert has reached and why those conclusions are correct.

3.5.1 The content of an expert's report

The rules of court contain provisions regarding the content of expert's reports. The provisions are virtually identical regardless of whether the report is prepared for criminal, civil or family proceedings, and require that an expert's report must:

1. give details of the expert's qualifications;
2. give details of any literature or other material which has been relied on in making the report;
3. contain a statement setting out the substance of all facts and instructions that are material to the opinions expressed in the report or on which those opinions are based;
4. make clear which of the facts stated in the report are within the expert's own knowledge;
5. say who carried out any examination, measurement, test or experiment which the expert has used for the report, give the qualifications of that person, and say whether or not the test or experiment has been carried out under the expert's supervision;
6. where there is a range of opinion on the matters dealt with in the report, summarise the range of opinions and give reasons for the expert's own opinion;
7. contain a summary of the conclusions reached;
8. if the expert is not able to give an opinion without qualification, state the qualification.

The Family Procedure Rules 2010, Practice Direction 25B (The duties of an expert, the expert's report, and arrangements for an expert to attend court – paragraph 9.1), provides additional guidance in respect of the approach an expert should take when expressing his/her opinion, noting that the expert must:

1. answer the questions about which the expert is to give an opinion and which relate to the issues in the case;
2. take into consideration all of the material facts, including any relevant factors arising from ethnic, cultural, religious or linguistic contexts at the time the opinion is expressed, identifying the facts, literature and any other material including research material that the expert has relied on in forming an opinion;

3. describe their own professional risk assessment process and process of differential diagnosis, highlighting factual assumptions, deductions from the factual assumptions, and any unusual, contradictory or inconsistent features of the case;
4. indicate whether any proposition in the report is an hypothesis (in particular a controversial hypothesis), or an opinion deduced in accordance with peer-reviewed and tested technique, research and experience accepted as a consensus in the scientific community;
5. indicate whether the opinion is provisional (or qualified, as the case may be), stating the qualification and the reason for it, and identifying what further information is required to give an opinion without qualification;
6. where there is a range of opinion on any question to be answered by the expert, in addition to summarising the range of opinion:

   - identify and explain, within the range of opinions, any 'unknown cause', whether arising from the facts of the case (e.g. because there is too little information to form a scientific opinion) or from limited experience or lack of research, peer review or support in the relevant field of expertise; and
   - give reasons for any opinion expressed: the use of a balance sheet approach to the factors that support or undermine an opinion can be of great assistance to the court.

Again, you would be well advised to comply with the additional guidance contained in Practice Direction 25B regardless of whether you are undertaking criminal, civil or family work.

3.5.2 Drafting your reports: Some suggestions

All expert witnesses approach report writing differently, and you will, of course, develop your own style. Set out below are some suggestions to assist you in developing an effective approach to report writing.

Avoid technical language

Remember that you are writing for an audience that does not possess your technical knowledge in relation to the subject matter of your report. You should, therefore, avoid technical language and jargon, which a non-expert reader would find difficult to understand. In *Re F (Children: DNA evidence)* [2008] EWHC 3235 (Fam), the High Court noted that expert witnesses should bear in mind that they were addressing lay people, and reports should provide analysis in clear language.

If your report includes technical terms, you will usually need to include a glossary. Where the definitions and the explanations are short, best practice is to highlight the term in bold and define it in the body of the report when first used, and then to also include it in the glossary for reference.

Avoid errors

It is essential that you check your reports carefully to ensure that they are correct and error-free. A report that contains errors, whether they be factual or grammatical, is likely to give the court cause for concern regarding the rigour and thoroughness of the expert's approach. In *Re C (Care: Contact)* [2009] EWCA Civ 959, the Court of Appeal was critical of the fact that there were a number of inaccuracies in the social worker's affidavit, noting that the 'disturbing tally of damaging inaccuracies ... indicate a deplorably casual and inappropriately hostile approach to a sensitive and responsible task on which that fate of families can depend'.

Keep your reports to a reasonable length

A common complaint among the judiciary is that experts' reports are often too long. One way to keep your reports to an appropriate length is to avoid simply repeating information the court has available to it from other sources. While an expert must always set out the facts and information on which he/she has relied, verbatim repetition of the contents of other documents that are available to the court is usually unnecessary. It is also good practice to make appropriate use of appendices. For example, if you have conducted an interview, then the detail of the interview could be provided in an appendix for reference, with the report noting the fact that the interview took place and referring to any key information arising from the interview, on which the expert wishes to rely.

Avoid offering an opinion on factual disputes

It is the role of the court, not the expert, to resolve any dispute of fact by making findings of fact. Where there is a dispute of fact, an expert should usually set out alternative opinions, making clear how the opinion would vary depending on the findings of fact ultimately made by the court.

Ensure that your opinion is clearly reasoned

An expert's report must be well-reasoned, and must draw on the available evidence in order to support the conclusions advanced. It is not sufficient to simply state facts followed by a conclusion; there must be analysis of why the facts suggest a particular conclusion. For example, in *R v T* [2010] EWCA Crim 2439, the Court of Appeal noted that 'it is simply wrong in principle for an expert to fail to set out the way in which he has reached his conclusions in his report'. Where there is a range of possible opinions, an expert is under an obligation to set out the applicable range and to explain where within that range their opinion falls.

There may be situations in which you wish to revise your opinion, for example when new information becomes available or following a meeting with another expert in the proceedings. Some experts worry that changing their opinion may undermine their credibility. Provided there is a good reason for the change, the court is unlikely to find that a change in opinion undermines an expert's standing, and experts are under a duty to keep their opinions under review. The court is far more likely to be concerned about the dogmatic expert who is unwilling to revise an opinion under any circumstances. For example, in *Re C and D (Children)* [2010] EWHC 3714 (Fam), the judge (HHJ Bellamy) criticised the overly dogmatic approach of a forensic odontologist, who expressed himself as being absolutely certain that a mark on a child's abdomen was a human bite, despite the fact that none of the health care professionals who had examined the child saw any teeth marks or abrasion of the skin. The court concluded that 'it would be surprising if a forensic odontologist viewing poor quality photographs was able to detect with such absolute confidence marks which others could not see with the naked eye with the child right in front of them'.

If you do find yourself in a situation where you wish to revise your opinion, you should contact your instructing solicitor immediately.

3.5.3 The required declarations

The rules of court also provide for reports to include a series of declarations regarding compliance with the expert's duties to the court. Unfortunately, the requirements differ according to whether the report has been prepared for criminal, civil or family proceedings. Table 3.2 summarises the declarations that are required in each of the jurisdictions.

Warranting that a false statement is true is punishable as a contempt of court. It is, therefore, essential that an expert understands and complies with each of the required declarations. The nature of each of the declarations is explored below, and any variance between the requirements for criminal, civil or family proceedings is highlighted.

Statement of truth

Any expert's report must be verified by a statement of truth. The wording of the statement in civil and family proceedings is the same, and is prescribed in the applicable

Table 3.2 Report writing: procedural requirements

Declaration	Criminal proceedings	Civil proceedings	Family proceedings
Statement of truth	Required (mandatory wording)	Required (mandatory wording)	Required (mandatory wording)
Declaration of compliance	Required	Required	Required
Declaration of awareness	Not to be included	Required	Required
Conflict statement	Recommended	Recommended	Required
Scope of instructions	Recommended	Required	Required

Practice Directions. The wording is mandatory and must state:

> I confirm that I have made clear which facts and matters referred to in this report are within my own knowledge and which are not. Those that are within my own knowledge I confirm to be true. The opinions I have expressed represent my true and complete professional opinions on the matters to which they refer.

For criminal proceedings, Rule 33.3(1)(j) requires that an expert's report must 'contain the same declaration of truth as a witness statement'. The recommended form of words is therefore:

> This report consisting of [XX] pages, is true to the best of my knowledge and belief and I make it knowing that, if it is tendered in evidence, I shall be liable to prosecution if I have wilfully stated in it anything which I know to be false or do not believe to be true.

The statement of truth must be verified by the expert's signature and date, and should usually appear as the final declaration in any report.

Declaration of compliance

As noted previously, the expert witness's overriding duty is to the court. All experts are required to include in their reports a declaration confirming that they understand the overriding duty and have complied with it. While there is no prescribed wording for the declaration, you may wish to consider using the following wording:

> I understand my duty as an expert witness to the court to provide independent assistance by way of objective unbiased opinion in relation to matters within my expertise. I will inform all parties and where appropriate the court in the event that my opinion changes on any material issue.

Declaration of awareness

Expert witnesses in civil and family proceedings must include a declaration of awareness in their reports. The declaration is designed to demonstrate that the expert is aware of the procedural rules applicable to the proceedings for which the report has been prepared. Again, there is no prescribed wording for the relevant declarations. In civil proceedings, you may wish to consider using the following wording:

> I confirm that I am aware of the requirements of Part 35 and Practice Direction 35, the Protocol for the Instruction of Experts to give Evidence in Civil Claims 2005, as amended, and the Practice Direction on Pre-action Conduct.

In family proceedings, the following wording should be sufficient:

> I confirm that I am aware of the requirements of Part 25 of the Family Procedure Rules 2010 and the accompanying Practice Directions.

There is no requirement for experts reporting in criminal proceedings to include a declaration of awareness, and therefore no declaration relating to compliance with Part 33 Criminal Procedure Rules should be included in reports prepared for criminal proceedings. However, expert witnesses instructed by the Crown Prosecution Service (CPS) will usually be required to warrant that they have complied with the disclosure requirements contained in the Criminal Procedure and Investigations Act 1996. The CPS produces a guidance booklet for expert witnesses, which all experts instructed by the CPS are required to read and follow (CPS, 2010).

Conflict statement

The inclusion of a statement in respect of any conflict of interest is mandatory only in family proceedings. However, it is recommended good practice in both civil and criminal cases (see *Toth v Jarman* [2006] 4 All ER 1276). Therefore, all experts should give consideration to including a conflict statement in their reports. Again, there is no prescribed wording for the statement, but the following should suffice:

> I confirm that I have no conflict of interest of any kind, other than any that I have already set out in this report. I do not consider that any interest I have disclosed affects my suitability to give expert evidence on any issue on which I have given evidence, and I will advise the party by whom I am instructed if, between the date of this report and the trial, there is any change in circumstances that affects this statement.

Any potential conflict of interests should be disclosed as early as possible, and so an expert should include details of any employment or other activity that might give rise to a conflict in the 'CV' provided to the parties. This will assist the parties, and ultimately the court, to decide whether it is appropriate for the expert to be instructed. In particular, an expert should always disclose any existing link with the parties to the litigation.

Source/scope of instructions

Expert witnesses are required to state the 'substance of all material instructions', whether written or oral. As noted previously, it is essential that the court knows what issues you have been asked to address, and also by whom you have been instructed. Therefore, any expert's report should make clear both the scope of the instructions received and by whom the expert was instructed (e.g. on behalf of the claimant, the defendant, as a single joint expert etc.).

3.6 Giving evidence at court

In the majority of cases an expert witness's involvement in proceedings will be limited to his/her report, as the expert's evidence will often be unchallenged and may lead to the litigation being resolved without the need for a fully contested hearing. However, there will still be a significant number of cases where it is necessary for the expert to give oral evidence. The following summary provides an overview of the key aspects of giving evidence at court.

3.6.1 The process of giving evidence

Before giving oral evidence all witnesses are asked to either take the oath or to affirm. The oath or affirmation is an important part of the evidence gathering process as it is a solemn promise by the witness to tell the truth. A witness who lies when giving evidence to the court could be prosecuted for perjury.

The process by which a witness gives oral evidence at court is usually divided into three stages:

- evidence-in-chief
- cross-examination
- re-examination.

Evidence-in-chief

Evidence-in-chief is the procedure by which an advocate facilitates the giving of evidence by their own witnesses. Therefore, an expert witness will usually be called to give evidence-in-chief by the party instructing them. The degree to which evidence-in-chief will be required will depend on the nature of the litigation. In all proceedings, a copy of the expert's report will have been provided to the other parties and to the court. In civil and family proceedings, the usual procedure is for the expert to adopt their report as being true and accurate. The report can then be accepted by the court as the expert's evidence-in-chief, and the expert may not be required to give much additional evidence-in-chief. However, in criminal proceedings the court usually requires witnesses to give all of their evidence orally, and therefore the advocate calling the expert will take them through their evidence-in-chief in detail.

The fact that, in civil and family proceedings, the expert's report will form the basis of their evidence-in-chief underlines how essential it is that the report sets out all the key evidence the expert is able to provide to the court, as the expert may have limited opportunity to expand on his/her written report when giving oral evidence.

Cross-examination

Cross-examination is the procedure by which an advocate challenges the evidence given by a witness for another party. A key difference between evidence-in-chief and cross-examination is that, during cross-examination, the advocate will usually be endeavouring to control the scope of the witness's responses and limit the witness's opportunity to 'tell their story'. Often this is achieved through the use of leading questions. A leading question is one which leads the witness towards a suggested response. For example, 'was he standing two feet away from you?' is a leading question, whereas 'how far away was he?' is non-leading. Leading questions often call for a 'yes' or 'no' response.

Re-examination

Re-examination is the procedure by which an advocate seeks clarification of matters arising during cross-examination. Re-examination is conducted by the advocate who calls the witness to give evidence-in-chief, and it provides an opportunity for the advocate to try to repair any damage done during cross-examination. As re-examination is restricted to matters arising during cross-examination, rather than being a further opportunity for a witness to give evidence-in-chief, it will not be required in every case.

3.6.2 Questioning

The majority of the questions that you will be asked at court will be asked by either professional advocates (barristers or solicitors), or perhaps by parties who are representing themselves. When giving evidence you should remember that, although questions are asked by the advocates, you should always direct your answers to the judge/magistrates who are hearing the case. You may also be asked questions by the judge/magistrates.

All advocates have their own styles, and it is impossible to provide you with a guide to dealing with each individual advocate's questioning techniques. However, it is very common for witnesses, including experts, to feel apprehensive about giving evidence. In order to familiarise yourself with the court process you should spend some time at your local courts observing cases and witnesses giving evidence. In particular, most criminal proceedings in the magistrates' courts and the Crown Court are open to the public, and some civil proceedings in the county courts are also open to the public.

While it is not possible to provide a guide to dealing with all the difficult questions you may be asked, there are some 'dos and don'ts' which you may find it helpful to follow.

Have a good knowledge of the relevant facts

There is likely to be a very long gap between writing your report and attending court to give oral evidence. It is essential that you re-familiarise yourself with the facts of the case before you give evidence. If you make errors in the basic facts of the case, this is likely to undermine the court's confidence in your evidence.

Give succinct and clear answers

The expert's role is to assist the court with matters outside of the court's expertise. An expert must give his/her evidence succinctly and clearly, so that it can be understood by – and therefore be of assistance to – the court. Lengthy answers which are difficult to follow should be avoided.

Avoid technical explanations

As with report writing, you should avoid using technical language when giving evidence. Matters that you may consider to be 'basic principles' may need to be explained, as the court will not possess your expertise. You should not assume that the court has a particular level of knowledge and, where appropriate, you must be prepared to provide basic explanations and clarification.

The 'yes'/'no' answer

One tactic that advocates sometimes employ is to demand a 'yes' or 'no' answer from an expert. You should never be afraid to explain to an advocate that the question requires a more detailed response, and that a yes/no answer is neither appropriate nor helpful. Similarly, if an advocate begins to talk over you and prevents you from fully answering a question, you should insist on completing your answer to the initial question before moving on to discuss the next issue. However, always retain your equanimity and never put yourself in a situation where you end up either arguing with an advocate or asking them questions. You should be protected from inappropriate questioning by the court, and always remember that the advocate is simply doing his/her job and there is nothing personal in tough cross-examination.

Never stray outside your expertise

It is essential that you limit your evidence to matters within your professional expertise. Advocates will often invite experts to speculate on issues in an attempt to undermine their credibility. If a question raises an issue that is outside your expertise, then you should explain the position and decline to answer the question unless requested to do so by the court.

Remember that your overriding duty is to the court

An expert witness should never be tempted to act as an advocate for the party instructing them. The court requires experts to give independent and objective evidence. If you are regularly instructed by the same party, for example undertaking only prosecution work in criminal proceedings, you should be prepared for an advocate to challenge your objectivity. It is essential that you are able to clearly explain the expert's overriding duty to the court, and that you are able to demonstrate that you have complied with the requirement to be objective. In *Re M (Adoption: Leave to Oppose)* [2009] EWHC 3643 (Fam), an expert was found to lack the detached objectivity expected in an expert witness, and it was noted that he gave evidence only on behalf of parents who have been accused of child abuse.

Where appropriate, you should be prepared to make concessions when giving your evidence. The court will place little confidence in the dogmatic expert who is not prepared to acknowledge any point of view other than his/her own. In *R v Hall* [2011] EWCA Crim 4, the Court of Appeal rejected the 'new' expert evidence advanced by the defendant and was particularly concerned by the expert's 'inflexibility towards reasonable scientific alternatives ... methodology and interpretation of spectra'. Where you are asked to consider a proposition that is credible, but with which you disagree, you should acknowledge the viability of the proposition and then go on to explain why you disagree with it.

Project confidently

Giving evidence is nerve racking. However, it is essential that an expert witness carries the confidence of the court. Therefore, you need to project confidently. Remember not to speak too quickly, as this may make you appear nervous and will also make it difficult for the court to take a note of your evidence. Try to avoid looking down or uncomfortable (e.g. grimacing), especially if you have been asked a difficult question. Remember that an expert should dress in a way consistent with his/her professional status, and the usual court dress is a business suit.

An excellent summary of what to do and what to avoid when giving expert evidence can be found in *Manning v King's College Hospital NHS Trust* [2008] EWHC 1838 (QB). In that case the judge, Stadlen J, noted that persuasive experts were 'authoritative, careful and straightforward in their evidence', but was critical of experts who:

- strayed 'into the territory of advocate rather than expert witness'
- were 'ready to volunteer opinions in areas outside his actual or apparent area of expertise'
- often volunteered 'by way of addition, answers to questions which he had not been asked which appeared to support the Defendants' case'
- created the impression that 'perhaps because he believed in the Defendants' case, he was somewhat inflexible in his answers and reluctant to concede points which on their merits were persuasive'.

3.6.3 Addressing the court

It is essential that you address correctly the judge/magistrates who are hearing your evidence. If in doubt about the appropriate form of address to use, you should ask your instructing solicitor before you begin giving your evidence. However, Table 3.3 should assist in ensuring that you use the correct terminology.

Who can you speak to at court?

If you are required to attend court to give evidence then this usually means that your evidence is not accepted by at least one of the parties in the case. Prior to

Table 3.3 Addressing the judiciary

Tribunal	Correct form of address
Magistrates	*Either* Your Worships (if addressed collectively) *or* Sir/Ma'am (when addressing the Chair of the Bench)
District Judge	Sir/Ma'am
Circuit Judge or Recorder	Your Honour (regardless of whether the judge is male or female)
High Court Judge	My Lord/Lady Your Lordship/Ladyship

giving your evidence, you can usually expect to be spoken to by the lawyer who commissioned your evidence, who should update you on any relevant developments that have occurred since your report was prepared. This is perfectly permissible.

If you are approached by any of the lawyers acting for the other parties (or by the parties themselves), then – other than exchanging the normal pleasantries – you should avoid discussing the case with them, unless you have been asked to do so by the lawyer who commissioned your evidence.

Once you have started giving your evidence, then it is not permissible for you to discuss your evidence with anyone. Therefore, if there is adjournment before your evidence is completed (e.g. for lunch or overnight) you cannot discuss your evidence with anyone. In practice, the lawyers will wish to avoid any possible suggestion that they have attempted to influence your testimony, and often will not engage in any discussion with you at all. This can make the witness box a very lonely place.

3.7 Ancillary topics

In addition to the key duties and skills already discussed, there are a number of other aspects of the expert's role about which any expert witness needs to be aware, and the principal ones are considered below.

3.7.1 Written questions to experts

Both the Civil Procedure Rules (Rule 35.6) and the Family Procedure Rules (Rule 25.10) allow the parties to put written questions to an expert following receipt of the expert's report. However, there are no corresponding provisions in the Criminal Procedure Rules, and so an expert witness instructed in criminal proceedings should not usually receive requests to answer written questions from the parties.

The purpose of any supplemental questions must be to clarify matters in the expert's report. Questions are not intended to be a form of 'paper cross-examination' to test the expert's opinion prior to trial. If you receive written questions you are obliged to answer them. Your answers to any questions will be treated as if they were part of your original report, and therefore, when answering written questions, you are bound by all the procedural declarations that must be included in a report.

3.7.2 Experts' meetings and 'hot tubbing'

Where more than one party wants to rely on expert evidence, the court may direct that the experts meet prior to trial. Experts' meetings represent an exception to the general position that witnesses should not discuss their evidence.

The purpose of an experts' meeting is to explore the level of agreement/ disagreement between the experts, with a view to reducing (or even eliminating) the need for contested, oral expert evidence. As with written questions, the purpose of the meeting is not for the parties to cross-examine the experts and test their evidence before trial, and the lawyers' input into the meeting should normally be limited to setting the agenda. At the conclusion of the meeting a Statement of Agreement and Disagreement will usually be prepared and signed by the experts.

Specific guidance about the conduct of experts' meetings in family proceedings is set out in Family Procedure Rules 2010, Practice Direction 25E (Discussions between experts in family proceedings), and you will probably find it useful to read Practice Direction 25E to help you prepare for any experts' meeting that you are required to attend even if you are undertaking civil or criminal work.

A recent development, which builds on the concept of the experts' meeting and which is likely to become more common in future, is 'hot tubbing'. Essentially, hot tubbing is a process that enables expert evidence to be considered in a more issues-based and discursive way. The first reported case in which the merits of hot tubbing were considered by the court was *A Local Authority v A (No. 2)* [2011] EWHC 590 (Fam), where three experts – two consultant psychiatrists and a clinical psychologist – were commissioned to provide evidence in relation to the child's future care. The High Court Judge (Ryder J) noted the potential benefits of hot tubbing when a court is hearing evidence from multiple experts:

> The three experts commissioned to analyse the key issues were heard in oral evidence by the court. Not for the first time this court was very greatly assisted by hearing their evidence concurrently. A device unfortunately and colloquially known as 'hot tubbing' was used with the agreement of all parties. This process has been tested in America and Australia but not in this jurisdiction. Out of the experts' reports and discussions the court derived an agenda of topics which were relevant to the key issues and to which counsel were asked to contribute. The witnesses were sworn together and the court asked each witness the same questions under each topic, taking a topic at a time. The experts were encouraged to add or explain their own or another's evidence so that a healthy discussion ensued, chaired by the court. Each advocate is permitted to examine or cross examine and where appropriate re-examine each witness after the court has elicited evidence on a topic.
>
> The resulting coherence of evidence and attention to the key issues rather than adversarial point scoring is marked. The evidence of experts who might have been expected to fill 2 days of court time was completed within 4 hours. The evidence can

conveniently be described under themes into which I have interpolated some of the written evidence which was not disputed in cross examination.

This strong endorsement suggests that the courts are likely to look to use hot tubbing in appropriate cases.

3.7.3 Obtaining directions from the court

Usually if an expert witness requires any clarification or assistance with their instructions or their role generally, the first port of call will be the instructing solicitor. Occasionally, an expert may encounter difficulties in obtaining a response from the instructing solicitor, or may be uncertain about the advice received. In such situations the expert is able to apply directly to the court for directions to assist them in carrying out their function.

As with written questions, only the Civil Procedure Rules (Rule 35.14) and the Family Procedure Rules (Rule 25.17) provide for an expert to apply to the court for directions, and there are no corresponding provisions in the Criminal Procedure Rules. Before an expert may file a request for directions with the court, he/she must provide copies of the request to:

- the party instructing them (at least 7 days before they file the request)
- all other parties (at least 4 days before they file the request).

When a request is filed at court, the court will consider it and make whatever directions are deemed to be appropriate. However, experts should use this power very sparingly, and should always endeavour to resolve any issues by liaison with the instructing solicitor.

3.7.4 Acting as a single joint expert

The court has the power to direct that any expert evidence needed in the case is given by a single joint expert. Effectively, this means that all of the parties seeking to rely on expert evidence must jointly instruct the same expert witness. In the event that the parties cannot agree on the identity of the single joint expert, the court may select the expert. This system has a number of attractions in terms of case management, as it limits the amount of evidence that the court has to consider, and also helps to control the costs of the litigation.

The power to direct that expert evidence is commissioned from a single joint expert is available to the court in all types of proceedings. The only exception is that in criminal proceedings the court cannot require the prosecution and defence to instruct the same expert. Therefore, if you receive joint instructions in a criminal case, they will be from co-defendants.

When you are instructed by a single party, your instructions will usually come from that party's solicitor. When you are instructed as a single joint expert, one of the parties' solicitors will usually be nominated as the lead solicitor and will take responsibility for instructing you. In some cases, where the parties cannot agree the scope of the expert's instructions, you may receive separate instructions from each party. However, such cases should be rare.

If you are instructed as a single joint expert, your duties and obligations are exactly the same as if you had been instructed by just one of the parties. Therefore, your overriding duty is still to the court. The principal difference between acting as a single joint expert and being instructed by just one party is that the single joint expert is usually the only expert in the proceedings. This means that there will be no other expert from the same discipline against whom you can compare your views. However, the decision-making process remains the same, and it is the court that decides, not the expert witness.

A single joint expert may be invited to meet with the parties to discuss his/her opinion. This is perfectly permissible, but you must always remember that, as you are jointly instructed, any meeting should include all the instructing parties. If you are invited to a meeting that does not include all of the instructing parties, you should seek confirmation, usually from your instructing solicitor, that all parties have agreed to the meeting taking place or that the meeting has been ordered by the court. This is essential to ensure that you remain objective and are not viewed by any of the parties as being biased against them.

3.7.5 Getting feedback on your work

Expert witnesses understandably like to receive feedback. Solicitors are notoriously bad at providing feedback to experts about how useful the court found the expert's evidence to be.

Experts instructed in family proceedings are entitled to receive feedback as the Family Procedure Rules (Rule 25.19) require the instructing solicitor to 'inform the expert in writing about the court's determination and the use made by the court of the expert's evidence', and to provide the expert with a copy of the court's final order. This should happen within 10 working days of the final hearing. Where a written judgment is produced, a copy of that judgment should be provided to the expert. While there are no equivalent provisions in either civil or criminal cases, one way of endeavouring to ensure that you get feedback on your performance would be to incorporate a requirement to provide feedback (similar to the provisions under Rule 25.19) into your standard terms and conditions when you accept instructions. This would place an obligation on the instructing solicitor to provide feedback. A more informal approach is simply to ask your instructing solicitors, particularly those who instruct you regularly, to give you feedback. Remember that lawyers are not permitted to coach witnesses or influence their evidence in any way, so always wait until a case has concluded before you ask for feedback.

3.7.6 Keeping up to date

Although expert witnesses are not expected to be lawyers, there will be times when the higher courts give judgments which impact on the role of the expert. It is, therefore, important that experts keep up to date with key court decisions. Subscriptions to legal databases are expensive. However, there are a number of free sources of information available, to which you may find it useful to refer.

Free law reports are available online from the British and Irish Legal Information Institute (BAILII; www.bailii.org) and the Judiciary of England and Wales (www.judiciary.gov.uk/media). Reports of family cases are available via the Family Law Week website (www.familylawweek.co.uk).

3.8 Things to avoid

As noted earlier, the purpose of this chapter is to provide you with the key information that you will require in order to be able to discharge the functions of an expert witness with confidence. However, acting as an expert witness is an important and responsible role, which means that there is always the possibility that things may go awry. The following summary endeavours to highlight the potential pitfalls that exist, in order to enable you to avoid getting into difficulties.

3.8.1 Being sued for negligence

Prior to 31 March 2011, witnesses (including expert witnesses) had 'immunity from suit in negligence', which meant that they could not be sued in relation to their evidence. The decision of the Supreme Court in *Jones v Kaney* [2011] UKSC 13 fundamentally altered the extent to which experts can be held liable for the evidence they give, both during, and in anticipation of, court proceedings.

The background to the litigation was that Mr Jones was injured in a road traffic accident, and instructed Dr Kaney (a clinical psychologist) to prepare an expert's report. Dr Kaney concluded that Mr Jones was suffering from post-traumatic stress disorder. Following a meeting with the expert instructed by the defendant, Dr Kaney agreed a joint statement which concluded that Mr Jones' reaction to the accident was simply an adjustment reaction, which did not reach the threshold for a diagnosis of a depressive disorder, and that Mr Jones' behaviour raised doubts about whether his subjective reporting was genuine. When challenged by the instructing solicitor regarding why she had changed her view so significantly, Dr Kaney made a number of admissions including the fact that the joint statement did not reflect her true opinion, and that she had felt under pressure to sign it. The court refused Mr Jones' application for permission to rely on another expert, and his claim had to be settled for significantly less than would have been awarded had the joint statement not been signed.

Mr Jones sued Dr Kaney in negligence. The claim was dismissed as the judge was bound by precedent to find that Dr Kaney was protected by immunity from suit. Given the importance of the issues raised by the litigation, permission was given for an appeal to take place in the Supreme Court. The Supreme Court held that there was no justification for continuing to hold expert witnesses immune from suit for breach of the duty to act with reasonable skill and care in either contract or negligence. However, the court also held that the absolute privilege in respect of claims in defamation should continue.

Although *Jones v Kaney* was a decision in civil proceedings, it applies to all expert witnesses, and thus immunity has been removed from all experts, whether they are involved in civil, criminal or family proceedings. Lord Brown attempted a definition of an expert witness, noting:

> For the purposes of this brief judgment I mean by 'an expert witness' a witness selected, instructed and paid by a party to litigation for his expertise and permitted on that account to give opinion evidence in the dispute. I am not referring, for example, to a treating doctor or forensic pathologist, either of whom may be called to give factual evidence in the case as well as being asked for their opinions upon it without their having been initially retained by either party to the dispute.

Therefore, a professional witness who becomes involved in the case by virtue of his/her day-to-day work and who is not paid for their evidence would not appear to be at risk of being sued. The Supreme Court also made clear that the loss of immunity relates only to a claim by the instructing party, so an expert witness cannot be sued 'by the other side'.

The principal impact of *Jones v Kaney* is that expert witnesses need to ensure that they have appropriate indemnity cover in place, and are likely to find that instructing solicitors will enquire about the nature of an expert's indemnity cover as part of their initial 'pre-instruction' enquiries. Lawyers will want to avoid any potential liability arising from the choice of expert, and are likely to be more diligent in their choice of expert witnesses. Experts, particularly those involved in substantial litigation, may find that they are asked to provide references and details of training undertaken in relation to the duties experts owe to the court. However, if an expert does his/her job properly and applies an appropriate level of skill and care to their work, while complying with the rules of court, then the risk of being sued should be minimal.

3.8.2 Being reported for misconduct

An expert witness who fails to discharge his/her role appropriately is at risk of being reported to their professional body. Such a complaint is most likely to be made by a disgruntled party, but, in appropriate circumstances, could be made by an instructing solicitor or even the court. For example, in *A London Borough Council v K* [2009] EWHC 850 (Fam), the trial judge, Baker J, was so concerned about a doctor's failure to confine his evidence to matters within his expertise and to approach his evidence objectively that he gave permission for the judgment to be released to the General Medical Council.

Unfortunately, there is very little that any professional can do to prevent a vexatious complaint. However, as with negligence claims, provided you comply with the duties that an expert witness owes to the court and remain within your sphere of competence, it is very unlikely that you will be at risk of any justifiable complaint.

3.8.3 Wasted-costs orders

A wasted-costs order is an order that a legal representative pay a specified sum in respect of costs to a party, or that the costs relating to work undertaken by a legal representative be disallowed. Wasted-costs orders are rare, and will only be made where loss and expense have been caused by the unjustifiable conduct of the litigation. In extreme circumstances, where an expert witness has recklessly failed to comply with his/her duties, they may be ordered to pay any costs incurred as a result personally; see *Phillips v Symes (no. 2)* [2004] EWHC 2330 (Ch).

3.8.4 Contempt and perjury

Witnesses are under an obligation to give truthful evidence. All expert witnesses are under an obligation to verify the contents of their reports with a statement of truth, and will be required to take the oath or affirmation before giving oral evidence. Failing to give truthful evidence can have serious consequences.

In criminal proceedings, making a false statement in a report prepared for court is punishable as perjury. In civil and family proceedings verifying a document as true without an honest belief in its truth is a contempt of court. Contempt of court can also cover other activities, such as inappropriate behaviour in court and refusing to comply with court orders. Giving false oral evidence in any court is punishable as perjury. Both perjury and contempt are punishable by a fine or imprisonment.

Obviously, any suggestion that an expert witness has deliberately given false evidence is going to significantly undermine their credibility and the treatment of their evidence by the court. In *R v O'Shea* [2010] EWCA Crim 2879, the Court of Appeal noted that a forensic computer expert's evidence should be treated with caution, commenting that:

> Quite apart from other reasons, in our view his denial to us of having signed a confidentiality agreement in the case of Grout was a deliberate lie, maintained until his signed agreement was produced to him. It is also relevant that he has been convicted of perjury as a result of his misrepresenting his qualifications when giving evidence.

3.9 A final thought

It is hoped that the information contained in this chapter will have reassured you that, provided you only accept instructions within your sphere of competence and you comply with the procedural rules of court, you should not encounter any difficulties in discharging the role of expert witness. However, if you do decide to start working as an expert, please remember that, no matter how much training you undertake with regard to the expert's role or how much experience you acquire as an expert, you are not a lawyer and should not be taking decisions about any legal issues. You will develop working relationships with your instructing solicitors. Therefore, if you are in any doubt about your instructions or your role in the proceedings, you should always ask your instructing solicitor. The latter would much rather you seek clarification than take your own decision, which may prove to be incorrect and could compromise the litigation.

3.10 References

Crown Prosecution Service (CPS) (2010) Disclosure: Experts' Evidence, Case Management and Unused Material'. Available at: www.cps.gov.uk/legal/d_to_g/disclosure_manual/annex_k_disclosure_manual/#a12 (accessed 10 June 2013).

The Right Honourable Lord Justice Auld (2001) *A Review of the Criminal Courts in England and Wales*, Department of Constitutional Affairs.

The Right Honourable Lord Justice Wall (2007, 2nd edn) *A Handbook for Expert Witnesses in Children Act Cases, Family Law*, Jordan Publishing Limited.

The Right Honourable the Lord Woolf (1996) *Access to Justice: Final Report to the Lord Chancellor on the Civil Justice System in England and Wales*, Department of Constitutional Affairs.

4

Mortuary practice

Alison Anderson
NHS Greater Glasgow and Clyde Mortuaries, UK

4.1 Definitions of a mortuary

4.1.1 Permanent mortuary

A permanent mortuary is a building where the deceased are cared for by trained mortuary staff, Anatomical Pathology Technologists (APTs). The premises will offer secure storage for the deceased, in refrigerated conditions, and will have a discreet, dedicated egress. Additional services may be provided including autopsy and bereavement services.

The premises must have refrigerated body storage, an autopsy suite, viewing/waiting room for the bereaved, offices and showering/changing facilities. Guidance on providing these facilities is provided by National Health Service (2005) and National Health Service Scotland (2002).

The mortuary may be located within an NHS facility or be a public mortuary under the jurisdiction of the local Coroner or Procurator Fiscal.

4.1.2 Emergency mortuary

An emergency mortuary or disaster/temporary mortuary may be required if an incident has a great number of fatalities that will overwhelm the existing local mortuary. The purpose of the mortuary will be (London Mass Fatality Plan, version 3, January 2010):

1. to establish identity, through careful examination of the deceased and associated property, in order to obtain evidence that can be matched with data obtained by the ante-mortem team and casualty bureau;
2. to facilitate establishment of the precise cause of death through proper examination of the deceased by pathologists;

Forensic Odontology: An Essential Guide, First Edition.
Edited by Catherine Adams, Romina Carabott and Sam Evans.

3. to facilitate collection of evidence of crime – not only in the cause of death but by examination of clothing and other exhibits recovered from the deceased (e.g. bomb fragments).
4. to allow for the preservation and recording of personal effects of the deceased;
5. to provide facilities for preparation of the deceased victims for release to family members by reconstructive techniques where necessary (embalming may be appropriate in some cases – particularly in the case of repatriation overseas).

Arrangements for the emergency mortuary will be predetermined as part of a local emergency plan which will pinpoint land, premises/demountable structure and locally sourced equipment and consumables. The arrangements may simply involve a retainer contract with a commercial disaster management company. For a larger number of fatalities, the National Emergency Mortuary Arrangements (NEMA) may be deployed. The structure requires a local authority to have predetermined a suitable site within the locality.

The emergency mortuary will require the same facilities and provide the same services as that of a permanent mortuary.

4.2 The Human Tissue Act and the Human Tissue Authority

In England, Wales and Northern Ireland, the Human Tissue Act (Act, 2004) requires that all premises where post-mortems are to be carried out must be licensed. Permanent and emergency mortuaries must comply with the regulations set by the Human Tissue Authority.

The Human Tissue Act 2004 and the Human Tissue Act (Scotland) 2006 (Act, 2006) consolidate earlier legislation, the Human Tissue Act 1961, the Anatomy Act 1984 and the Human Organ Transplants Act 1989. This was mainly brought about as a consequence of the Alder Hey inquiry (Redfearn *et al.*, 2001) and the Kennedy inquiry at the Bristol Royal Infirmary (DH, 2001). These inquiries demonstrated that body parts were being retained after post-mortem examinations without the consent or knowledge of the next of kin. The Human Tissue Acts aim to make *consent* a fundamental principle underpinning the use and storage of human tissues.

The Human Tissue Authority (HTA) was established under the Human Tissue Act 2004. It regulates the removal, storage, use and disposal of human bodies, organs and tissues. The following are illegal:

- removing, storing or using human tissue without consent
- DNA 'theft' – taking and testing DNA without consent
- organ trafficking
- storing tissues or organs for a purpose not stated.

The penalties range from a fine to three years' imprisonment, or both.

Post-mortem examinations, whether authorised by the coroner or not, must take place on HTA licensed premises. In the pathology sector the following activities (taken from the HTA website) will need to be licensed:

- carrying out of an anatomical examination
- making of a post-mortem examination
- removal of relevant material from a deceased person
- storage of relevant material from a deceased person (other than for a specific ethically approved project)
- storage of anatomical specimens
- storage of relevant material from a living person for research (other than for a specific ethically approved project) or for human application
- public display of a body or material from a deceased person.

The Scheduled Purposes (as written in the Human Tissues Act 2004) which apply to this storage licence are as follows:

- determining the cause of death
- obtaining scientific or medical information about a living or deceased person which may be relevant to any other person (including a future person)
- research in connection with disorders, or the functioning, of the human body
- clinical audit
- quality assurance
- establishing after a person's death the efficacy of any drug or other treatment administered to him/her
- education or training relating to human health
- public health monitoring.

4.3 Legal requirements for licence issue

The legal requirements for licence issue (taken from the HTA website) are as follows:

1. The HTA must have received an application (HTA compliance report).
2. The HTA must be satisfied that the proposed *designated individual* (DI) is a suitable person.
3. The HTA must be satisfied that the proposed *licence holder* (LH) is a suitable person/entity.

4. The HTA must be satisfied that the premises are suitable.
5. The licence and any conditions must be acknowledged in writing by the DI and LH.

The Human Tissue Act 2004 specifies several statutory roles that must be filled by named personnel in order for a licence to be granted. In particular, DIs and LHs both have significant roles in the licensing arrangements under the Act.

4.3.1 Designated individuals

A designated individual is the person under whose supervision the licensed activity is authorised to be carried out. He/she has legal responsibility under Section 18 of the Act to ensure:

- that suitable practices are used in undertaking the licensed activity
- that other persons working under the licence are suitable
- that the conditions of the licence are complied with.

The HTA is not prescriptive about who should take on the role of the DI. However, it is important that it be a person who is in a position to ensure that activities are conducted properly, by people who are suitable to carry out those activities, and that all the necessary requirements are complied with. The DI could be a head of department, pathologist, or mortuary manager.

4.3.2 Licence holders

The licence holder is usually a corporate body where possible (e.g. an NHS Trust). The corporate body should provide the contact name of an individual (more senior than the DI) who will act as a representative for the corporate body. The HTA is required to provide all notices of licence decisions to both the LH and the DI.

4.4 Mortuary facilities

4.4.1 Mortuary layout

As previously stated, guidance for the provision of mortuary facilities is provided in the design and briefing guidance.

The design of the mortuary must be conducive to safe working practices. A good mortuary layout allows an organised methodical workflow, thus avoiding or minimising unnecessary movement or manual handling (Figure 4.1).

In line with health and safety regulations, the mortuary facility must have clear demarcation between areas that are considered 'clean' (dry) or 'dirty' (wet). If possible,

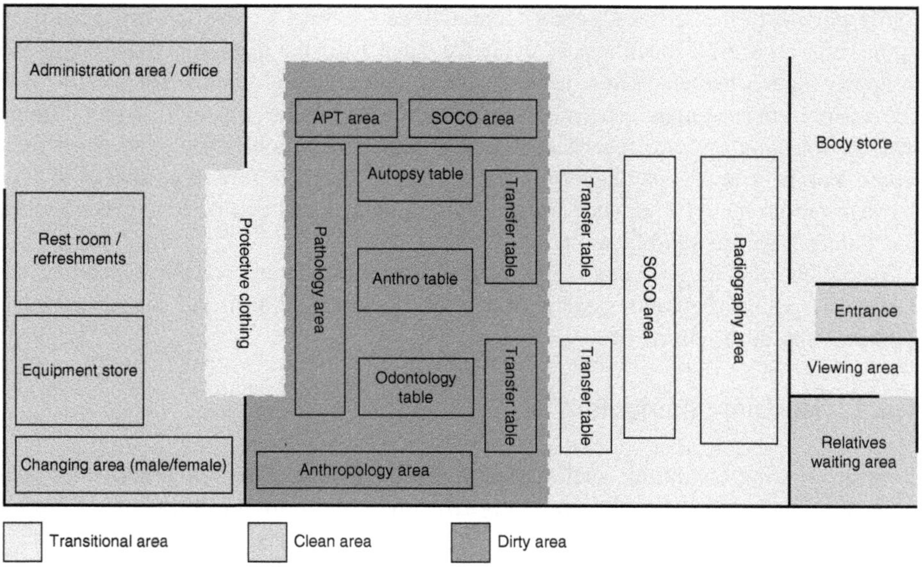

Figure 4.1 Delineation of clean, dirty and transitional areas in a temporary mortuary. APT, Anatomical Pathology Technologist; SOCO, Scenes of Crime Officer

a physical boundary should clearly designate the areas, so promoting awareness and ensuring that no cross-contamination occurs.

Clean areas include:

- reception, waiting and viewing areas
- storerooms
- offices
- post-mortem visitor observation areas.

No protective clothing is required in these areas, but soiled clothing must be appropriately disposed of before entering designated clean areas.

The mortuary facility will also have a *transitional area.* This includes washing, showering and changing facilities and a stock of protective clothing. The area will be set up to allow removal and disposal of soiled protective clothing (dirty) before moving into the washing area (clean).

Dirty areas include:

- post-mortem room
- soiled protective clothing discard area.

The appropriate protective clothing for use in the dirty areas will be detailed in *standard operating procedures*.

All work with the deceased, organs and unfixed specimens must be carried out only in the dirty area. Any specimens or evidence taken from the dirty area must be placed in appropriate containers which are then surface cleaned and disinfected.

Post-mortem specimens are generally transported to laboratories in fixative solutions such as formalin and are regarded as being free of infectious agents. As such they would not be considered dangerous for transport and therefore not subject to any carriage requirements. Guidance for transporting specimens can be found in a Health and Safety Executive publications (2003a,b).

Specimens that may contain infectious agents have their carriage controlled by dangerous goods regulations (Department of Transport, 2009) and the appropriate guidance should be followed.

4.4.2 Mortuary equipment

General working conditions such as temperature, lighting, ventilation and floor surfaces are detailed in a Health and Safety Executive publication (1992).

- *Ventilation*. There must be a fresh air flow throughout the mortuary and post-mortem room. Down-draught ventilation is preferable as this draws air into the mortuary at a high level and discharges at a low level away from staff, and also plays an important role in odour control.
- *Floor, work surfaces, fittings and furnishings*. Floors must be hard wearing, impervious and resistant to chemical damage. Slightly sloping a floor into the drainage area makes for easier cleaning and disinfection. Post-mortem tables and dissecting benches should again be hard wearing and easily cleanable.

4.5 The Anatomical Pathology Technologist

Anatomical Pathology Technologists (APTs) are professionals who staff both NHS and local authority mortuaries in the UK.

APTs are represented and supported by a professional body, the Association of Anatomical Pathology Technology (AAPT; www.aaptuk.org). AAPT is acknowledged, by all major stakeholders allied to anatomical pathology technology, as the principal voice for the profession. It was formed in 2003 with the support of the Royal College of Pathologists (RCP; www.rcpath.org), the Institute of Biomedical Science (IBMS; www.ibms.org) and the Royal Society of Public Health (RSPH; www.rsph.org.uk).

The AAPT was set up with several objectives, one of which was to pursue state registration for APTs. APTs are one of the healthcare science professions who are at the moment unregulated. Regulation is extremely important as a tool for ensuring that the public receive excellent services provided by professionals who can be held accountable for their actions.

The first stage to compulsory regulation is available to APTs in the form of a voluntary registration scheme offered by the Voluntary Registration Council (VRC; www.vrcouncil.org). The sole aim of any registration process is to provide protection for the public.

4.5.1 Training and qualifications of APTs

There are currently no minimum entry qualifications for a trainee APT, although the AAPT recommend that a student of anatomical pathology technology should have attained at least five passes at GCSE (or the Scottish equivalent) to include English, Maths and a Science (preferably Biology).

An APT will have a period of workplace-based training, practical assessment (usually about 2 years) and mandatory attendance at an approved training course with a view to presenting for the RSPH Certificate examination in Anatomical Pathology Technology. The examination covers topics such as:

- anatomy and physiology
- post-mortem examination techniques
- health and safety
- medico-legal legislation and codes of practice
- administration and documentation.

For advancement to more senior positions and a higher level of skill and proficiency, APTs may continue for a further 2 years of workplace-based training and practical assessment, finally presenting for the RSPH Diploma examination in Anatomical Pathology Technology.

Both Certificate and Diploma examinations include a written and oral component with a pass required in both.

NHS and local authority employers will usually have mandatory training in:

- manual handling
- infection control
- health and safety;

and others such as violence and aggression, as required by the employer.

4.5.2 Responsibilities of APTs

APTs have very varied roles, but in essence they are the staff who deal with all aspects of after-death care. They provide assistance to all service users. Duties of an APT include:

- reception, storage and subsequent release of the deceased
- coordination of the necessary legal certificates required for release of the deceased
- accurate record keeping of the dead and their property
- liaison with medical, nursing and administrative staff

- liaison with outside agencies (e.g. funeral directors, local authorities, religious representatives, police and the Coroner/Fiscal)
- assisting bereaved relatives and arranging viewing appointments
- preparing the deceased for post-mortem, including the coordinating of next of kin consent (post-mortems can include HM Coroner/Procurator Fiscal, forensic, paediatric and hospital consented)
- assisting the pathologist at autopsy and reconstituting bodies to a high standard
- taking samples for histology, toxicology, DNA
- enucleation and tissue retrieval
- training of junior pathologists and trainee technicians
- maintaining stocks of instruments and disposable of materials
- maintain or arranging maintenance of all equipment
- ensuring compliance with health and safety requirements, as recommended by the Health and Safety Advisory Committee.

All visitors to the mortuary who are not fully aware of local rules and regulations should report to the senior APT who will facilitate local induction.

4.6 The odontologist in the mortuary: Specialist resection techniques

The APT can assist with the dental examination by performing, if required, specialist jaw resection or facial dissection, allowing effective examination when rigor mortis is present. The procedure should be carried out only on the instruction of the Coroner or Procurator Fiscal.

The following brief description of a jaw resection is taken from the American Board of Forensic Odontology *Diplomates Reference Manual* (2013). The procedure is conducted in a way that facilitates reconstruction and viewing. Restricted opening due to rigor may require:

- intraoral incision of masticatory muscles, with or without fracture of the condyles
- breaking the rigor with bilateral leverage on jaws in the retromolar regions
- waiting until rigor subsides
- inframandibular dissection, with or without mandibular resection.

Removal of the larynx and tongue at post-mortem may facilitate visual examination of the teeth and placement of intraoral films.

Dissection and resection techniques

Facial dissection using the inframandibular approach

- Bilateral incisions are made across the upper anterior neck and extend to points posterior and inferior to the ears.
- The skin and underlying tissue is then reflected upward over the face to expose the mandible and maxilla.

Jaw resection using an oscillating electric saw

- The soft tissue and muscle attachments on the lateral aspect of the mandible are dissected away by incisions which extend through the mucobuccal fold to the lower border of the mandible.
- Lingual attachments are similarly incised to include the internal pterygoid attachments to the medial aspect of the rami and the masseter attachments on the lateral aspect.
- On the maxilla, facial attachments are incised high on the malar processes and superior to the anterior nasal spine.
- Saw cuts are made high on the rami to avoid possible impacted third molars. Alternatively, the mandible may also be removed by disarticulation at the temporomandibular joints.
- Bony cuts on the maxilla are made high on the malar processes and above the anterior nasal spine to avoid the apices of the maxillary teeth.
- A surgical mallet and chisel inserted in the saw cuts in the malar processes and above the anterior nasal spine are used to complete the separation of the maxilla.
- Remaining soft tissue in the soft palate and fauces are then dissected free.

4.7 Health and safety in the mortuary

Safe working in a mortuary and post-mortem facility requires a high standard of training and education, and visitors should be guided in all aspects of health and safety by the APT. Mortuaries should follow the guidance from Health and Safety Executive publications (2003a,b). The guidance was prepared by the Health Services Advisory Committee in consultation with the HSE and represents what is considered to be good practice. Following the guidance generally ensures compliance with health and safety laws such as Management of Health and Safety at Work Regulations (MHSWR) published by the HSE (1999) and the Control of Substances Hazardous to Health Regulations (COSHH) published by the Department for Work and Pensions (2002).

Table 4.1 Hazard groups

Hazard group	Definition	Example
1	A biological agent unlikely to cause human disease.	Lactobacillus
2	A biological agent that can cause human disease and may be hazardous to employees. It is unlikely to spread to the community and there is usually effective prophylaxis or effective treatment available.	Seasonal influenza
3	A biological agent that can cause severe human disease and presents a serious hazard to employees. It may present a risk of spreading to the community, but there is usually effective prophylaxis or treatment available.	Mycobacterium tuberculosis
4	A biological agent that causes severe human disease and is a serious hazard to employees. It is likely to spread to the community and there is usually no effective prophylaxis or treatment available.	Lassa fever

Those in charge of health and safety in the mortuary should be able to:

- identify and assess risks
- ensure such risks are avoided or adequately controlled
- prepare comprehensive standard operating procedures specific to the facility.

There is a potential, through poor hygiene, to transmit infections to the environment outside the mortuary setting. Adherence to the appropriate health and safety principles greatly reduces this risk.

4.7.1 Safe working practices

Forensic dentists/odontologists working in the mortuary will be advised how to conduct their examinations safely. A risk assessment is required for each case and the precautions to be followed are decided. Factors to consider include the following:

- *Known or suspected infection hazards.* Guidance on infection hazards can be found in an Advisory Committee on Dangerous Pathogens (ACDP) publication (2004). The approved list classifies biological agents into hazard groups (Table 4.1).

- *Timing of the post-mortem examination*. Examples are: allowing appropriate time for each case to avoid rushed examinations, and carrying out high-risk cases in isolation or dealing with them last.
- *Staff requirements*. Consider the number of staff required to perform the examination safely, and the appropriateness of allowing access to visitors/observers.

Other considerations for safe working are:

- strictly controlled access using ID badges
- an organised methodical workflow to prevent excess manual handling
- restricted movements between clean and dirty areas
- appropriate cleaning and disinfection of instruments, workstations and floors
- designated working hours and rest breaks to prevent human error due to tiredness
- appropriate use and disposal of personal protective equipment (PPE) – discussed further below
- radiation protection.

4.7.2 Hygiene

Standard operating procedures in the mortuary will set out strict standards of personal hygiene which all staff must follow. Measures for personal hygiene include the following:

- Change into protective clothing before carrying out any post-mortem examination.
- Always wear the correct protective clothing. High-risk cases may require respiratory protection.
- Remove protective clothing when leaving the post-mortem area, and dispose of it appropriately.
- Open wounds, cuts, skin abrasions or active dermatitis on exposed skin should have the area adequately protected by waterproof dressings.
- Actions that bring the hands (gloved or otherwise) into contact with face, eyes, nose and mouth should be avoided.
- Hands should be thoroughly washed prior to leaving any of the designated dirty work areas of the mortuary, and showering ensures that skin and hair are free from contamination.
- Smoking, drinking and eating are strictly prohibited in areas that are not specifically designated for that use.

4.7.3 Personal protective equipment (PPE)

Standard operating procedures will stipulate what protective clothing is required during the post-mortem examination. Prior to entering the post-mortem area, staff will be required to use the changing facilities to don the appropriate PPE. Protective clothing usually supplied is:

- surgical shirt and trousers (scrubs)
- long-sleeved surgical gown or coverall (TYVEK)
- plastic apron which extends outside boots
- waterproof boots with non-slip soles
- disposable surgical gloves (double gloving may be appropriate in high-risk cases)
- visor or mask with goggles (a ventilated visor/hood should be used for high-risk cases).

Disposal of PPE is strictly controlled and the changing area should have a dirty and clean side. Reusable PPE such as scrubs should be placed in an appropriately labelled laundry container on the dirty side. Reusable PPE such as visors or boots should be cleaned and disinfected at the end of each session as detailed in standard operating procedures (see below). Disposable PPE such as gloves, aprons or gowns/overalls can be disposed of in a clinical waste bin on leaving the post-mortem area.

4.7.4 Cleaning and decontamination

The mortuary and post-mortem room environment must be regularly cleaned and disinfected so that all infectious agents are kept to a level which is not harmful to health. Blood, tissues and other factors can adversely affect disinfection, so all surfaces should be washed down with detergent and rinsed prior to application of the disinfectant.

The most commonly used disinfectants in the mortuary and post-mortem room are clear soluble phenolics, chlorine-based hypochlorites, quaternary ammonium compounds ('quats') and halogenated tertiary amines (Table 4.2).

Standard operating procedures (SOPs) will specify the disinfectant to be used, the appropriate dilutions, and instructions on safe usage. The disinfectants must be used in accordance with manufacturer's instructions and should be accompanied by a manufacturer's safety data sheet (MSDS) giving all the relevant information about the product. The use of chemical disinfectants is controlled by 'COSHH', the Control of Substances Hazardous to Health Regulations (Department for Work and Pensions, 2002).

Instruments, after use, can be decontaminated using a washer–disinfector that complies with the requirements of Department of Health (DH) guidance (DH, 1997). As mentioned earlier, non-disposable protective equipment such as visors and boots should also be cleaned and disinfected at end of each session.

Table 4.2 Summary of properties of commonly used disinfectants

Disinfectant	Efficacy
Chlorine-based	• Effective against many biological agents • Agent of choice for blood-borne viruses • Readily inactivated by organic material
Phenolics	• Effective against *Mycobacterium tuberculosis* • Effective against only a limited range of viruses
Hypochlorites	• Effective against vegetative bacteria • Effective against blood-borne viruses • Limited effect on bacterial spores • Corrosive, therefore not used for disinfecting metal instruments
Quaternary ammonium compounds ('quats')	• Effective against wide range of microorganisms • Odourless • Non-corrosive
Halogentated tertiary amines	• Effective against vegetative bacteria, spores, mycobacterium and viruses • Low toxicity • Low irritation • Detergent properties • Non-corrosive

4.7.5 Waste disposal

Waste generated from the post-mortem room is classified as *clinical waste*. Standard operating procedures will detail a waste policy, but all clinical waste is required to be contained within the correct sack and appropriately sealed and labelled.

Contaminated *sharps* which are disposable should be discarded in a solid container that meets the requirements of the sharps injury-protection standard (British Standards Institution, 2012). Other clinical waste is disposed of in accordance with a Department of Health publication (DH, 2013).

Protective clothing that is reusable is divided into three categories as directed by NHS executive guidelines (DH, 1995):

- used (soiled and foul)
- infected (infectious agents in hazard groups 3 and 4 – see Table 4.1)
- heat-labile (fabrics that would be damaged by normal heat disinfection processes and likely to be damaged at thermal disinfection temperatures).

4.7.6 Immunisation

All those working in the mortuary should be immunised, as a minimum, against hepatitis B, tetanus and tuberculosis. Immunisation procedures for staff are based on guidance in several relevant Department of Health publications (DH, 1993, 1996, 1998, 2000, 2005).

4.8 References

Act (2004) *Human Tissue Act*, Chapter 30. London: The Stationary Office. Available at www.legislation.gov.uk/ukpga/2004/30/contents (accessed: 29 April 2013).

Act (2006) *Human Tissue Act* (Scotland), Chapter 4. London: The Stationary Office. Available at www.legislation.gov.uk/asp/2006/4/contents (accessed: 29 April 2013).

Advisory Committee on Dangerous Pathogens (2004) *Approved List of Biological Agents*. Available at www.hse.gov.uk/pubns/misc208.pdf (accessed: 29 April 2013).

American Board of Forensic Odontology Inc. (2013) *Diplomates Reference Manual*. Available at www.abfo.org/wp-content/uploads/2012/08/ABFO-Reference-Manual-1-22-2013-revision.pdf (accessed: 29 April 2013).

British Standards Institution (2012) BS EN ISO 23907:2012 – *Sharps Injury Protection, Requirements and Test Methods: Sharps Containers*.

Department of Health (1993) *Protecting Health Care Workers and Patients from Hepatitis B*: HSG(93)40 and addendum EL(96)77. Available at http://webarchive.nationalarchives.gov.uk/+/www.dh.gov.uk/en/Publicationsandstatistics/Lettersandcirculars/Healthserviceguidelines/DH_4084234 (accessed: 29 April 2013).

Department of Health (1995) *Laundry Arrangements for Used and Infected Linen*: HSG(95)18. Available at http://webarchive.nationalarchives.gov.uk/20100702173605/http://dh.gov.uk/prod_consum_dh/groups/dh_digitalasset/@dh/@en/documents/digitalasset/dh_4012310.pdf (accessed: 29 April 2013).

Department of Health (1996) *Joint Committee on Vaccination and Immunisation against Infectious Disease*. London: DH/The Stationery Office (ISBN 011321815X); see paragraph 137.

Department of Health (1997) *Washer–Disinfectors: Design Considerations*. Health Technical Memorandum 2030.

Department of Health (1998) *The Management of Health, Safety and Welfare Issues for NHS Staff*: HSC(98)064. Available at. http://webarchive.nationalarchives.gov.uk/+/www.dh.gov.uk/en/Publicationsandstatistics/Lettersandcirculars/Healthservicecirculars/DH_4004185 (accessed: 29 April 2013).

Department of Health (2000) *Hepatitis B Infected Health Care Workers*: HSC2000/020. Available at http://webarchive.nationalarchives.gov.uk/+/www.dh.gov.uk/en/Publicationsandstatistics/Lettersandcirculars/Healthservicecirculars/DH_4004553 (accessed: 29 April 2013).

Department of Health (2001) 'Learning From Bristol: report of the public inquiry into children's heart surgery at the Bristol Royal Infirmary 1984–1995', presented in July 2001. Available at www.bristol-inquiry.org.uk (accessed: 29 April 2013).

Department of Health (2005) *HIV-infected Health Care Workers: Guidance on Management and Patient Notification*: DH 269675. Available at http://webarchive.nationalarchives.gov.uk/20130107105354/http://www.dh.gov.uk/prod_consum_dh/groups/dh_digitalassets/@dh/@en/documents/digitalasset/dh_4116416.pdf (accessed: 29 April 2013).

Department of Health (2013) *Safe Management of Healthcare Waste*: Technical Memoranum 07-01. Available at www.gov.uk/government/uploads/system/uploads/attachment_data/file/167976/HTM_07-01_Final.pdf (accessed: 29 April 2013).

Department of Transport (2009) *The Carriage of Dangerous Goods (Classification, Packaging and Labelling) and Use of Transportable Pressure Receptacles*: Regulations SI 2009/1348. London: The Stationery Office (ISBN: 9780111480120). Available at www.legislation.gov.uk/uksi/2009/1348/contents/made (accessed: 29 April 2013).

Department for Work and Pensions (2002) *The Control of Substances Hazardous to Health Regulations* (COSHH): SI 2002/2677. London: The Stationery Office (ISBN 0110429192). Available at www.legislation.gov.uk/uksi/2002/2677/pdfs/uksi_20022677_en.pdf (accessed: 29 April 2013).

Health and Safety Executive (1992) *Workplace (Health, Safety and Welfare) Regulations: Approved Code of Practice and Guidance*: L24. HSE Books (ISBN 0717604136). Available at www.hse.gov.uk/pubns/priced/l24.pdf (accessed: 29 April 2013).

Health and Safety Executive (1999) *The Management of Health and Safety at Work Regulations* (MHSWR): SI 1999/3242. London: The Stationery Office (ISBN 0717624881). Available at www.hse.gov.uk/pubns/priced/l21.pdf (accessed: 29 April 2013).

Health and Safety Executive (2003a) *Safe Working and the Prevention of Infection in the Mortuary and Post-mortem Room*. HSE Books (ISBN 0717622932). Available at www.hse.gov.uk/pubns/priced/mortuary-infection.pdf (accessed: 29 April 2013).

Health and Safety Executive (2003b) *Safe Working and the Prevention of Infection in Clinical Laboratories and Similar Facilities*. HSE Books (ISBN 0717625133). Available at www.hse.gov.uk/pubns/priced/clinical-laboratories.pdf (accessed: 29 April 2013).

National Health Service (2005) *Facilities for Mortuary and Post-mortem Room Services*. London: The Stationary Office (ISBN 0113227159).

National Health Service Scotland (2002) *Mortuary and Post-mortem Room: Scottish Hospital Planning Notes* (Management Executive 20), London: The Stationery Office (ISBN 011495187X) and Supplement 1, 1994 (ISBN 0114952337).

Redfearn M., Keeling J. and Powell E. (2001) *Report of the Royal Liverpool Children's Inquiry*. Available at www.rlcinquiry.org.uk (accessed: 29 April 2013).

5

Dental human identification

Romina Carabott
expertFORENSICS Ltd, Cardiff, UK

5.1 Introduction

> Under most conditions occurring in nature, the teeth are the least destructible part of the body and they may readily survive all of these changes ... Fire, putrefaction or prolonged immersion in water. (Whittaker and McDonald, 1989)

The need to identify the deceased can arise in a variety of scenarios ranging from motor vehicle accidents, suspected suicide and murder investigations, natural death and natural disasters. This chapter will be looking at the various means of identifying a single individual using dental information – which is what dental human identification relies on. The role of the forensic dentist in multiple fatality scenarios is discussed in detail in Chapter 6, but it is relevant to note here that all the aspects that will be described in this chapter are applicable to dental identification in multiple fatality scenes.

5.1.1 Why is human identification necessary?

Very often a triad of reasons are put forward to justify identification of a deceased individual: social, legal and forensic reasons. The first of these comes as no surprise to most of us, although it may not always apply in the same manner in all cultures. It is generally accepted in society that providing tangible proof to the relatives of the deceased that this is, in fact, their cherished family member is an essential part of the grieving process, thereby bringing closure to the surviving relatives. There are then legal aspects, such as will executions, debt payments, life insurances and remarriage, which can only be set into motion once a particular person is certified dead.

If a dead body is found in suspicious circumstances, an investigation as to how that person came about their death will be triggered. Without the identity of the victim, the investigative team are not able to establish who the possible suspects may be. On the other hand, a murder suspect linked to a missing person cannot be charged with the crime until the body of the missing person is found.

Forensic Odontology: An Essential Guide, First Edition.
Edited by Catherine Adams, Romina Carabott and Sam Evans.

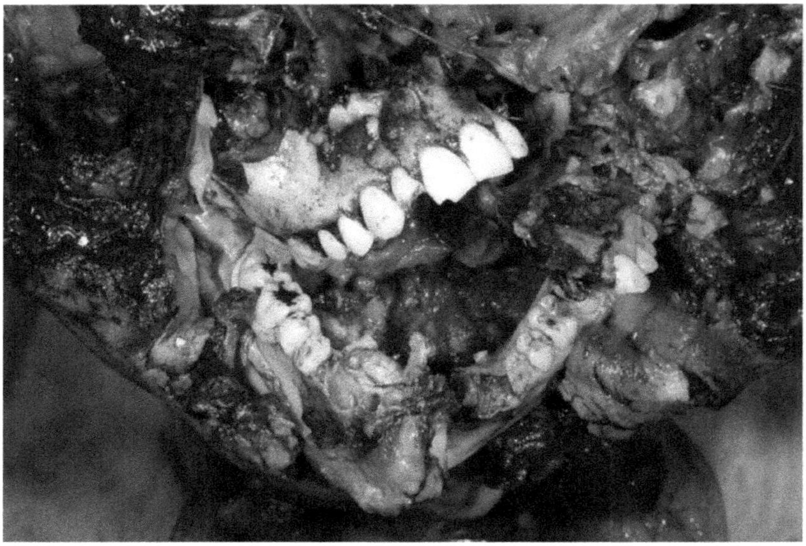

Figure 5.1 Severe facial trauma. Courtesy of Dental Illustration Unit, Cardiff University (For colour details, please see colour plate section.)

A scientific method of identification is often necessary because the way the victim died or the advanced state of decomposition render visual identification unreliable. An example of such a scenario is a suicide victim who came by his death by jumping in front of a train or setting fire to his car; the severe trauma from the impact with the train or incineration from the high temperatures reached in a car fire render visual identification impossible (Figure 5.1 and colour plate). Another example is an individual who dies from natural causes alone in his house and is not discovered for a few days, or sometimes weeks. The resultant decomposition necessitates a scientific means of identification.

Even though the recommendations of Lord Justice Clarke (2001) were directed towards mass fatality scenarios, the general principles should be borne in mind whenever we are identifying the deceased:

- respect for the deceased and the bereaved, and
- the avoidance of mistaken identification.

5.1.2 Why comparative dental analysis?

Nowadays, there are four accepted scientific primary methods of human identification:

- fingerprint analysis
- comparative dental analysis
- DNA analysis
- medical devices.

All of these can play a role in identifying a particular deceased individual. The method or methods of choice will often be dictated by the state of decomposition or fragmentation of the body, the amount and quality of ante-mortem records available, and (at least in the UK) the preference of the Coroner who has jurisdiction. There are also secondary methods of identification, such as personal descriptions, medical findings, clothing and other documents and evidence. These are often used to support an identification established by one or more of the primary identifiers.

Out of the above list of primary methods, comparative dental analysis is in all likelihood the quickest, easiest and cheapest method of human identification – with the added benefit that it is less invasive to the family of the presumed deceased individual. All the family need to provide is the name of their presumed dead relative's dentist, as opposed to the samples and/or personal belongings required for fingerprint or DNA analysis.

One other well-documented advantage is that, as a general rule, it is accepted that an individual may have attended a dental clinic at least once in his/her lifetime. It therefore follows that the obvious limiting factor to the use of dental identification becomes the availability of ante-mortem dental records of the presumed deceased individual. Even if such dental records are in fact available, their quality (clarity and completeness) may still preclude a definitive identification, as will be explained later in this chapter.

5.1.3 What if there is no presumptive identification?

Comparative dental identification, whereby we compare dental information of the deceased with known dental information of the missing person, assumes that we have some idea of who the person might be – that we have a lead. Consider the following scenario.

Case scenario 1

One fine evening you are walking your dog on the local beach, as you do every other evening when the weather and the tide permit. But today there is something different, and as you get closer to whatever has piqued the interest of your dog, you discover what looks like a human lower jaw. You call the police and a few hours and a search party later you are told that more human body parts were discovered in the area, mostly completely skeletonised.

The police have no reports of a person missing within the last few months. It is not known whence the body came before it was washed up in that location, so the Coroner has no lead, no presumptive identity, no relatives to approach to ask for ante-mortem information for comparison. Therefore one might think that a forensic dentist cannot be of assistance in this case, at this stage. It could be one of a large number of individuals who are on missing persons lists not only in the UK but also abroad. Where does the Coroner start from?

> The teeth can provide considerable information to assist in building up a profile of the deceased which, together with information from other forensic experts, such as forensic anthropologists, can help narrow down the large pool of possible identities. Dental analysis can therefore be also used in a reconstructive identification.

The most useful and reliable piece of information that can be derived from the teeth is age estimation. This is dealt with in detail in Chapter 7. However, there are other useful aspects of dental information – such as the type and quality of dental treatment, the types of materials used for fillings and fixed prosthesis, developmental anomalies, ethnic traits, and trace elements present in the enamel and dentine – all of which will be discussed later in this chapter.

5.1.4 When does the forensic dentist 'come on the scene'?

In the UK, the HM Coroner is responsible for all deceased found in his/her jurisdiction and on most occasions it is a Coroner's Officer who will call on the forensic dentist on behalf of the Coroner. Generally the forensic dentist is called in at a later stage of the investigation, often once the body has been recovered from the scene, transported to the mortuary and a post-mortem, if one is necessary, completed or well under way.

There are, however, few scenarios – in fact the author would venture to say only two types of scenario – when it is of benefit for the forensic dentist to be called out to the location where the body is found, ideally before the body is moved. These are cases related to fire and incineration of the body, and when foetal or newborn remains are suspected.

Incinerated remains

In cases where the body has been subjected to high temperatures, the teeth will suffer changes from incineration, eventually turning into ash.

Even in these times when smoking indoors is not allowed in public places, most of us can probably bring to mind the image of a cigarette between the smoker's fingers, forgotten in the middle of a heated argument or interesting conversation. As the cigarette continues to burn, it will turn into ash but will maintain its original cigarette-shape until someone bumps into the person holding the cigarette, and the ash falls off.

The situation is somewhat similar with incinerated teeth. As the body is subjected to the high temperatures of a house fire or fuel fire in a motor vehicle, train or airplane, the soft tissues of the lips will shrink away, exposing the anterior teeth to the heat. These teeth will subsequently burn and turn into ash. As long as the body remains untouched the ash will maintain its 'tooth shape', but as soon as the body is moved all the ash will fall away and important information will be lost for good. The forensic dentist's job at such scenes is therefore to stabilise these teeth before the body is moved, ensuring preservation of possibly vital identification evidence.

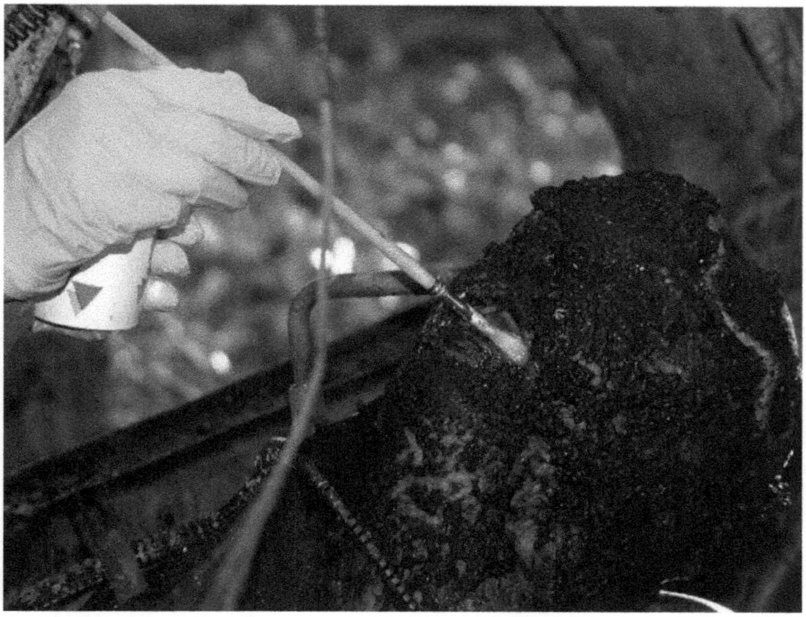

Figure 5.2 Applying a runny mix of cold cure acrylic using a horsehair brush

A number of materials have been used in the past to achieve this, such as hairspray or cyanoacrylate glue. However, a more manageable material that gives an excellent result – and is easily found in most dental surgeries – is clear cold-cure acrylic. The powder and liquid monomer can be carried to the scene and mixed to a very runny consistency that can be delivered to the 'ash teeth' using a horsehair brush and dripped gently (Figure 5.2). The runny polymer will seep through the ash and eventually set. This then allows movement of the body without the risk of losing any of the teeth.

Fetal material

Occasionally skeletal material is found and the forensic dentist alongside the forensic anthropologist can assist with identification by comparative or reconstructive means. In cases where it is suspected that fetal material is among the skeletonised remains, the forensic dentist should be called to the scene during excavation and recovery (Figure 5.3).

Deciduous teeth start calcifying at 6 weeks *in utero* and the level of calcification of each tooth can assist in age estimation of the fetus or newborn. Examination of sectioned teeth may also shed some light on the question of whether this had been a live birth or a stillborn, by looking for the presence or otherwise of the neonatal line.

As the teeth are developing, they consist of thin, small, calcified shells suspended within a soft tissue follicle. Hence, in circumstances where there is advanced decomposition and skeletonisation of the remains resulting in loss of all soft tissue, the

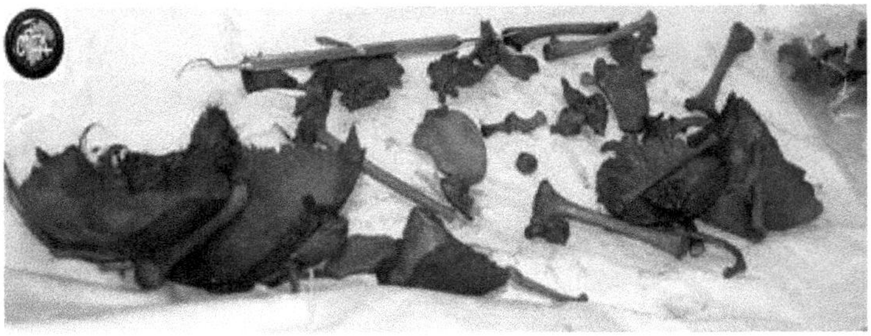

Figure 5.3 Collection of fetal bones, with a standard dental instrument to illustrate scale

minute calcified crowns or cusps come loose and will easily fall out of the bony crypts that normally surround the follicle. Depending on the age of the fetus/newborn, pin-head sized separate cusps of deciduous or permanent molars may be present since calcification has not yet advanced to the stage of coalescence of the individual tooth cusps into the occlusal surface of the molar crown.

It is these small tooth fragments that the forensic dentist would assist with recovering when called at the scene of skeletal fetal/infant material, making sure they are adequately stored and documented.

5.2 Comparative dental identification

Comparative identification is in essence a comparison of two dental records. One is the post-mortem dental record – i.e. the state of the dentition of the unidentified body after death. The other is the ante-mortem dental record – i.e. the state of the dentition of a missing individual before death or, more accurately, before he/she went missing. There may be more than one ante-mortem dental record, compared to one post-mortem dental record, if a number of individuals are missing and the authorities suspect that the unidentified deceased could be any one of the indicated missing persons. However, in a comparative dental identification scenario the authorities often have a suspicion of who the deceased is likely to be and the dental identification is more for confirmatory reasons.

5.2.1 Post-mortem examination

In effect, this is the same as a basic dental examination carried out on a new patient in the dental clinic. The difference is that this may be the only chance available for collecting the information, so the examination should be as thorough as necessary to avoid re-examination of the body at a later date. Examination should aim to collect:

- dental photographs
- a complete full-mouth dental examination including an odontogram
- a full-mouth dental radiography series.

One difficulty with a post-mortem dental examination often arises in gaining adequate access. Depending on the post-mortem interval, the body may be in such rigor mortis that achieving adequate access will require incision of the soft tissues or resection of the jaws. It is recommended to discuss achieving such access with the pathologist responsible in the particular case. He/she will be in charge of the body while it resides in the mortuary and should be notified of any plans to expose the jaws for access. In fact, the pathologist will often prefer to do what is necessary to allow adequate access for examination of the jaws. The correct method of achieving access is described in Chapter 3.

The dignity of the individual should be kept in mind at all times. Once identified, the individual will be viewed by his/her next of kin and any incisions applied to allow access to the jaws should be done with this in mind and placed in a location where they can be concealed in the best way possible.

Complete resection of the jaws and removal from the body should be avoided unless absolutely necessary. In the rare situations when such necessity arises – such as the need to take dental radiographs when no radiographic facilities are available in the mortuary – permission from the Coroner should be sought. The pathologist responsible should again be informed and the jaws should be repatriated as soon as possible. In the UK, the Human Tissue Act 2004 will apply in these situations; if you are unfamiliar with the legislation, guidance from the mortuary staff and/or the lead pathologist should be sought (see also Chapter 3).

Photographs should be taken *before* any soft tissue is incised, soft tissue flaps raised or jaws resected. These photographs will record the gross findings, including the extent of decomposition and/or trauma to the soft tissues and jaws before commencement of examination.

Once adequate physical access to all aspects of the teeth is secured, the teeth should be thoroughly cleaned of any debris or decomposed material that may hinder adequate examination of the teeth. The use of a toothbrush, water, alcohol, swabs/gauze and some patience is often all that is required.

At this stage it is relevant to comment that a post-mortem dental examination may require an element of improvisation. This is necessary not only in order to maintain the mouth and jaws in an accessible position for examination, but also to make up for the lack of 'dental chair comforts' the dentist is accustomed to. In a clinic a patient sits on the dental chair and the dentist or dental nurse presses the foot pedal to obtain the perfect ergonomic position for the examination with least effort. The examiner reaches for the light and aims it at the open mouth, and reaches for the 3-in-1 syringe to wash and dry the teeth. It is only when the dentist is by the mortuary gurney that the lack of these 'comforts' is first noticed.

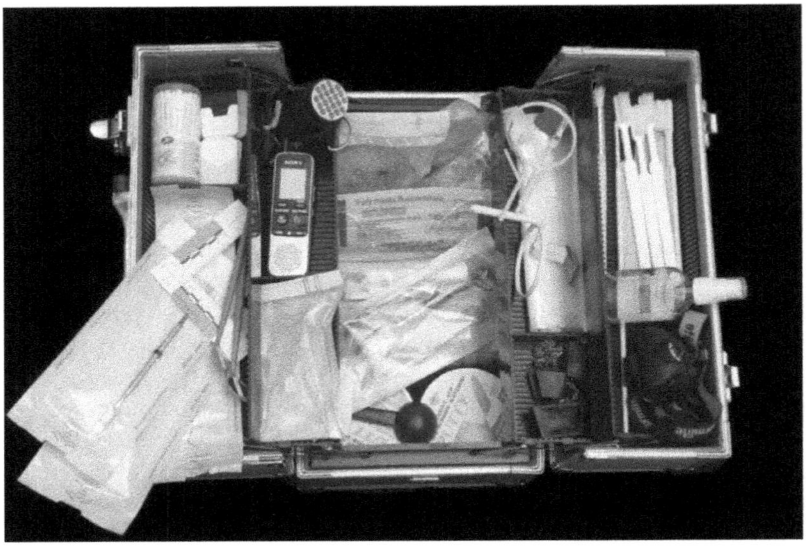

Figure 5.4 Some of the dental kit in a mobile hard-wearing case (for full details of the dental kit, refer to Table 5.1). Courtesy of Dental Illustration Unit, Cardiff University

These are not insurmountable problems and a little bit of foresight can ensure that the right 'bits of kit' are in the equipment case to assist in the hour of need (Figure 5.4 and Table 5.1). A head torch can easily replace the dental light without the necessity of an extra pair of hands to aim a pen light. Toothbrush, alcohol (in a squeezy bottle) and swabs to replace the 3-in-1 syringe have already been mentioned. Cotton buds may also assist in the cleaning and drying process. Utilising the neck blocks available in the mortuary will provide some help in positioning the head backwards, which assists in keeping the jaws open as well as giving better access to the maxillary teeth if the soft tissues are lax enough. If the jaws need to be kept open, a mouth prop can be used and hands-free lip/cheek retractors can keep the soft tissues out of the way as well.

Each forensic dentist will develop his/her own way of working around these little problems or 'inconveniences' and will also have a preferred brand or style of equipment/instruments that will be changed and developed with experience.

Disposable gloves, visor and mask are worth having in the kit, although if working in the mortuary the necessary personal protective equipment (PPE) will be provided and the forensic dentist will be expected to abide by the mortuary's health and safety protocols (Health and Services Advisory Committee, 2003). If in doubt, always refer back to the mortuary manager.

The author also recommends having a small selection of extraction forceps available, particularly molar ones. The Coroner may request that DNA tests also be carried out, particularly if the dental records have not been located yet or are of poor condition. Molar teeth can be a very good source of DNA in skeletonised or severely decomposed bodies, as will be discussed later in this chapter. Also discussed later and in Chapter 7 is dental age assessment as part of a reconstructive identification. The more accurate adult dental age estimation methods will require a tooth from the

Table 5.1 Kit for dental identification

- Visor/goggles
- Gloves
- Mask
- Head torch or portable light source
- Disposable toothbrushes
- Cotton buds
- Swabs/gauze
- Alcohol (in a squeezy bottle)
- Mouth props (various sizes)
- Camera with macro lens and ring flash (or two-point flash)
- Hands-free lip/cheek retractors
- ABFO no. 2 scales
- Photography mirrors
- Mirrors, probes, forceps
- Small selection of extraction forceps
- Dental radiographic films
- Dental film-holders
- A selection of dental impression trays
- Addition silicone impression material
- Paperwork and pens
- Disposable bags
- Ultraviolet LED portable light
- Cold-cure acrylic

deceased to be sectioned (assessment of translucent dentine) or chemically treated (amino acid racemisation). For these cases, canine or upper incisor teeth may be the teeth of choice.

Considering the aesthetic and prominent position of canine and incisor teeth, it is wise to once more bear in mind that the next of kin may have to view the deceased at a later stage; and that, were other methods of identification are unsuccessful, facial comparison may be necessary and may be reliant on a distinctive smile line.

Any tooth removal should take place at the end of the post-mortem dental examination. In addition to photography, examination and radiography, silicone dental impressions should be taken prior to removal of any teeth. If removing an anterior tooth, before the tooth is sent to the laboratory for analysis, a replica should be produced and repatriated to the body.

In the UK, removal of a tooth for analysis must be compliant with the Human Tissue Act and permission to remove teeth should be sought from the Coroner.

Once adequate access is secured and the teeth are cleaned and isolated as best possible, dental photographs should be taken. Frontal, buccal and occlusal views should be taken, as well as close-ups of specific fillings or dental anatomy that may be unusual or unique and hence assist in the identification. If any appliances have been recovered with the body, such as dentures, photographs should be taken, with and without such dentures *in situ* as well as photographs of the appliance outside the mouth with a scale. Further detail about dental photography in identification scenarios can be found in Chapter 10. Although of more relevance in multiple fatality scenarios, it is good practice to include a small card with the forensic dentist's case reference number in the photographs to ensure there is no mixing up of photographs. Also note the possibility of needing facial mapping/comparison for the purpose of supporting identification. Further details are provided at the end of this chapter and in Chapter 10.

A full dental examination should then take place, noting the status of each tooth in words/code as well as completing an odontogram. Figure 5.5 shows an example of a post-mortem chart which is based on an Interpol Postmortem F1 form (further detail in Chapter 6). There is no unique internationally recognised post-mortem examination form for individual unidentified bodies and the form shown here can be adapted to the individual's preferences, the main aim being to facilitate recording a detailed dental examination. The amount of detail recorded should be such that the need for re-examination at a later date is avoided if at all possible, especially if no putative identification exists at the time of examination. The internationally accepted colour for post-mortem records is pink and these forms are generally referred to within disaster victim identification (DVI) teams as 'the pink forms'.

Quality assurance ideally would dictate that two individuals with knowledge of dental nomenclature and treatment undertake dental examination and recording. This could be two dentists, or a dentist and a dental care professional. One professional would undertake the examination of the teeth and call out the findings while the assisting professional takes notes and records the charting, akin to what happens during an initial routine dental examination in dental practice. Roles would then be swapped (if two dentists are working together) or the record read back to the examining dentist, to ensure that all teeth and related dental work have been recorded accurately. Unfortunately, this is not always possible. Often a forensic dentist is working on his/her own, so photographs are of vital importance as they can act as a reference to ensure that the records from a direct dental examination are correct.

There is the added difficulty of removing and replacing gloves when a single dentist needs to conduct an examination and make records at the same time. An audio recorder such as a Dictaphone can resolve this problem.

Another problem that may be encountered during charting is clearly identifying tooth-coloured fillings. Current trends of minimally invasive dentistry and the exceptional colour-matching qualities of modern resin filling materials create a challenge to the forensic dentist attempting to identify all tooth-coloured fillings. A portable LED light in the kit can come in handy, as the tooth-coloured fillings fluoresce when illuminated by wavelengths close to the ultraviolet (UV) range (Figure 5.6).

Finally, after photography and the written record, a radiographic examination should be undertaken. It is recommended that a full-mouth, 18-film radiographic series be done to ensure that full details of dental anatomy and dental treatment are recorded.

POSTMORTEM IDENTIFICATION FORM
MISSING PERSON

Date:........................ Time:........................ Location:..

Our Case No:..................... Male / Female Photographs taken YES / NO X-rays taken YES / NO

Gross Exam Build:... Facial features:...

Facial injury:.................................... Occlusion:...

Other: ....

51	11			21	61
52	12			22	62
53	13			23	63
54	14			24	64
55	15			25	65
	16			26	
	17			27	
	18			28	

18 17 16 15 14 13 12 11 21 22 23 24 25 26 27 28

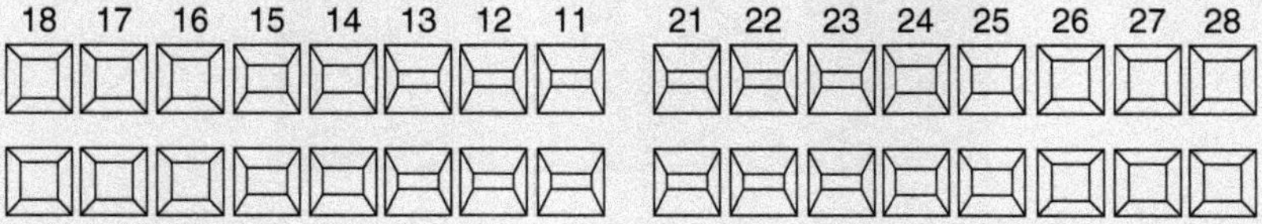

48 47 46 45 44 43 42 41 31 32 33 34 35 36 37 38

	48			38	
	47			37	
	46			36	
85	45			35	75
84	44			34	74
83	43			33	73
82	42			32	72
81	41			31	71

Specific data

Crowns, bridges, dentures, RCT etc.
(use diagram on back of form if necessary)

Other data

Occlusion, attrition, smoker, anomalies, staining, OH, perio status etc.

Ethnicity

Age estimate *(approximate)*

Dentist	Exam by	Charted by
1		
2		

Figure 5.5 Example of a dental identification post-mortem form (printed on pink paper)

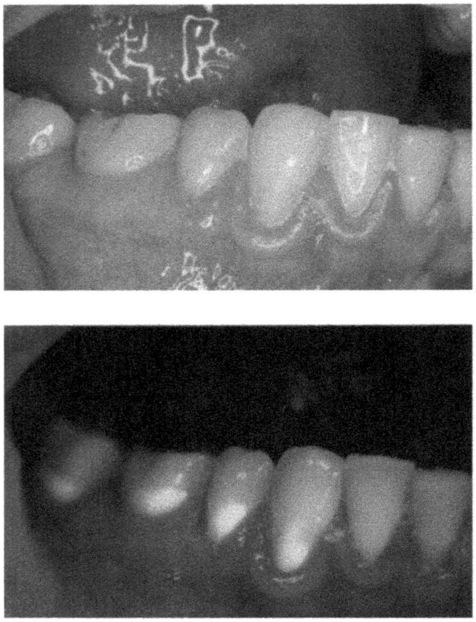

Figure 5.6 Composite fillings seen in normal light and with ultraviolet (395 nm) illumination (For colour details, please see colour plate section.)

This ensures that all dental information is recorded and available if/when required, in particular when there is no indication as to who the deceased individual might be. However, if the requirement is to confirm a presumptive identity, the ante-mortem records are likely to be available at the time that the post-mortem dental examination is taking place. The dentist should check which, if any, radiographic views are available and take the post-mortem equivalent views for comparison. In fact, the post-mortem views should attempt to reproduce the ante-mortem radiographs as closely as possible in film type, x-ray tube angulation and any technique errors. This ensures comparison of 'like with like' can be done. Occasionally, additional radiographs may be useful to confirm features recorded in the ante-mortem dental records for which radiographs have not been taken and which are noted at post-mortem, such as periodontal disease.

It is becoming increasingly common for radiographic facilities to be available in the mortuary – either as a permanent piece of mortuary equipment or through the availability of a mobile unit – and radiographers who can be called to assist. If you are attending a particular mortuary for the first time, mortuary staff should be asked what facilities are available before attending, to make sure that the necessary arrangements are made either for the mobile radiography unit to be notified, or for permission for jaw removal to be requested from the Coroner for radiographic examination at an alternative site.

Handheld x-ray devices are available, albeit arguably at prohibitive cost for the purpose of the individual forensic dentist conducting a few identifications a year. These can make radiographic dental examination in the mortuary much easier. Further detail is given later in this chapter.

5.2.2 Incinerated remains

Severely incinerated remains present unique problems. Exposure to explosion or longstanding extreme fires (akin to cremation) will lead to destruction of the dental structures. Various studies have been published detailing the effect of heat on teeth and dental restorations (Fairgrieve, 1994; Myers *et al.*, 1999; Merlati *et al.*, 2002; Savio *et al.*, 2006; Bush *et al.*, 2007; Bonavilla *et al.*, 2008; Fereira *et al.*, 2008; Karkhanis *et al.*, 2009).

At temperatures beyond 800°C all organic material burns and the remains are described as *calcined.* Calcined bones and teeth appear white and will be very fragile. At this point the crown part of the teeth will have been shattered and lost as a result of expansion of the tissues of the pulp complex. Roots will often still be retained within the sockets.

Calcined material is very fragile and should be recovered with great care. As mentioned earlier, the forensic dentist should be present at the scene before recovery of the remains starts to ensure that photographs, visual examination, stabilisation and (if possible) radiography is done prior to moving the remains. It is highly likely that further fragmentation will occur once the remains are moved, leading to loss of useful anatomical information.

All debris surrounding the victim should be recovered and careful sieving and sifting of the material conducted at the mortuary to ensure that all dental material is recovered. Porcelain, metal and some parts of composite resin materials used in dental prostheses and restorations have high melting temperatures and can be resilient to cremation conditions, surviving after the tooth tissue has turned to ash.

It is also important to note that calcined material will have shrunk considerably (as much as 20–25% (Bush and Bush, 2011), so anatomical features visible on a radiograph may not be as useful for comparison to ante-mortem radiographs.

Dental materials could provide some leads for investigation in themselves, particularly if there is little else dental information to work with. The microstructure of dental materials (apart from amalgam) can be unique to the brand. When analysed by energy-dispersive x-ray spectroscopy, an elemental fingerprint is generated that is virtually unchanged by incineration (Bush *et al.*, 2006). This can assist in identifying the brand of the material if a complete database of x-ray spectra for dental materials exists. This technology is reported to have assisted in identifying incinerated victims of a plane crash (Bush and Miller, 2011). X-ray fluorescence spectrometry (XRF) is also reported to identify brands of dental resin restorative materials (Bush *et al.*, 2007), the advantage of this technique being the portability of the scanners providing an immediate readout at the scene.

In a comparative scenario, the above information is of assistance only if the brand of composite resin or root filling material has been recorded in the dental records. Although some dental schools may advise denoting brands of dental materials, this is unlikely to be widespread routine practice in dental surgeries. Nonetheless, it is a practice to be encouraged – particularly when digital dental records make it easy to include the list of materials used in the practice in a drop-down menu for quick data entry.

5.2.3 Ante-mortem data collection

Comparative dental identification will depend on the availability and quality of the dental records of the presumed deceased victim. If the Coroner or police have no idea who the deceased might be, then a comparative dental identification cannot take place. Having said this, the forensic dentist may still be asked to conduct the full post-mortem examination for record purposes. Such a record will then be included in the file of the deceased until such time when putative ID(s) come to light and the relevant ante-mortem records available.

In a considerable number of cases a presumptive or tentative ID can be derived from property found on or with the body, or in the vicinity of the body, and from circumstantial evidence. Consider the following case.

Case scenario 2

Two women go to have their regular evening stroll, at a brisk 'keeping fit' pace, in the local public park. As they walk through the gate to the park they notice a small backpack hanging on the gatepost. From the way it is hanging it is clear that it is not empty. The women decide to do their usual hour-long walk and, if the bag is still hanging there unclaimed, they will take it to the local police station.

However, their walk is not without incident. As they pass a clearing in some woods they see a burning car. They call the police who attend as soon as possible with the fire services. As the women relate how they came across the car they happen to mention the abandoned backpack they saw on the gatepost about 100 metres before the path takes a sharp turn.

The police search the bag. As well as a wallet complete with driving licence, a diary and some other personal effects, they find a handwritten letter addressed to 'Dear Mum', with all the characteristics of a 'suicide note'.

With this tentative lead, the police will confirm that the individual is missing and the Family Liaison Officer (FLO) will then contact the family of the individual. Depending on the state of decomposition or fragmentation of the body and the recommendation of the Coroner, the FLO will gather from the family all necessary ante-mortem data related to the missing person. There might be a toothbrush for DNA analysis, or a glass on the bedside table for latent fingerprints. There will almost certainly be details of the missing person's dentist. In fact, the latter may be the only thing requested of the family.

One of the advantages of conducting a dental comparison for identification is the reduced invasiveness during liaison with the family of the missing person (presumed dead). No personal belongings have to be removed from the house. The name of their latest dentist or dental clinic is all that is required.

Table 5.2 Items making up a complete dental record

- Written/digital record (complete with glossary of abbreviations/acronyms)
- Radiographs – hard copies and/or digital
- Photographs – hard copies/digital
- Dental Casts
- Old appliances:
  orthodontic
  prosthetic
- manufacturer's receipts (as per the Medical Devices Directive)
- Referral letters:
  hospital
  specialists – endodontics, orthodontics, aesthetics, implantology

Most often the police or Coroner's officer will contact the forensic dentist after the dental records have been recovered. It is important to ensure that all the original dental records have been recovered, including radiographs, photographs, dental casts or appliances (Table 5.2). The FLO may need to be informed that further radiographs, photographs, or other records at a hospital are available, and occasionally the forensic dentist may need to liaise directly with the treating dentist to justify requirement of the full original records.

There may also be more than one dental record for the same missing person, if he/she has attended different dental clinics. Then the forensic dentist has the sometimes arduous task of trawling through the various notes, odontograms and radiographs to come up with a composite dental chart, which represents the state of the teeth just before the person went missing.

Case scenario 3

An upper molar tooth may have been recorded as having an occlusal amalgam filling in 1990 when the dentist first examined Jane Doe. A year later she had a new cavity on the distal surface. In 2000, she moved to a different county and presented with a fractured lingual cusp in a lower molar tooth at a new dentist (private clinic) in her area. Subsequent treatment involved a root canal treatment and a full crown. She has also developed decay in her partially erupted wisdom tooth and the new dentist refers Jane Doe to the local hospital for surgical removal of this wisdom tooth. She attends for the surgical extraction but never goes back for any further dental treatment. In 2003, Jane Doe goes missing.

In an ideal world, all three records of Jane Doe in the above case should be collected and provided to the forensic dentist so that the composite updated chart can be created.

This may not always be possible, because dental records do not 'follow' the individual to their subsequent dentist. Furthermore, particularly in the UK since the NHS dental contract changes in 2006, more individuals have their dental treatment at a private dentist and have no centralised NHS record. Therefore, unless the next of kin know the details of all dentists that their relative may have attended, tracing all dental records will prove difficult.

Once the dentist of the missing individual is located, he/she may not feel comfortable about releasing dental records owing to the associated data protection issues. In the UK, the General Dental Council's guidance on patient confidentiality advises:

> In exceptional circumstances, it may be justified to make confidential patient information known without consent if it is in the public interest or the patient's interest.

The same document further specifies:

> If you cannot persuade the patient to [give permission to release information], or it is not practical or appropriate to do so, get advice from an appropriate source, such as your defence organisation, before you release the information. ... In any circumstance where you decide to release confidential information, be prepared to explain and justify your decision and any action you take.

Ultimately, a court could order release of all required dental records.

Once all dental records are available, the composite dental chart can be compiled using an ante-mortem dental record form – or, as often referred to in DVI scenarios, the 'yellow form'. Figure 5.7 shows an example of such a form, which is again based on the Interpol DVI ante-mortem F1 form.

5.2.4 Reconciliation: The comparative process

Once all post-mortem and ante-mortem dental data have been recorded and compiled on the appropriate forms, the two can be compared and scrutinised for any discrepancies and for concordant points.

There is no set minimum number of concordant points required for a positive identification. The complexity of certain dental treatments, as well as the virtual uniqueness associated with certain treatments such as root canal fillings and the floor of restorations, means that in certain cases treatment in only a few particular teeth is sufficient to establish identification. In contrast, a series of multiple small occlusal isolated restorations may not lend sufficiently strong support to establish a positive identification owing to their high incidence in the general population. The forensic dentist will need to consider each case individually, making note of concordant features and their relative weight, individually or in combination, based on their knowledge and experience of dental treatments.

Table 5.3 is adapted from Pretty and Sweet (2001) and provides a list of features that can be used during comparative dental identification if recorded in the ante-mortem dental records.

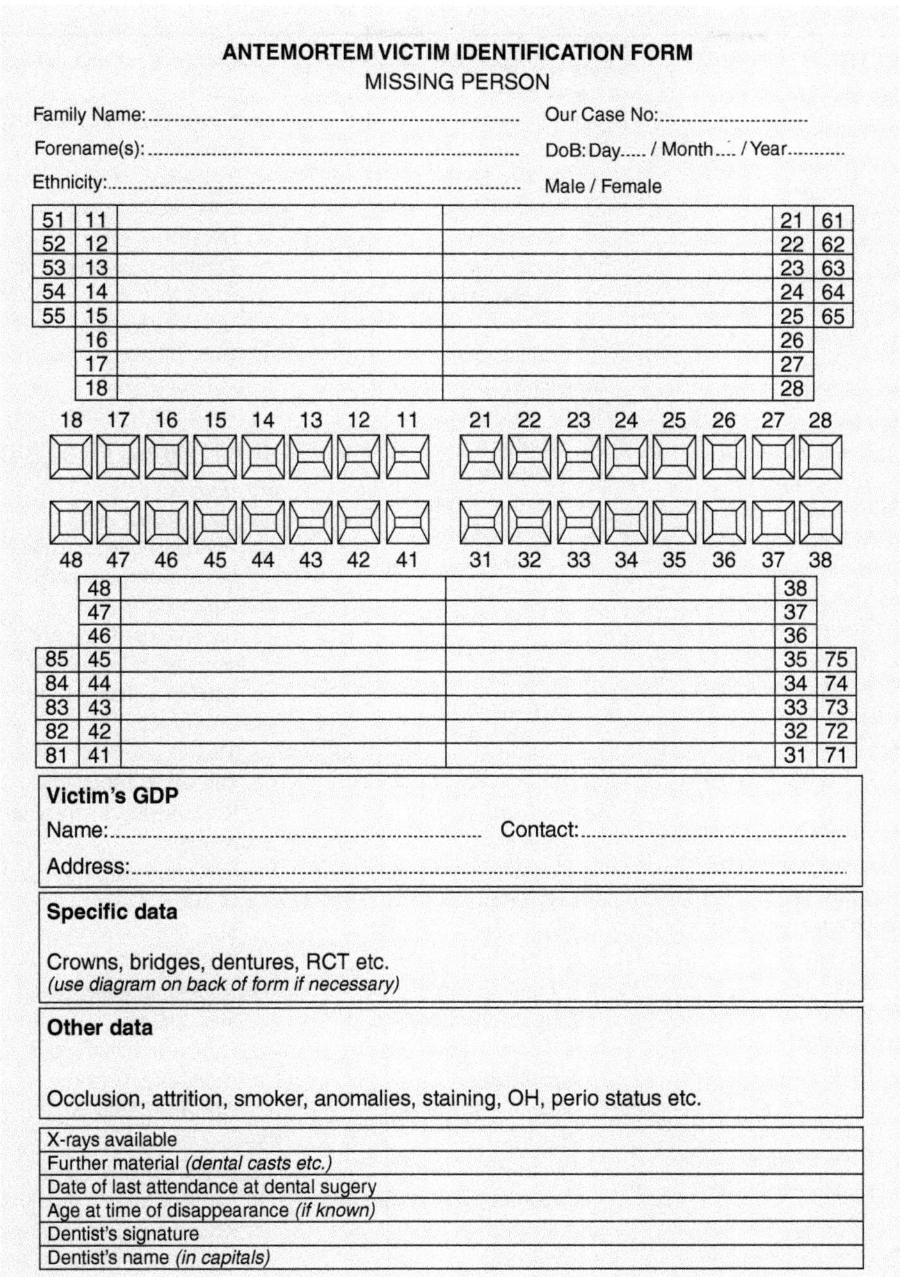

ANTEMORTEM VICTIM IDENTIFICATION FORM

MISSING PERSON

Family Name:.. Our Case No:..............................

Forename(s):.. DoB: Day...... / Month..... / Year...........

Ethnicity:.. Male / Female

51	11			21	61
52	12			22	62
53	13			23	63
54	14			24	64
55	15			25	65
	16			26	
	17			27	
	18			28	

18 17 16 15 14 13 12 11 21 22 23 24 25 26 27 28

48 47 46 45 44 43 42 41 31 32 33 34 35 36 37 38

	48			38	
	47			37	
	46			36	
85	45			35	75
84	44			34	74
83	43			33	73
82	42			32	72
81	41			31	71

Victim's GDP

Name:.. Contact:..

Address:..

Specific data

Crowns, bridges, dentures, RCT etc.
(use diagram on back of form if necessary)

Other data

Occlusion, attrition, smoker, anomalies, staining, OH, perio status etc.

X-rays available
Further material *(dental casts etc.)*
Date of last attendance at dental sugery
Age at time of disappearance *(if known)*
Dentist's signature
Dentist's name *(in capitals)*

Figure 5.7 Example of a dental identification ante-mortem form (printed on yellow paper)

Table 5.3 Features that can be used during comparative dental identification. This extensive list represents the complexity of these cases, particularly in instances in which restorative treatment is absent or minimal. Adapted from Pretty and Sweet (2001)

TEETH

Teeth present
- a. Erupted
- b. Unerupted
- c. Impacted

Missing teeth
- a. Congenitally
- b. Lost ante-mortem
- c. Lost post-mortem

Tooth type
- a. Permanent
- b. Deciduous
- c. Mixed
- d. Retained primary
- e. Supernumerary

Tooth positioning
- a. Malpositions

Crown morphology
- a. Size and shape
- b. Enamel thickness
- c. Contact points
- d. Racial variations

Crown pathology
- a. Caries
- b. Attrition, abrasion, erosion
- c. Atypical variations, enamel pearls, peg laterals, etc.
- d. Dentigerous cyst

Root morphology
- a. Size
- b. Shape
- c. Number
- d. Divergence of roots

Root morphology
- a. Dilaceration
- b. Root fracture
- c. Hypercementosis
- d. Root resorption
- e. Root hemisections

Pulp-chamber/root-canal morphology
- a. Size, shape and number
- b. Secondary dentine

Pulp-chamber/root-canal pathology
- a. Pulp stones, dystrophic calcification
- c. Root canal therapy
- d. Retrofills
- e. Apicectomy

Periapical pathology
- a. Abscess, granuloma or cysts
- b. Cementomas
- c. Condensing osteitis

Dental restorations
1. Metallic
   - a. Non-full coverage
   - b. Full coverage
2. Non-metallic
   - a. Non-full coverage
   - b. Laminates
   - c. Full coverage
3. Dental implants
4. Bridges
5. Partial and full removable prostheses

PERIODONTAL TISSUES

Gingival morphology and pathology
- a. Contour, recession, focal/diffuse, enlargements, interproximal craters
- b. Colour: inflammatory changes, physiological (racial) or pathological pigmentations
- c. Plaque and calculus deposits

Periodontal ligament morphology and pathology
- a. Thickness
- b. Widening
- c. Lateral periodontal cysts and similar

Alveolar process and lamina dura
- a. Height, contour, density of crestal bone
- b. Thickness of inter-radicular bone
- c. Exostoses, tori
- d. Pattern of lamina dura
- e. Bone loss (horizontal/vertical)
- f. Trabecular bone pattern and bony islands
- g. Residual root fragments

ANATOMICAL FEATURES

Maxillary sinus
- a. Size, shape, cysts
- b. Foreign bodies, fistula
- c. Relationship to teeth

Anterior nasal spine
- a. Incisive canal (size, shape, cyst)
- b. Median palatal suture

Mandibular canal
- a. Mental foramen
- b. Diameter, anomalous
- c. Relationship to adjacent structures

Coronoid and condylar processes
- a. Size and shape
- b. Pathology

Temporomandibular joint
- a. Size, shape
- b. Hypertrophy/atrophy
- c. Ankylosis, fracture
- d. Arthritic changes

Other pathologies
- a. Developmental cysts
- b. Salivary gland pathology
- c. Reactive/neoplastic
- d. Metabolic bone disease
- e. Focal or diffuse radio-opacities
- f. Evidence of surgery
- g. Trauma: wires, surgical pins etc.

Discrepancies identified during comparison of ante- and post-mortem dental charts should be considered individually and a decision made as to whether these discrepancies are explainable or unexplainable. An 'explainable discrepancy' is one that can be illustrated by referring back to case scenario 3 above.

Case scenario 3 (continued)

In 2004, a body is discovered in woods not far from the last known address of Jane Doe. An inscribed pendant and tattoo suggest that the body could be that of the reported missing Jane Doe. The relatives provide Jane Doe's dentist details and the dental records from her dentist are recovered. They span from 1980 to 1997, the last entry being a note that three letters for recall appointments had been sent to Jane's address but she had failed to attend. The family, the FLO and the forensic dentist have no knowledge of – and therefore no access to – the subsequent treatment that Jane Doe received at a private dentist and the hospital in the area of her latest known address.

The forensic dentist identifies three discrepancies between the dentition of the deceased and the dental records of Jane Doe, as seen in the odontograms taken for the pink and yellow forms for this case (Figure 5.8)

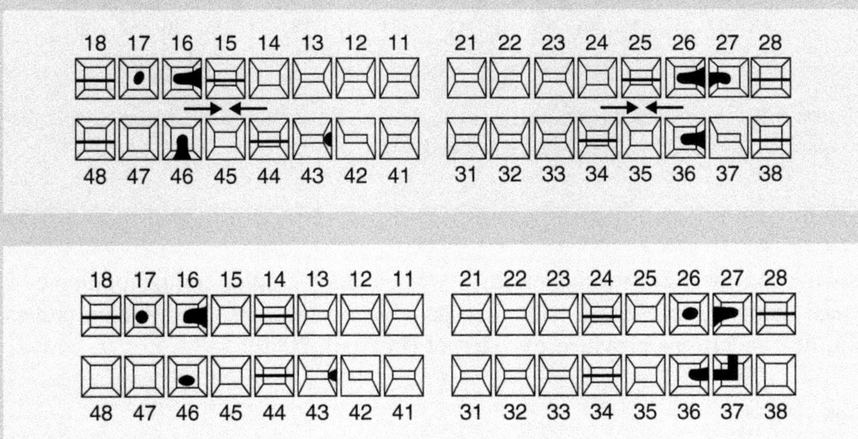

Figure 5.8 Ante-mortem and post-mortem dental charts illustrating explainable discrepancies (compare teeth 15, 14, 24, 25, 26, 38, 37 and 46)

Seven years have passed since Jane Doe saw a dentist (longer if we consider the failed appointments). Jane had also moved location and had been living there for the three years prior to her disappearance. All other features are concordant. It is possible for further treatments to have occurred subsequent to 1997, making the discrepancies *explainable*.

Take into consideration another scenario. A missing individual's dental records show missing upper left and right premolars and a full crown on an upper left premolar tooth, but the post-mortem dental examination shows that all four upper premolars are present and sound in the mouth of the deceased as well as fillings on certain teeth which are smaller in the deceased than they appear on the dental records (Figure 5.9). Tooth tissue and whole teeth cannot be regenerated (to date), and so here we have an example of *unexplainable* discrepancies

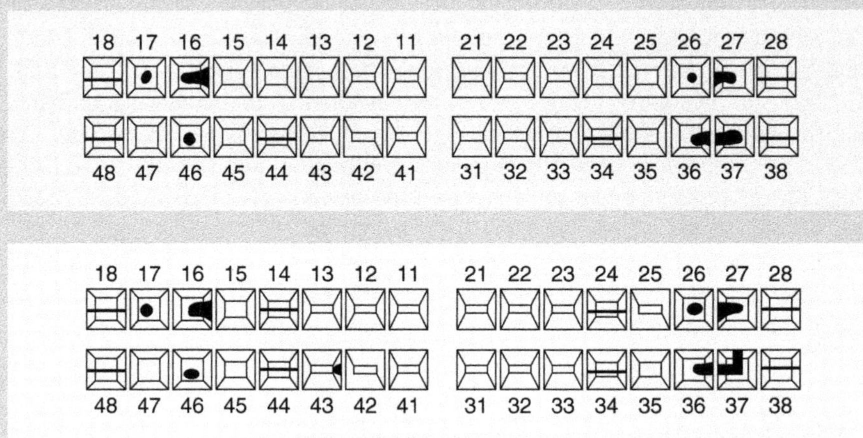

Figure 5.9 Ante-mortem and post-mortem dental charts illustrating unexplainable discrepancies (compare teeth 14, 24 25, 37 and 43)

Having considered all available data – written, photographic and radiographic – the forensic dentist is presented with four possible conclusions. The author prefers to adopt the conclusions provided by Interpol (Interpol, 2009):

1. exclusion
2. identity possible
3. identity probable
4. identity established.

The American Board of Forensic Odontology (2012) provides conclusions in different terminology but to a similar effect.

1. positive identification
2. possible identification

3. insufficient evidence
4. exclusion.

5.2.5 Problems with comparative dental identification

Comparative dental identification relies on:

- the availability of ante-mortem dental records
- the accuracy and completeness of those records.

Depending on where one is in the world, access to a dentist may not be easy. In some countries, a rural location, long distances and poor infrastructure make reaching a dentist nearly impossible. In other areas, varying levels of poverty and no national free dental service result in no dental treatment and records. In developed areas where dentists per capita make access relatively easy, the perceived lack of importance of maintaining dental health may still result in poor attendance, if any. In the UK, underfunding of the NHS and subsequent changes in dental NHS contracts resulted in a decrease of about 8 million patients on the NHS dental registers (Hardy, 2006). Some of these people have sought treatment through a private dental practice, but the majority have simply not accessed dental treatment. Whatever the reason, there are individuals in every country who will go through life without having a dental record, and these individuals cannot be identified by dental means if the need arises.

However, trouble finding a dental record is only part of the problem. An incomplete, unclear or inaccurate dental record could easily be as 'good' as not finding a dental record at all. The first problem with manual dental records is illegible handwriting. This is then compounded by the dentist's own acronyms and shorthand which can sometimes mean that the dental record is not far from being unintelligible to anyone outside that particular practice.

Different charting systems are a common problem, particularly if dealing with records from different countries. The FDI World Dental Federation system was an attempt to have a single international charting system, but to date dentists worldwide may still use alternative systems that they are familiar with, and this can cause confusion in communicating dental information. For example, 'tooth 16' in the FDI system refers to the upper right first permanent molar, whereas 'tooth 16' in the Universal System refers to the upper left third permanent molar. Obviously, viewing a completed odontogram would resolve the issue in situations of this kind.

Or maybe not! A recent MSc research project showed that use of different charting systems is only a part of the problem (Manica, 2011). Table 5.4 gives a snapshot of some of the findings. Language, codes and acronyms – and even diagrammatic representations of dental work such as bridges and crowns – vary widely between countries and within countries. The project contacted largely national dental associations and organisations. The author's prediction is that the diversity might be even wider if individual dentists were to be surveyed.

Ultimately, although it can translate the written word in a pictorial, more understandable manner, the odontogram will still suffer from the same problems as the

Table 5.4 Excerpt from the results tables of a master's research project illustrating the varying symbols that countries use to denote a 'missing tooth' (Manica, 2000)

M – missing (Libya)	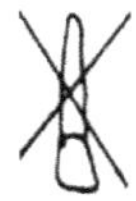 (Saudi Arabia)
Mis – missing tooth (Australia) **dente ausente** (Brazil) **ελλείπων δόντι** (Greece)	***Rule a line on odontogram*** (Australia, Barbados, Colombia, England, Finland, Jordan, Malaysia)
AB – tooth absent **f** – fehlender zahn (Germany) **MT** (Japan) **diente faltante ó ausente** (Chile)	***Draw a square around the missing tooth*** (Canada)
dent manqué (France) **Mam** – missing ante mortem **M** (Pakistan, United Arab Emirates)	⊕ (Croatia)
Mis (Thailand) **zub extrahiran** (Croatia) **LPM** – lost post-mortem	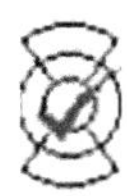 ***Tick on the tooth*** (Colombia) # (Greece) ***Horizontal lines crossing the crossing the missing tooth*** (Germany)
	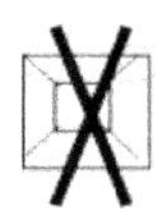 (Indonesia)
	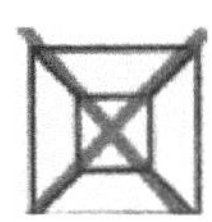 = missing AM (Indonesia)
	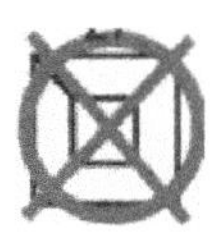 = missing PM (Indonesia)

written records – incompleteness and inaccuracies. The author's experience suggests that not every dentist routinely charts in detail the status of the mouth when examining a patient for the first time. The records of the dentist may be thorough in recording every episode of treatment that he/she subsequently undertakes, but without a full dental chart at initial examination the dental records will be inadequate for dental identification. A full radiographic dental survey could replace the information from an odontogram, but again this is not always undertaken.

A degree of human error will be present in almost any dental chart. Charting is normally completed by the dental nurse while the dentist examines the patient and dictates the findings. The reality is that most dental practices are busy and scrutinising charting is not always possible. After all, the dentist is there to treat current problems and an accurate record of past treatment is only of limited value.

Digital dental records have improved the efficiency and quality of dental record keeping, at least in as far as illegible handwriting is concerned. Proprietary dental software makes it quick to maintain the record, with odontograms often being completed automatically from the typed data. Treatment updates are quick to record and simultaneously reflected in the odontogram, making the forensic dentist's compilation of the composite dental chart much easier.

An MSc research project (Clarkson, 2011) looked at the use of manual dental records and computerised dental records in the military. Among other things, one of the advantages of the computerised system over the written record was that it allowed for a larger amount of information to be recorded in text format. This meant that conditions like tooth wear and tooth developmental anomalies were more often recorded. Current technology makes it easier to take photographs of the teeth and these can be easily stored 'attached' to the digital dental record and digital radiographs.

There are, however, multiple software packages available, and each can have its own key codes both for dental treatment acronyms and colour-coded filling materials. If a digital record is to be used for dental examination, a colour printout should be provided as well as the associated key for the particular software.

Human errors in dental charting are not just related to a busy clinic or communication breakdown. Every dentist will be able to recall numerous cases when a premolar is missing, its space is now closed and it is extremely difficult to tell whether the premolar present is the first or the second. And the same can apply to molars. Once again radiographs of these teeth often can shed some light, but that is not always the case.

5.3 Radiography in dental identification

The usefulness of radiographs in identification cannot be over-emphasised and has been documented on numerous occasions. The advantages apply to any medical radiograph but are much more evident in dental radiographs owing to the amount of inert, clearly visible anatomical structures and any associated dental treatment.

The adage 'a picture is worth a thousand words' has never been more appropriate. No matter how detailed the description of a filling in the written dental records, no words could describe the unique outline of the floor of the cavity dictated by the

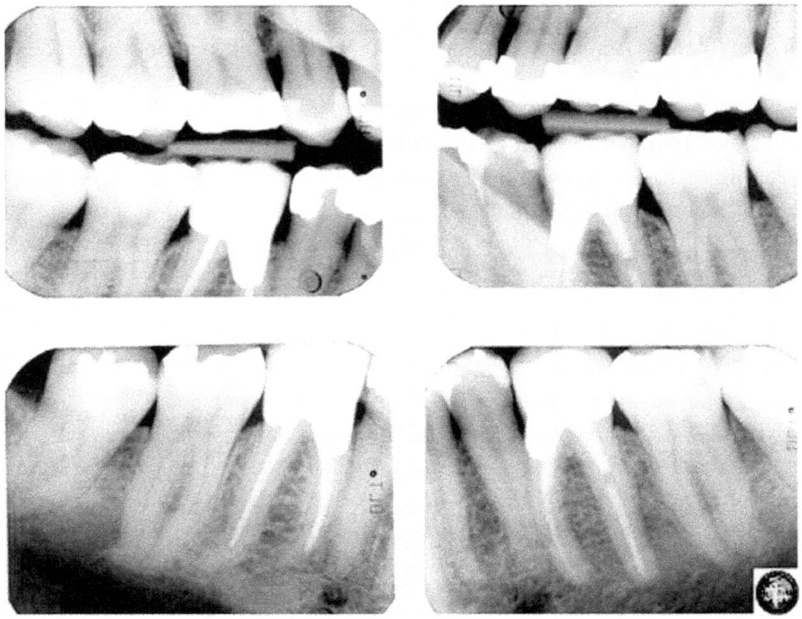

Figure 5.10 Radiograph illustrating uniqueness of amalgam restoration floors and root canal fillings

extent of caries before the filling was applied. This is even more evident with root canal fillings, posts, amalgam pins and dental implants (Figure 5.10).

Less than ideal dental treatment can be even more valuable than the perfectly executed treatment in an identification scenario. A broken endodontic instrument, over-filled root canals and amalgam filling overhangs are all essentially 'unique' because of their randomness.

But even in a situation when no dental treatment has been administered, a full-mouth radiographic survey could provide sufficient information to allow a positive identification. Unerupted wisdom teeth, supernumerary teeth, root morphology and maxillary sinus floors are all mostly biologically inert anatomical features with the added advantage of being essentially unique in their pattern and conformation. Table 5.5 lists some useful features in radiographs.

The ante-mortem radiograph increases the amount of information available exponentially because it reveals a whole host of detail that would otherwise not be charted and not be visible. The added advantage of comparing patterns and shapes of fillings and anatomical features other than just location and presence of fillings and teeth is immense and can change a possible identification to an established one.

A good set of radiographs can be sufficient, on their own, to provide a comprehensive picture of the ante-mortem dental status of the missing person, making up for all other problems that arise from incomplete, inaccurate or illegible manual or digital dental records (Pretty *et al.*, 2003). Van der Meer *et al.* (2010) showed a similar success rate in 'positive identifications' using digital periapical radiographs cropped so as to leave only untreated root morphology and anatomical patterns visible for

Table 5.5 Features visible in dental radiographs which assist dental identification

- Outline of restorations
- Root fillings
- Metal posts/pins
- Implants
- Root anatomy
- Pulp/root canal anatomy
- Inferior alveolar nerve canal
- Mental foramen
- Maxillary sinus floor
- Supernumerary teeth
- Unerupted teeth
- Plates and screws

comparison. Although the study is not based on actual cases, it highlights the value of anatomical features and pattern recognition and comparison.

5.3.1 Post-mortem radiography

When a dental identification is requested for confirmatory purposes, it is important to find out what radiographs are present with the ante-mortem dental records and ensure that any post-mortem records reflect the same technique used when the ante-mortem radiographs were taken: x-ray tube position and angulation, film size and location/angulation should be reproduced as closely as possible in the post-mortem radiographs, including any detectable errors in technique.

A radiograph is a flattened 2-dimensional image of 3-dimensional structures, complicated by the fact that the x-ray tube and the film lie on opposite sides of the structures in question. The appearance of restorations and root morphology on the film can change drastically even with a slight change in angulation of the x-ray tube to the film. The more widespread use of film-holders in dental practices has gradually standardised the quality of films and one sees less coning of films and fewer distorted images. This then facilitates somewhat the post-mortem imaging, with post-mortem use of the film-holder producing a more comparable image to the ante-mortem radiographs.

Taking radiographs of the deceased can be tricky. The author is not aware of a proprietary jig on the market that allows appropriate positioning of the head in relation to the x-ray tube and film and keeps them in place while the x-ray is taken. The limit to how this is achieved in the mortuary is one's own imagination and enterprising ability. Small sandbags, foam or paper tissues can be used to hold the film in place and/or to hold the mouth closed with the film in position (Figures 5.11 and 5.12).

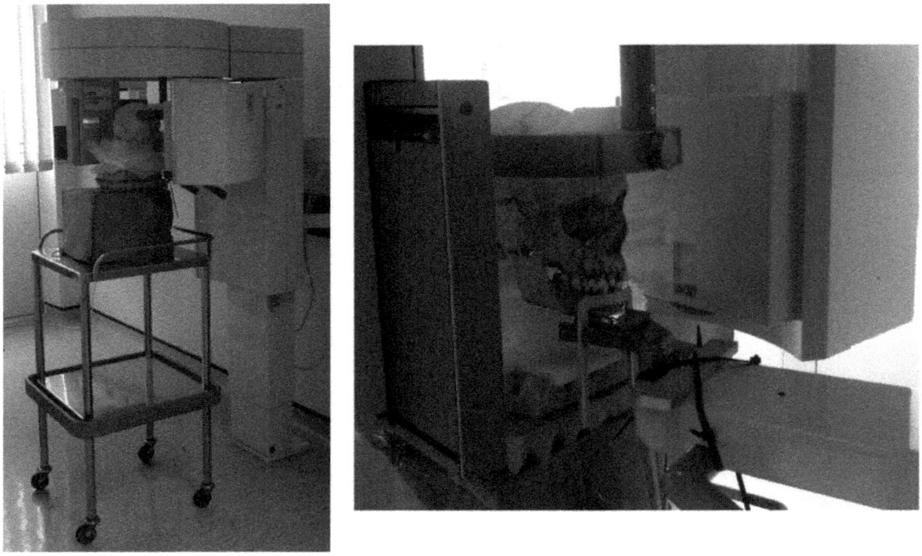

Figure 5.11 Improvised stand to aid in holding a dry skull in the correct position for an orthopantomogram

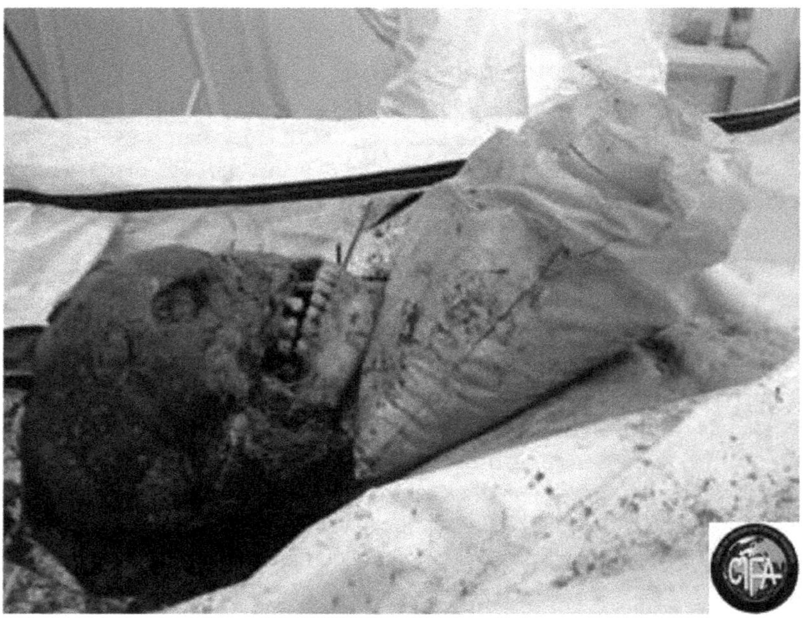

Figure 5.12 Using a small sandbag to hold the jaws in occlusion with an intraoral periapical radiograph held in position with a dental x-ray holder

When radiographs of skeletonised remains are being taken, voltage (kV) and exposure time will need to be reduced to compensate for the loss of intervening skin, fat or muscle tissue. Some trial and error may be required to achieve the correct exposure levels, a process much simplified by the advent of digital radiography which allows near instantaneous assessment and retaking if necessary. Even with the use of a film-holder, positioning the film appropriately and capturing the relevant detail can be difficult and a number of retakes may be necessary.

Excision of the jaws for radiography is never ideal, although it is possible if necessary and with the appropriate permissions. A portable platform that can be rested on the dental chair arms, or a stand, can be useful when taking radiographs of resected jaws or skeletonised materials, but other means can be improvised (Mincer *et al.*, 2008). In these cases and when the circumstances allow for excision, a panoramic post-mortem radiograph should be taken as it is likely to provide the most information and is easier to execute.

Portable radiography facilities do exist, albeit at a considerable expense, which may be prohibitive to the individual forensic dentist. First employed in a forensic dental setting during the 2004 tsunami victims identification, the NOMAD® handheld x-ray system has now been approved for use in the dental setting, and publications suggest that operator exposure is well below the annual maximum permissed dose of 50 mSv (Gray *et al.*, 2010; Danforth *et al.*, 2009). Use of a handheld unit in the mortuary setting should not be done without seeking advice from the Health Protection Authority (HPA) or the National Radiation Protection Board (NRPB) in the UK or the equivalent authorities in another country. It is also advisable to seek permission from the mortuary manager.

As long as the necessary health and safety regulations are adhered to, a handheld x-ray unit, dental digital sensors and portable computer with the relevant digital x-ray software would be the ideal package for a comprehensive dental examination of the deceased for the purpose of identification. If such facilities are available, a full radiographic survey should be done to ensure that all relevant information is recorded.

5.3.2 Ante-mortem radiographs

While the forensic dentist can strive to achieve the ideal scenario for capturing the best quality post-mortem full digital dental radiographic survey, a dental identification may still not be possible if the ante-mortem radiographs are of inadequate quality.

Any radiographic dental view can be useful. Ideally we compare like with like, but useful information can still be revealed from any ante-mortem radiographic view. When a considerable number of restorations are present, bitewing radiographs will provide most of the necessary information. On the other hand, when few or no restorations are present, an orthopantomogram view will be the most useful, providing a whole array of anatomical features, such as maxillary sinus floor, to compare and rely on. These two views are probably the most commonly utilised in dental practice, followed closely by peri-apical views, and are therefore the most encountered in an identification scenario. It must be noted, however, that any radiographic view including the jaw area could be of assistance if available.

Digital radiography is becoming more widespread in dental practices but there are still a large number of practices that have not yet made the leap. Mauthe and Eaton (2011a) reported that just fewer than 50% of general dental practices in the West Kent Primary Care Trust area in the UK were using digital radiography. The likelihood is that there is a good chance that the forensic dentist will need to rely on wet-film ante-mortem radiographs, if available. There is a suggestion that there is an under-use of bitewing radiographs for the detection of caries (Mauthe and Eaton, 2011b); although it is possible that the reported under-use is compensated by an over-use of orthopantomogram radiography, which from a dental identification point of view is more informative.

Problems unique to wet-film processing in conventional radiography include damage from inappropriate storage, over- and under-exposure, and improper chemical processing. Textbooks and some published articles suggest means of salvaging information from affected radiographs (Mincer *et al.*, 1997; Winstanley, 1996; Dailey and Furue, 1988). But such techniques are now rarely employed, and often the radiographs are just deemed inadequate to assist with the identification.

When ante-mortem wet-film developed radiographs are available, it is essential to work from the originals. This is the only way to ensure the maximum amount of information is available and the radiographs are viewed in the appropriate orientation. While it may seem unnecessary, the forensic dentist should emphasise that scans, faxed or photocopied radiographs are next to useless. The possibility of films getting muddled during filing should also be kept in mind, especially if information from the radiographs and the written dental record appear disparate.

Digital ante-mortem radiographs are, of course, immune to the above problems. Most exposure issues can be compensated to some extent through contrast and brightness enhancement (it is important to ensure that only enhancements are applied and no manipulation of the image). The advantage of electronic transfer, by secure network or on digital media, is obvious.

Digital radiographs also lend themselves to the idea of computerised or 'automated' comparison (Santoro *et al.*, 2009; Flint *et al.*, 2009; Jain and Chen, 2004). While this is an attractive, objective means of supporting or otherwise an identification, the author is of the opinion that it is essential for a trained dentist to assess the comparison – particularly when the number of restorations is low and the identification relies on the knowledge of anatomical landmarks and morphology. A number of studies have shown that trained odontologists, or expert groups, will perform better than the novice groups (Pretty *et al.*, 2003; Scholl and Moody, 2001).

As with any kind of image comparison, the geometric projection of ante-mortem and post-mortem radiographs will need to be taken into account since this can lead to false-negatives. If such differences are adjusted by manipulation of the image through the software, then we will be entering a minefield. When comparison relies on pattern recognition and such patterns include small detail, it is imperative not to conduct any manipulation to a digital image without knowing precisely the effect that such manipulation has on the image. As noted earlier, there are a number of elements involved in producing an x-ray and any slight change in their relationship to each other could change the geometric projection and hence produce an altered image. An experienced dental radiologist may be able to detect such changes and have a good idea of how to correct the technique to achieve the correct projection. However, in the author's opinion, calculating the exact extent of digital manipulation necessary to achieve a similar effect is still not sufficiently understood. In a controlled scenario, research may give promising results; but when applying these manipulations to ante-mortem radiographs of 'unknown origin' and post-mortem radiographs taken in less than ideal situations, great caution should be applied. In the author's opinion this is a space to be watched for future developments, but any such 'automated' digital methods of comparison should be considered carefully before being applied in live cases – particularly if they don't recommend the necessity of a trained dentist/odontologist for execution.

5.3.3 Computed tomography

Correcting distortions that result from a 2-dimensional representation of a 3-dimensional structure may not be necessary in the future if the use of computed tomography (CT) in post-mortem examination becomes more widespread. This imaging system produces undistorted, 3-dimensional images of the area under examination. Widespread use is unlikely to happen in the near future for routine dental identifications, but the literature has reported the use of multi-slice CT (MTCT) for some time (Thali *et al.*, 2003), and in recent years the application to multiple-fatality situations has also been explored (Sidler *et al.*, 2007).

The application of MTCT to dental identification has so far been very limited owing to the poor clarity of the detail in the dentition recorded by this method, particularly when metal restorations are present (Kirchoff *et al.*, 2008). Having viewed both 3-dimensional and CT-OPT reformatted images of the jaws from multi-slice CT, the author does not deem it safe to base identification on such data.

The use of cone-beam CT (CBCT) is a major improvement and, in the author's opinion, utilising such data for identification is as good as using conventional dental radiographs, with the added advantage of the third dimension and the ability to reformat images comparable to the ante-mortem conventional radiographs available. A preliminary study (Murphy *et al.*, 2012) looked mainly at CT-OPT reformations from CBCT images and the results are promising. The clarity of the image in CBCT is decidedly better than MTCT; however, the practical issues of acquiring CBCT scans for a deceased individual in a mortuary setting are still prohibitive, unless the jaws are excised and scanned in a dental clinic.

Some familiarity with CBCT imaging and the viewing software would still be advantageous to the forensic dentist. The systems need some familiarisation which is not beyond the basic capabilities of standard computer literacy. CBCT is found in hospital settings and in a slowly increasing number of dental practices, particularly specialist clinics providing implant surgery. The possibility of having an ante-mortem CBCT to consider during dental identification could soon become a reality.

5.4 Dental appliances in identification

A number of appliances can be provided to patients, some being temporary and others more permanent. Table 5.6 lists a few of these.

Table 5.6 Examples of devices/appliances that a dentist may provide for patients

- Acrylic denture (partial or complete)
- Chrome cobalt denture
- Crown (porcelain/metal)
- Bridge (tooth or implant supported)
- Orthodontic appliance
- Sports mouth guard
- Bleaching tray
- Occlusal splint
- Mandibular advancement device (MAD)

5.4.1 Dental models (casts)

There is a common denominator in the provision of all of the listed appliances: at some stage a dental impression of the patient's teeth needs to be taken and dental models cast in plaster or stone. In some instances, more than one set of dental casts is produced for a given course of treatment – implant treatment with a temporary removable denture being a case in point. Strictly speaking, dental casts form part of the dental record and should be stored by the dentist in the same way as the written, radiographic and digital records. In practice, in most instances dental casts are either destroyed as part of the appliance production method, such as with production of dentures, or at the end of the relevant course of treatment.

Alternatively, the dentist may give the dental casts to the patient once the course of treatment is finished. It is likely that on the majority of occasions the patient will discard these dental casts, with the exception of patients who underwent orthodontic treatment. This treatment may provide the most appeal for an individual to want to keep a record of the appearance of his/her teeth before the arduous dental treatment. On the other hand, certain appliances, such as bleaching trays or protective splints worn at night, may at times be provided to the patient with the dental cast to help with safe-keeping of the appliance when not in use.

If the dental records show production of an appliance, it is always worth asking the treating dentist or the family whether the dental casts are still available. The dental casts are essentially a replica of the teeth and can therefore disclose considerable 3-dimensional information that could be used to support, if not establish, an identification. The shape of palatal surfaces of anterior teeth can have distinctive features such as an enlarged cingulum, talon cusp, dens invaginatus or evaginatus, palatal fissures. These features are not distinctive on their own, although incidence figures can be found in the textbooks; but they can become very relevant in combination with other concordant features. Such features are rarely clearly recorded in the written record; and if they are, their particular shape, which is what makes them distinctive, cannot be described accurately.

Similarly any anatomical feature affecting the labial aspect of the teeth, or the position of the teeth themselves, would be clearly visible on the dental cast and could assist in facial comparison, covered later in this chapter.

Before using the dental casts for any identification work it is of great importance to note when these casts were taken and what type of dental treatment was undertaken subsequently. Dental casts before orthodontic treatment or before implant surgery are of less value compared to dental casts produced during production of a night guard or a bleaching tray, the latter being more likely to represent the state of the mouth at the time that the individual went missing.

5.4.2 Palatal rugae

Another important anatomical feature that the dental casts give access to are the palatal rugae. There is conflicting evidence in the literature about their uniqueness, stability and usefulness in establishing identification, but it is generally accepted that they can be useful in assisting with identification (De Angelis *et al.*, 2012). The palatal rugae are very well protected from external trauma owing to their position, and from thermal injury by the tongue and surrounding soft tissues. High palatal rugae integrity has been recorded in cases of incineration and decomposition (Muthusubramanian *et al.*, 2005).

Most of the published studies hinting at stability of palatal rugae before and after orthodontic treatment, individuality and even sex and racial distinction, rely on relatively small sample sizes (Shukla *et al.*, 2011; Jibi *et al.*, 2011; Santos and Caldas, 2012) and should be considered more as pilot studies rather than evidence for the uniqueness and stability of the palatal rugae.

There is also a variety of suggested classifications and methods of comparison for analysing palatal rugae, and to date the author is not aware of a single universal classification.

Having considered all this, if dental casts (or appliances covering the palatal surface) are available as part of the ante-mortem record, palatal rugae should be utilised to support or otherwise the identification, particularly when there is insufficient number of restorations or radiographic views available.

In these cases, dental impressions of the deceased should be obtained, paying particular attention to the reproduction of the palate. Close-up photographs of the palatal rugae should also be taken before the dental impressions are taken, owing to the potential disturbance of the remains when removing the impression from the mouth. Careful choice of the impression material is also important. The longevity and stability of the impressions are of utmost importance, so silicone materials are best. However, the strength of such materials may render removal of the impression from the mouth difficult, particularly if the remains are fragile. Alginate may be more appropriate for these circumstances, bearing in mind its lack of stability and the need for models to be poured as soon as possible.

The reader may think that the pattern of the palatal rugae could be most useful in the identification of the edentulous individual. In these cases the palatal rugae could be used to establish that a particular denture belongs to the deceased, if the denture had not been recovered *in situ* with the body. Knowing who the denture belonged to could provide support to confirming a suspected identity.

Stronger support could be provided if dental casts produced during the process of making the full dentures were still stored and available as part of the ante-mortem dental records. If present these could be compared to the palatal pattern obtained from an impression of the mucosal surface of a denture found in the mouth of the deceased, as well as with the pattern of the palatal rugae taken directly from the hard palate of the deceased.

However, in one study, Ohtani *et al.* (2008) encountered problems with palatal height, poorly demarcated eminences of the rugae, and changes from atrophy of the alveolar bone with resultant changes in the apparent pattern of the rugae closest to the maxillary ridge. Atrophic changes in the edentulous mouth are continuous; and so, although use of the palatal rugae in identification of the edentulous deceased would be most welcome, this is probably when it is the least reliable and should not be used as the sole means of establishing identity.

To the author's knowledge, no published study has considered a large enough sample to be able to provide reliable statistical data of the probability of finding two similar patterns of palatal rugae. Neither is there a tested, accepted, reliable comparison method that established how many points of concordance need to be present to be certain that the two palatal patterns being compared are from one individual and couldn't be from anyone else. Most of the studies documenting high percentage figures of positive identifications used an experimental model based on 'finding the match' within a random set of casts which included all of the matching pairs of casts. This is hardly a representation of the real scenario where a forensic odontologist has a 'stand alone' pattern of palatal rugae and has to decide whether the pattern seen on the deceased could belong *only* to the person from whom the ante-mortem dental casts were produced.

Until such studies are presented in the literature the author remains somewhat sceptical and feels that palatal rugae can provide only *supportive* evidence to a forensic dental identification, particularly in edentulous individuals.

5.4.3 Removable appliances

Dental appliances made for a specific patient fall under the 'custom-made devices' for the purpose of the Medical Devices Directive 93/42/EC. This directive was amended by the European Commission and such amendments came into effect on 21 March 2010. The Medical and Healthcare Products Regulatory Agency (MHRA) is responsible for enforcing the directive in the UK, and as the regulatory body the General Dental Council (GDC) provides guidance through its standards guidance.

A dental appliance can be anything from a full removable denture to fixed prosthdontics, with anything in between including removable orthodontic appliances, sports gumshields and bleaching trays.

The standards on commissioning and manufacturing dental appliances state that every patient receiving an appliance must be provided with a statement of manufacture compliant with the legal responsibilities of the 'manufacturer'. The statement must include the following information:

- the name and address of the manufacturer and, if outside the EU, their authorised representative
- data allowing identification of the device
- a statement that the device is a custom-made dental appliance and intended for exclusive use by a particular named patient
- the name of the practitioner or other authorised person who made out the prescription and, where applicable, the name of the practice concerned
- specific characteristics of the product as indicated by the prescription
- a statement that the device conforms to the essential requirements set out in Annex I of Medical Devices Directive 93/42/EC and, where applicable, indicating which essential requirements have not been fully met, together with the grounds.

The dentist prescribing and fitting the appliance has a legal obligation to clearly inform the patient that this statement of manufacture is available for him/her to take away. If the patient declines taking this statement, then the dentist must keep it with the patient's record for the lifetime of the appliance. If the patient requests the statement, then they should sign for it and thish signature record retained with the dental records.

What does this mean to a forensic dental identification? In the past, identifying the manufacturer and the prescriber of a particular removable denture found at the scene required an element of investigative work, with a heavy dose of guesswork and trial and error. With the production of the statement of manufacture, information is available that can link the denture to its owner, its prescriber and its manufacturer. If the patient chooses not to take the statement, it should come to the forensic dentist with the dental records and may make recognising and identifying the denture as the same one that was custom-made for a particular individual a little easier.

Before the directive came into effect, a dentist complying with recommended good practice most likely kept the prescription of the denture with the dental records in any case. This prescription included most of the details required in the statement of manufacture and so would have been of some use to the forensic dentist. What the amendments to the directive have done is made the requirement to keep the statement with the patient's dental record (if the patient does not request it) a legal requirement.

If the patient does request the statement, he/she has no legal obligation to keep it, so in these cases the forensic dentist may still be missing a piece of useful information.

5.4.4 Denture marking

In a dentate individual, establishing that a particular appliance or removable denture belongs to a specific patient may not be crucial to the identification, particularly if the appliance fits well in the mouth. In an edentulous individual this is much more relevant, highlighting the importance of denture marking. Hardy (2006) states that in the UK the reasons given for not making denture marking mandatory relate to a perception of infringement of personal liberty by the denture wearer, as well as a cost implication. Hardy urges: 'perhaps it is time the dental profession in the UK became more persuasive about the importance of denture marking and explained the beneficial reasons more fully to their patients'. The author shares Hardy's sentiments and believes that legal obligations of the directive have maybe made this the opportune time to push for denture marking to become a mandatory requirement in the UK.

The statement of manufacture must include 'data allowing identification of the device in question'. If this were a unique identifying number, it could be included in the denture with the prescriber's and/or the manufacturer's GDC registration number, making the particular denture retraceable to the dental record without including the patient's personal data on the appliance itself – hence overcoming the issues with having personal data on a removable appliance that can be lost.

Harvey (1966) reports that identification utilising dentures occurred as early as 1193 when the Raja Chandra was identified from his denture after his death in battle. The indestructibility of dentures has been well documented (Haines, 1972; Olsson *et al.*, 1993). Moreover, numerous disasters are also documented highlighting the prevalence of denture wearers, the majority of which have unlabelled dentures and cannot be identified by this simple means (Clarke, 1994; Ayton *et al.*, 1985; Haines, 1972).

Peterson and Yamamoto (2005) reported that the 2003 WHO figures for edentulous people aged 65 years or older in Europe were between 12% and 78%. It is unlikely that we will have a denture-free society in the immediate future.

The requirements of a denture marking system can be summarised as (Johansen and Eckman, 1984):

- fully and easily legible
- capable of withstanding high temperatures (up to 1300°C) and strong acidity
- easy to apply
- inexpensive
- not weakening the denture
- allowing subsequent relining and repair
- radio-opaque
- aesthetically acceptable.

Various methods have been described in the literature, most of which are variations of the same two themes: surface identifiers and inclusion methods (Heath *et al.*, 1988; Tabak, 1993; Bernitz and Blignaut; 1998; Rötzscher *et al.*, 1999; Rajan and Julian, 2002; Richmond and Pretty, 2009a).

MacEntee and Campbell (1979) tested the heat resistance of eight different inclusion materials for denture marking. More recently, Richmond and Pretty (2009b) subjected ten different denture markings to a variety of assaults, including acid, soil, naked flame and crematorium furnace. A stainless-steel orthodontic band was the most resilient in both studies, with radio-frequency ID (RFID) tagging a close second (Figure 5.13).

The use of an embedded RFID tag was the preferred method of denture marking in a sample of 100 edentulous patients in the UK (Richmond and Pretty, 2007). The same

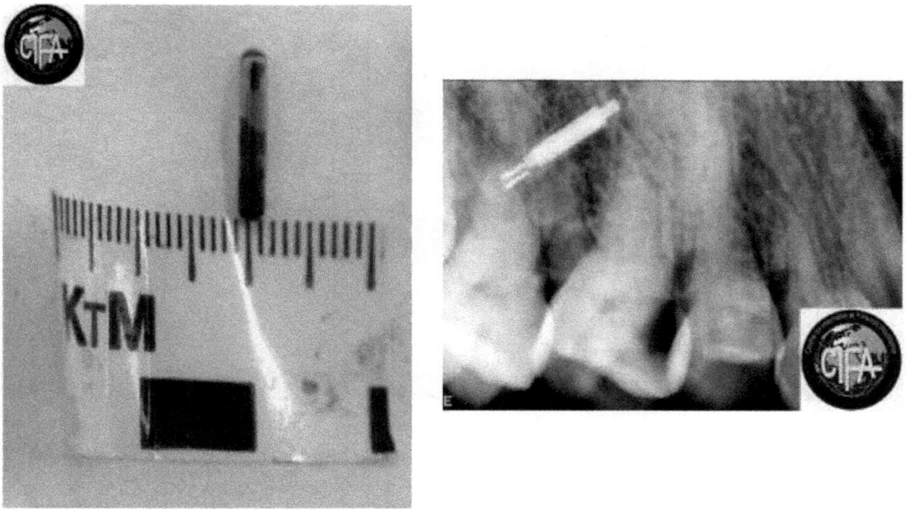

Figure 5.13 Radio-frequency ID tag used during recovery of deceased victims of the Boxing Day tsunami that hit Thailand in 2004. On the right is a radiograph of the RFID *in situ*

cohort was also reportedly unanimously happy to have their dentures marked once they understood its involvement. This was also reflected in an earlier study (Cunningham and Hoad-Reddick, 1993) where compliance was more than 90% once the availability and advantages of denture marking were explained.

Denture marking systems, including RFID tags, are already in use in care homes in a number of countries (Madrid *et al.*, 2012; Richmond and Pretty, 2009a). The author believes that a change of attitude and appreciation of the advantages of denture markings by the dental community and willingness to educate patients is what is needed to ensure an increase in the prevalence of marked dentures among wearers of full dentures.

5.4.5 Bleaching trays

Tooth bleaching treatments have become increasingly common over the last decade, including home treatments. If constructed by the dentist, these trays will be custom-made for the individual patient. A perfect fit of the tray over the teeth of the deceased can be sufficient to establish identity, particularly if there are any imbricated or irregularly positioned teeth.

5.4.6 Fixed prostheses

Although a means of marking metal fixed prostheses using copper vapour laser has been suggested in the literature (Ling *et al.*, 2003), it is unlikely that such practice will become routine. The usefulness in dental identification of post and core crowns,

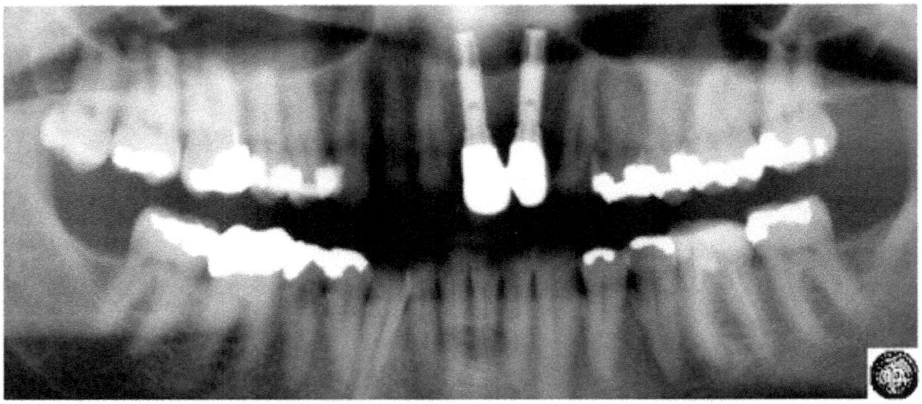

Figure 5.14 Dental implants and crowns provide additional features for comparison

fixed bridges and dental implants is mainly through radiographic comparison. Each element in the dentition adds a feature useful for comparison (Figure 5.14).

Replacement of missing teeth with dental implants and implant-supported dentures is becoming increasingly common. Unfortunately, in contrast to other surgically implanted devices such as hip and knee replacements and fixation plates, dental implants are machine-made and to date manufacturers do not include an individual serial number on each dental implant.

Berketa *et al.* (2010) have reported that the Straumann™ Company (Waldenburg, Switzerland) have released information that their implants will have laser-etched batch numbers on the internal chambers. They stated that the number of implants with the same batch number varies from 24 to 2400, and such batch numbers were still identifiable on an implant and abutment submitted to 1125°C in a furnace. According to the authors, this temperature is above that seen in crematoria, burning vehicles, and the 9/11 World Trade Centre disaster.

In a similar study, the same authors (Berketa *et al.*, 2011) have shown that, apart from oxidation on the surface of the implants, all four tested implants from three different manufacturers were virtually unchanged with no sagging visible on the radiographic images taken pre- and post-incineration.

5.5 Dental profiling

This chapter has so far considered mainly comparative dental identification which relies on the availability and accuracy of ante-mortem dental records. There are instances, however, as described in case scenario 1 earlier in the chapter, when no clue exists as to who the deceased may be – and therefore it is not possible, even if they do exist, to locate and acquire ante-mortem dental records for comparison. Dental profiling – also known as 'reconstructive dental identification' – describes the process of extracting information from the teeth in an attempt to piece together a profile of the deceased individual. Gender, ethnicity, geographical provenance, habits, nutritional deficiencies and indicators of past severe illness are bits of information that can be derived to some extent from teeth. Each piece of information narrows down the pool of missing individuals, one of which could be the deceased.

Case scenario 1 (continued)

The set of recovered bones consists of a skull, a mandible, parts of a rib cage and a scapula. The pathologist assesses the remains and, from features in the skull and mandible, he suggests that they are of a female. Police look at their list of missing persons and, considering the location where the body was found, make a presumptive identification. Dental records are provided. A forensic dentist is called. Examination of the teeth of the deceased is completed. Comparison with the available dental records quickly reveals that this person can be excluded from being the deceased.

The missing persons database shows that the number of possible females that went missing in the area in the last few years was considerable and the police therefore ask the forensic dentist for help to narrow the possibilities down.

5.5.1 Gender

Establishing gender in these situations is an essential first step as this immediately almost halves the possibilities. The pelvis (as a consequence of the female role of childbirth) and the skull and mandible are two parts of the skeleton that show the highest level of sexual dimorphism and should be relied on for this purpose when available.

It has been reported that teeth also show sexual dimorphism in their mesiodistal, buccolingual (İşcan and Kedici, 2003) and diagonal crown dimensions (Zorba *et al.*, 2012), as well as in cuspal diameter (Macaluso, 2010). The significant differences are often of low order, are based on reasonably small samples and are population-specific. The value of using the teeth to determine gender in skeletal material is questionable and should be used with caution, if at all.

Apart from reducing the pool of possible missing persons for comparison; establishing gender is relevant for subsequent information that is to be derived from the teeth (and the skeleton). Age estimation tables (and tables of stature from long bones) are usually gender-specific.

5.5.2 Ethnicity

Having established gender as reliably as possible, the next piece of the puzzle is ethnicity. In current times when intercontinental travel is as easy as going to the city centre, populations are subject to gene flow such that no 'pure' race actually exists; instead there is a continuous flow (Duray *et al.*, 1999).

As with gender, the bones of the skull, in the hands of experienced professionals such as anthropologists or odontologists, are likely to give the best indications of ethnicity. For example, the shape of the upper arch can give some indication of ethnicity, being more likely horseshoe shaped in Asians and U-shaped in Caucasians.

Teeth may provide indicators of ethnicity or ethnic descent. Morphometric variations in teeth have been described for more than 100 years, and systems exist that can identify the variants and measure the level of variation. The most widely used scheme, and the standard recommended by anthropologists working in the field, is the Arizona State University dental anthropology system which provides plaques for scoring the level of variation of a particular trait (Turner *et al.*, 1991). Some examples are:

- shovelling of upper incisors most frequently found among Asians and Native Americans
- enamel extensions on the facial surfaces of molars in Asians
- Carabelli's trait most commonly seen in Europeans
- prominent canine mesial ridge in Bushman Africans
- Uto-Aztecan premolar – where the buccal cusp of upper first premolars bulges out to the buccal – seen only in Native Americans, with the highest frequency in Arizona.

Most of these variations present differently in different populations with only a few being present exclusively in one population. Identification of the features during a dental profiling exercise can provide an indication of ethnic ancestry of the deceased but should not be considered definitive in isolation.

5.5.3 Age assessment

Age estimation is arguably the most useful piece of information that can be derived from the teeth. It is accepted that dental age estimation is the most reliable age estimation method even through adulthood, the assessment being more reliable if the gender and ethnicity are known. The various methods are dealt with in detail in Chapter 7.

5.5.4 Habits

Occupational, social and dietary habits can be reflected in the appearance of the teeth. Extrinsic staining of the teeth can suggest tobacco smoking or consumption of tea and/or coffee or red wine. Depending on its distribution and location, severe tooth surface loss due to erosion can suggest heavy consumption of acidic foods and drinks or conditions like bulimia or anorexia. Horse jockeys are known to suffer from acid erosion on the palatal surfaces of upper incisors, in an attempt to keep their body weight down through vomiting.

Specific areas of abrasion may give indications of occupation-related habits. For example, a groove in the incisal edge of the central incisors may be the result of holding an implement between the teeth or using the teeth for cutting – seamstresses biting thread, electricians biting plastic casing from electrical wire (Hardy, 2006), fishermen fixing fishing nets. Chemical erosion of the labial surfaces of incisors was also commonly seen in those working in the chemical industry before health and safety in the workplace was enforced.

5.5.5 Developmental tooth anomalies

Development of the teeth can be affected in a variety of ways and the resultant appearance of a tooth may be of value in constructing the profile of the deceased.

- Inherited traits like amelogenesis imperfecta or dentinogenesis imperfecta will be visible on examination and on radiographs and can link a deceased individual to his relatives who will also present with similar tooth anomalies.
- Conditions like scurvy as a result of vitamin C deficiency are less commonly seen these days but should also be kept in mind and can manifest in the appearance of the teeth.
- Severe illness disturbances both at birth and in later stages during enamel formation of the permanent teeth will affect ameloblasts and result in hypoplasias which will remain visible in the teeth throughout lifetime. Childhood fevers like chickenpox, measles, pneumonia or gastroenteritis occurring in the first year or two of life are often the cause. Because of the sequential development of enamel, the location of the area of hypoplasia on the crowns of the teeth can be translated to the time of development of that particular area of the tooth, and hence the chronological age of the individual when he/she suffered the traumatic or febrile episode can be established and linked to medical records.
- Hutchinson's insicors or barrel-shaped incisors are a specific developmental anomaly, less commonly seen in recent years, associated with congenital syphilis.

5.5.6 Fluorosis

Exposure to fluoride concentrations in excess of 2 parts per million (ppm) during dental development may cause varying degrees of fluorosis, from small opaque patches to enamel hypoplasias and dark staining (Figure 5.15).

The relevance to dental profiling is correlating the fluorosis with the geographical distribution of naturally occurring fluoride in water. This is not as straightforward as one may think. Not only must fluoride supplements including fluoridation of water be taken into account, but one must also bear in mind that the clinical presentation of fluorosis can vary from individual to individual even when there is the same exposure

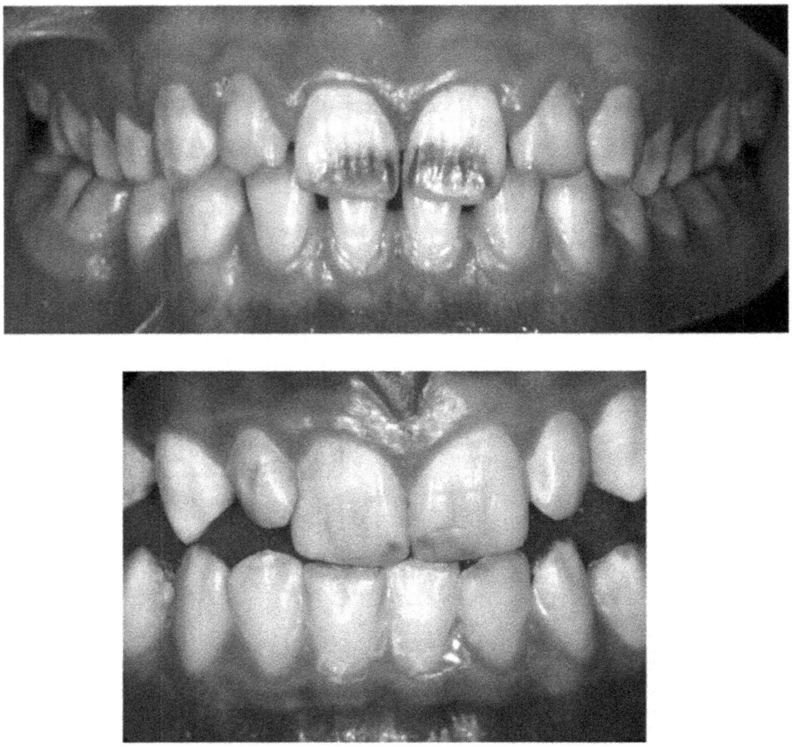

Figure 5.15 Moderate and mild fluorosis with distinctive discoloration of the anterior teeth. Courtesy of Professor Barbara Chadwick (For colour details, please see colour plate section.)

to the same level of fluoride. There are also suggestions in the literature that other external factors like a high average daily temperature will cause fluorosis even at low levels of fluoride (<1 ppm) (Louw *et al.*, 2002). Therefore, a particular appearance of teeth affected by fluorosis as seen during visual examination does not always correspond to exposure to a particular concentration of fluoride.

Thus fluorosis is useful to indicate provenance only in extreme cases such when effecting deciduous teeth. Deciduous teeth develop *in utero* and so it is extremely rare for these teeth to present with fluorosis. However, this does occur in certain parts of India where the fluoride content is in excess of 8 ppm. At other times, visible fluorosis can assist only by highlighting certain geographical areas as possible areas of provenance.

Fluoride content as part of elemental analysis of ground teeth is likely to be more informative. Fluoride is locked in once enamel maturation is complete. Apart from outer surface enamel, the level of fluoride in enamel will remain constant as when the teeth first completed development. Therefore analysis of fluoride content in ground enamel could give a better indication of where the individual resided at the time of tooth development.

5.5.7 Tetracycline staining

The side-effects of administering tetracycline to developing children and during pregnancy are well known and this drug is now very rarely administered to these cohorts. If seen, tetracycline staining will be in the form of a band of discoloration on all or a number of teeth – the number of teeth affected and the location of the band corresponding to the stage of tooth development at the time of tetracycline administration (Figure 5.16). The age at which the individual suffered a serious illness can then be deduced.

5.5.8 Isotope and trace element analysis

Studies of isotope ratios and trace elements in human tissues have been conducted in isolation for some years with some promising results. Hair, bone and nails can be used to give the short- to medium-term provenance of the individual. These tissues

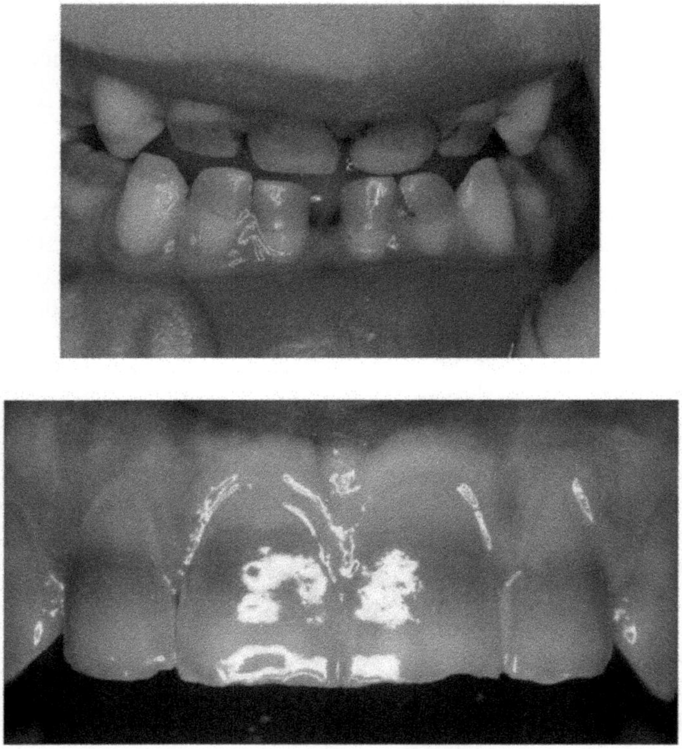

Figure 5.16 Tetracycline staining in deciduous and adult dentition (unrelated cases). Courtesy of Professor Barbara Chadwick (For colour details, please see colour plate section.)

turn over in a matter of days to months or few years with a continuing changing picture of the component elements. Teeth are biologically inert; once mineralisation of the roots is complete the composition of tooth tissue remains unchanged except for a few micrometers of surface enamel and secondary and tertiary dentine. As with the case of fluoride (see earlier), any isotope or trace element information derived from teeth will give information about the early years of life. Analysing different teeth or micro-sampling from different parts of an individual tooth can give diet and living environment information on an annual or seasonal basis (Pye, 2004).

There are various methods of sampling and analysis: scanning electron microscopy with energy-dispersive x-ray spectroscopy (SEM/EDS), laser ablation or solution, inductively coupled mass spectrometry (ICP-MS), to mention but a few. Neodymium, strontium, lead, carbon, oxygen, hydrogen and radioactive isotopes ratios as well as major and trace element concentrations have been studied with varying levels of success. The utility of these methods to dental profiling is restricted by the availability of appropriate database information that can be used for comparison purposes. The data are scattered in the literature and interpretation is difficult owing to the array of different methodologies of pre-sampling and analysis used in different laboratories (Pye, 2004).

If considering the use of such techniques, careful discussions with the laboratories conducting the analysis should be undertaken to ensure that the correct tooth is harvested and that it is stored and transported in the appropriate manner.

5.5.9 Dental restorations

The general condition of the mouth could be an indicator of socioeconomic status: the level of oral hygiene, the ratio of restored teeth to decayed unrestored teeth, the quality and type of restorations. Severe neglect of the mouth can also be suggestive of mental or physical disability or even dental phobia. This information can educate the dental profile but is also likely to be relevant as corroborative information to identification.

Elemental analysis of the dental materials by x-ray fluorescence spectrometry or SEM/EDS could also provide some useful information. This can only be of assistance if a database of the spectra for brands of dental materials used in the country is available. If a brand of resin is identified, depending on how widely distributed it is, it may be possible to work backwards and narrow down the number of practices that use that particular brand.

5.5.10 Facial reconstruction

In cases where no manageable number of missing individuals can be compared, or when there is no information whatsoever to point to the presumptive identifications, information gathered during profiling of the deceased can assist facial reconstruction. Reconstruction can be 2- or 3-dimensional, the latter being either manual or computer-generated. The intention of a facial reconstruction is often a last-ditch attempt for the police to bring up new leads for investigation.

The reconstruction in itself is not a means of identification but acts as an aid to jog the memory of people who might have known the victim. The police can then look into whether these proposed individuals fit the profile and if so recover dental records for a comparative dental identification.

Information about gender, ethnicity and age will influence the final appearance of the reconstruction. The forensic dentist can also advise on the position and shape of the teeth and how they would affect the position of the adjacent soft tissues.

5.5.11 Craniofacial superimposition

In cases where no dental records are available, superimposition can aid identification if an ante-mortem photograph of the face is available. The forensic dentist can be of assistance in these cases if the ante-mortem photograph shows a clear smile. Dependent on the position and shape of the anterior teeth, sufficient evidence can be available to at best strongly support identification or exclude identification, or at worse act as corroborative information.

It is beyond the scope of this chapter to discuss in detail the techniques of superimposition, forensic or otherwise. More detailed texts are available, such as İşcan and Helmer's (1993) *Forensic Analysis of the Skull: Craniofacial analysis, reconstruction, and identification.* The principles of the technique have been around for about 130 years (Glassman, 2000) and continuously developed ever since, mainly with the application of new technology to help overcome technical difficulties. The earliest documented use of this technique in a medico-legal setting was the 1935 identification of Isabella Ruxton by Glaister, Smith and Brash in Edinburgh, which subsequently led to the conviction of Dr Buck Ruxton for the murder of his wife and maid (Taylor, 2000).

Whether the superimposition is photographic, video or computer-aided, the principles (and technical difficulties) remain the same. Ante- and post-mortem photographs are projected over each other using bony landmarks on the unidentified skull and the ante-mortem photograph/video as guidance. The landmarks are chosen because the thickness of soft tissue is at its lowest in these areas and they are easiest to locate on the ante-mortem material. The advantage of a clear wide smile in the ante-mortem photograph is obvious – unchanging hard contours unobstructed by soft tissue.

It is essential to compare like with like. The closest possible orientation of the head in all three planes is essential to ensure that any result lends strong support to an identification.

5.6 Teeth as a source of DNA

Enamel, with its 96% of mineral composition, is the hardest tissue in the body. It therefore protects the soft tissues of the pulp against all manner of assault and degradation from the effects of humidity, temperature, bacterial and fungal action. Molar teeth are also further mechanically protected by the tongue, buccinator muscle and facial soft tissues.

The literature reports various successes of extracting DNA from the teeth, including from archaeological material (Ricaut *et al.*, 2005; Sosa *et al.*, 2012). In fact, genomic ancient DNA from the teeth often proves better for amplification of a full DNA profile than DNA from bones. Application of the techniques to mass fatalities, both natural disasters or mass graves, has also been well documented (Andelinović *et al.*, 2005; Parsons *et al.*, 2007; Hinchcliffe, 2011).

Numerous specialised texts are available describing the technical details of DNA analysis. This chapter will look at the basic aspects of harvesting teeth for human identification and the scenarios when this may be of assistance.

The best teeth for DNA extraction are unrestored molar teeth as they have the largest pulp chambers, although usable DNA has been extracted from all types of teeth, even those with restorations. Some forensic DNA analysis texts will recommend removal of a canine. This recommendation is likely based on the fact that this is the largest single-rooted tooth – allowing easy removal with minimal compromise to the quantity of pulpal tissue available. Viewing by the relatives of the deceased should be kept in mind. It is also possible that other means of identification, such as photographic comparison, will be required if amplication of good-quality DNA from the tooth were to fail. Anterior teeth should therefore be harvested for analysis only as a last resort and first preference given to more posterior teeth.

The DNA is normally sampled by one of two methods:

- dissection of the pulp tissues from the tooth
- pulverisation of the whole tooth by cryogenic grinding.

Although the majority of the DNA is within the pulp tissue, mitochondrial and arguably nuclear DNA will reside within dentinal tubules and on the inner surface of the dentine. Cryogenically grinding of the whole tooth ensures that all possible DNA material is harvested.

DNA material is inherited half from the mother and half from the father. Mitochondrial DNA is passed on only along the maternal line while the Y-chromosome is passed on only along the paternal line. Therefore, DNA identification can not only be achieved by directly comparing the DNA from the tooth to an ante-mortem sample but also by an indirect comparison with DNA from members of the family.

As little as 20–70 pg of good-quality DNA is required for DNA identification, and even smaller amounts for mitochondrial DNA analysis since mitochondria are present in abundance in each cell. Polymerase chain reaction (PCR) allows amplification of even the smallest amounts of DNA evidence to a level adequate for profiling. A variety of kits are commercially available which will then detect and measure 13 (or 16 depending on the kit used) different lengths of DNA tracts. The areas of interest consist of short non-coding sequences on the genome which are highly repetitive and variable, termed *short tandem repeats* (STRs). A DNA profile will therefore consist of peaks corresponding to 13–16 different lengths of DNA as seen in Figure 5.17.

Because each STR is polymorphic (variable), it will be slightly different for each individual. Therefore each profile of 13–16 STRs will be different for each individual. A DNA profile is produced from reference ante-mortem samples and then compared to the DNA profile from the post-mortem sample. Matching a profile of 13–16 STRs from the deceased to the profile of 13–16 STRs in a reference ante-mortem sample establishes identity.

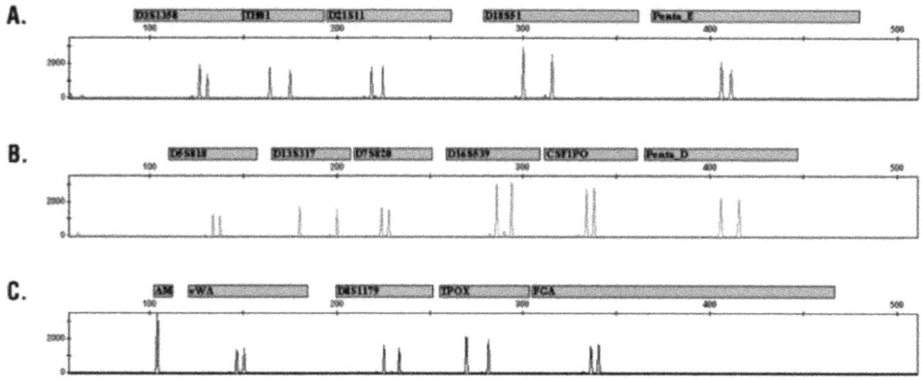

Figure 5.17 Diagram showing the 16 loci produced from standard DNA using the PowerPlex® 16 System (Promega). Adapted from the technical manual of the PowerPlex system

In highly degraded DNA it is likely that the larger lengths of STR are broken down and, despite PCR amplification, it is not possible to generate a complete DNA profile. This problem has been surmounted by targeting shorter fragments of DNA, termed *mini-STRs*. The smaller the target lengths of DNA, the higher is the chance that they will still be intact despite degradation, and therefore available for amplification.

This highly sensitive feature of DNA analysis makes the technique very susceptible to contamination. To ensure reliable results, sample collection should follow strict protocols that safeguard against scene-to-sample, person-to-sample and sample-to-sample contamination. If collecting tooth samples for DNA analysis, the forensic odontologist should contact the laboratory that will be undertaking the analysis, comparison and evaluation and take instructions on the standardised protocols and documentation expected by the laboratory.

Some common sense and basic principles will always apply:

- Wear disposable coveralls, masks and disposable gloves.
- Use single-use items whenever possible.
- Use a different extraction forceps if extracting teeth from more than one body.
- Transfer the tooth directly from body to container and seal appropriately.
- Store at minus 20°C in a sealed container.
- Label the container with the same unique reference number assigned to the deceased, the date and the name of the person who collected the sample.
- Complete relevant documentation.

In the UK, it is essential to acquire the Coroner's permission before removing any teeth for DNA analysis.

It is important to ensure that the tooth is accurately and clearly labelled in a way that it can only be linked to that one specific body. It is also important to maintain a chain of custody. If a contamination issue arises, the DNA analyst may be able to achieve a usable result by taking reference samples from those who handled the sample and subtracting their DNA profiles from that of the post-mortem sample.

Reference samples for direct comparison could be acquired from the toothbrush or hairbrush of the missing person. Reference samples from relatives for indirect comparison (or from staff to exclude contamination) will normally be in the form of a buccal scrape. It is important that the reference samples and the 'questioned' post-mortem sample be transported separately and do not come into contact with each other.

5.7 Conclusion

It has been stated that, statistically, there are over two billion possibilities in the charting of the adult dentitions, and it has been documented that even identical twins are not necessarily dentally identical (Furness, 1970; cited in Hardy, 2006, p. 178). Comparative dental identification relies on this principle and is in essence a comparison of shapes and data between post-mortem dental information and ante-mortem dental records of the missing person presumed dead.

Comparative dental identification is the cheapest, quickest and easiest means of scientific human identification, with one major limitation – the availability of ante-mortem dental records, and their accuracy and clarity.

Even when dental records are not available or no presumptive identity exists, the teeth can still provide useful information that neither of the other scientific methods of identification can. Dental profiling allows a reconstruction of a picture of who the missing person could be, which allows narrowing down to a manageable number the pool of missing persons who could be the deceased in question. Leads from the dental profiling can make it easier to acquire dental records of the missing persons if these are available, leading to an established identity by comparative dental identification.

The author believes that a better understanding of the usefulness of day-to-day dental record keeping and practices, such as routine denture marking by the general dental practice community, could help put back dental identification as the top scientific method of human identification, which in recent years has been challenged by DNA analysis.

5.8 References

American Board of Forensic Odontology Inc. (2012) *Diplomates Reference Manual*. Available at www.abfo.org/wp-content/uploads/2012/08/ABFO-Reference-Manual-August-2012-revision1.pdf (accessed: 6 December 2012).

Anđelinović S., Sutlović D., Erceg Ivkosić I., Skaro V., Ivkosić A., Paić F., Rezić B., Definis-Gojanović M. and Primorac D. (2005) Twelve-year experience in identification of skeletal remains from mass graves, *Croatian Medical Journal* **46**(4): 530–539. DOAJ Directory of Open Access Journals [Online]. Available at www.cmj.hr (accessed: 10 September 2012).

Ayton F. D., Hill C. M. and Parfitt H. N. (1985) The role in the identification of the victims of the Bradford city football ground fire, *British Dental Journal* **159**(8): 262–264.

Berketa J., James H. and Marino V. J. (2010) Survival of batch numbers within dental implants following incineration as an aid to identification, *Journal of Forensic Odontostomatology* **28**(1): 1–4. Journal of Forensic Odontostomatology Online [Online]. Available at www.iofos.eu/JFOSOnline2.html (accessed: 3 September 2012).

Berketa J., James H. and Marino V. (2011) Dental implant changes following incineration, *Forensic Science International* **207**(1–3): 50–54. ScienceDirect [Online]. Available at www.sciencedirect.com (accessed 10 September 2012).

Bernitz H. and Blignaut J. (1998) An inclusion technique for marking dentures, *Journal of Forensic Odontostomatology* **16**(1): 14–16.

Bonavilla J. D., Bush M. A., Bush P. J. and Pantera E. A. (2008) Identification of incinerated root canal filling materials after exposure to high heat incineration, *Journal of Forensic Sciences* **53**(2): 412–418. Swetswise [Online]. Available at www.swetswise.com (accessed: 10 September 2012).

Bush P. J. and Bush M. A. (2011) The next level in victim identification: materials properties as an aid in victim identification. In: Bowers C. M. (ed.), *Forensic Dental Evidence*. California: Elsevier, pp. 55–72.

Bush M. and Miller R. (2011) The crash of Colgan Air flight 3407: advanced techniques in victim identification, *Journal of the American Dental Association* **142**(12): 1352–1356. Highwire Press American Dental Association [Online]. Available at http://jada.ada.org (accessed: 10 September 2012).

Bush M. A., Bush P. J. and Miller R. G. (2006) Detection and classification of composite resins in incinerated teeth for forensic purposes, *Journal of Forensic Sciences* **52**(3): 636–642. Swetswise [Online]. Available at www.swetswise.com (accessed: 10 September 2012).

Bush M. A., Miller R. G., Prutsman-Pfeiffer J. and Bush P. J. (2007) Identification through X-ray fluorescence analysis of dental restorative resin materials: a comprehensive study of noncremated, cremated, and processed-cremated individuals, *Journal of Forensic Sciences* **52**(1): 157–165. Swetswise [Online]. Available at www.swetswise.com (accessed: 10 September 2012).

Clarke D. H. (1994) An analysis of the value of forensic odontology in ten mass disasters, *British Dental Journal* **44**: 241–250.

Clarke, Lord Justice (2001) *Public Inquiry into the Identification of Victims following Major Transport Accidents*. London: The Stationary Office.

Clarkson M. (2011) Primary dental in the military: written documentation versus the defence medical information capability programme. Unpublished MSc dissertation (part fulfilment), University of Glamorgan.

Cunningham M. and Hoad-Reddick G. (1993) Attitudes to identification of dentures: the patients' perspective, *Quintessence International* **24**(4): 267–270.

Dailey J. C. and Furue T. J. (1988) A photographic technique for the restoration of damaged radiographs, *Journal of Forensic Sciences* **33**(5): 1273–1277.

Danforth R. A., Herschaft E. E. and Leonowich J. A. (2009) Operator exposure to scatter radiation from a portable hand-held dental radiation emitting device (Aribex NOMAD) while making 915 intraoral dental radiographs, *Journal of Forensic Sciences* **54**(2): 415–421. Swetswise [Online]. Available at www.swetswise.com (accessed: 10 September 2012).

De Angelis D., Riboli F., Gibelli D., Cappella A. and Cattaneo C. (2012) Palatal rugae as an individualising marker: reliabiity for forensic odontology and personal identification, *Science and Justice* **52**(3): 181–184. ScienceDirect [Online]. Available at www.sciencedirect.com (accessed 20 August 2012).

Duray S. M., Morter H. B. and Smith F. J. (1999) Morphological variation in cervical spinous processes: potential applications in the forensic identification of race from the skeleton, *Journal of Forensic Sciences* **44**(5): 937–944.

Fairgrieve S. I. (1994) SEM analysis of incinerated teeth as an aid to positive identification, *Journal of Forensic Sciences* **39**(2): 557–565.

Fereira J. L., Fereira A. E. and Ortega A. I. (2008) Methods for the analysis of hard dental tissues exposed to high temperatures, *Forensic Science International* **178**(2–3): 119–124. ScienceDirect [Online]. Available at www.sciencedirect.com (accessed 10 September 2012).

Flint D. J., Dove S. B., Brumit P. C., White M. and Senn D. R. (2009) Computer-aided dental identification: an objective method for assessment of radiographic image similarity, *Journal of Forensic Sciences* **54**(1): 177–184. Swetswise [Online]. Available at www.swetswise.com (accessed: 16 August 2012).

General Dental Council (2005) *GDC Standards Guidance: Principles of Patient Confidentiality*. Available at http://gdc-uk.org (accessed: 25 August 2012).

General Dental Council (2011) *Standards on Commissioning and Manufacturing Dental Appliances*. Available at http://gdc-uk.org (accessed: 15 September 2012).

Glassman D. M. (2000) Methods of superimposition. In: Taylor K. T. (ed.), *Forensic Art and Illustration*. New York: CRC Press, pp. 477–498.

Gray J. E., Bailey E. D. and Ludlow J. B. (2010) Dental staff doses with handheld dental intraoral x-ray units, *Health Physics* **102**(2): 137–142.

Haines D. H. (1972) Dental identification in the Rijeka air disaster, *Forensic Science* **1**(3): 313–321.

Hardy J. H. (2006) Odontology. In: Black S. and Thompson T. (eds), *Forensic Human Identification: An Introduction*. New York: CRC Press, pp. 177–198. CRCnetBase [Online]. Available at http://crcnetbase.com (accessed: 15 September 2012).

Harvey W. (1966) Identity by teeth and the marking of dentures, *British Dental Journal* **121**(7): 334–340.

Health and Services Advisory Committee (2003) *Safe Working and the Prevention of Infection in the Mortuary and Post-mortem Room*, 2nd edn. London: HSE Books.

Heath J. R., Zoitopoulos L. and Griffiths C. (1988) Simple methods for denture identification: a clinical trial, *Journal of Oral Rehabilitation* **15**(6): 587–592.

Hinchliffe J. (2011) Forensic odontology. Part 2: Major disasters, *British Dental Journal* **210**(6): 269–274.

Interpol (2009). *Disaster Victim Identification Guide*.

İşcan M. Y. and Helmer R. P. (1993) *Forensic Analysis of the Skull: Craniofacial Analysis, Reconstruction, and Identification*. New York: Wiley-Liss.

İşcan M. Y. and Kedici P. S. (2003) Sexual variation in bucco-lingual dimensions in Turkish dentition, *Forensic Science International* **137**(2–3): 160–164. ScienceDirect [Online]. Available at www.sciencedirect.com (accessed 10 September 2012).

Jain A. K. and Chen H. (2004) Matching dental X-ray images for human identification, *Pattern Recognition* **37**(7): 1519–1532. ScienceDirect [Online]. Available at www.sciencedirect.com (accessed 20 August 2012).

Jibi P. M., Gautam K. K., Basappa N. and Raju O. S. (2011) Morphological pattern of palatal rugae in children of Davangere, *Journal of Forensic Sciences* **56**(5): 1192–1197. Swetswise [Online]. Available at www.swetswise.com (accessed: 25 August 2012).

Johanson G. and Ekman B. (1984) Denture marking, *Journal of the American Dental Association* **108**(3): 347–350. Highwire Press American Dental Association [Online]. Available at http://jada.ada.org (accessed: 10 September 2012).

Karkhanis S., Ball J. and Franklin D. (2009) Macroscopic and microscopic changes in incinerated deciduous teeth, *Journal of Forensic Odontostomatology* **27**(2): 9–19. Journal of Forensic Odontostomatology Online [Online]. Available at www.iofos.eu/JFOSOnline2.html (accessed: 3 September 2012).

Kirchhoff S., Fischer F., Lindemaier G., Herzog P., Kirchhoff C., Becker C., Bark J., Reiser M. F. and Eisenmenger W. (2008) Is post-mortem CT of the dentition adequate for correct forensic identification? Comparison of dental computed tomograpy and visual dental record, *International Journal of Legal Medicine* **122**(6): 471–479.

Ling B. C., Nambiar P., Low K. S. and Lee C. K. (2003) Copper vapour laser ID labelling on metal dentures and restorations, *Journal of Forensic Odontostomatology* **21**(1): 17–22.

Louw A. J., Grobler S. R. and van W. Kotze T. J. (2002) Degree of fluorosis in areas of South Africa with differing levels of fluoride in drinking water, *General Dentistry* **50**: 352–356.

Macaluso P. J. (2010) Sex discrimination potential of permanent maxillary molar cusp diameters, *Journal of Forensic Odontostomatology* **28**(1): 22–31. Journal of Forensic Odontostomatology Online [Online]. Available at www.iofos.eu/JFOSOnline2.html (accessed: 3 September 2012).

MacEntee M. I. and Campbell T. J. (1979) Personal identification using dental prostheses, *Prosthetic Dentistry* **41**(4): 377–380.

Madrid C., Korsvold T., Rochat A. and Abarca M. (2012) Radio-frequency identification (RFID) of dentures in long-term care facilities, *Journal of Prosthetic Dentistry* **107**(3): 199–202. ScienceDirect [Online]. Available at www.sciencedirect.com (accessed 10 September 2012).

Manica S. (2011) Guide to international dental chartings translated into English: decoding international ante-mortem dental chartings for Interpol disaster victim identification forms (F2). Unpublished MSc (part fulfilment) dissertation, University of Glamorgan.

Mauthe P. W. and Eaton K. A. (2011a) An investigation into dental digital radiography in dental practices in west Kent following the introduction of the 2006 NHS General Dental Services contract, *Primary Dental Care* **18**(2): 73–81. IngentaConnect Journals [Online]. Available at www.ingentaconnect.com (accessed: 20 August 2012).

Mauthe P.W. and Eaton K. A. (2011b) An investigation into the bitewing radiographic prescribing patterns of west Kent general dental practitioners, *Primary Dental Care* **18**(3): 107–114. IngentaConnect Journals [Online]. Available at www.ingentaconnect.com (accessed: 20 August 2012).

Merlati G., Danesino P., Savio C., Fassina G., Osculati A. and Menghini P. (2002) Observations on dental prostheses and restorations subjected to high temperatures: experimental studies to aid identification processes, *Journal of Forensic Odontostomatology* **20**(2): 17–24.

Mincer H. H. et al, (1997) In: Bower C. M. and Bell G. L. (eds), *Manual of Forensic Odontology*, 3rd edn. USA: American Society of Forensic Odontology, p. 38.

Mincer H. H., Chaudhry J., Blankenship J. A. and Turner E. W. (2008) Postmortem dental radiography, *Journal of Forensic Sciences* **53**(2): 405–407. Swetswise [Online]. Available at www.swetswise.com (accessed: 16 August 2012).

Murphy M., Drage N., Carabott R. and Adams C. (2012) Accuracy and reliability of cone beam computed tomography of the jaws for comparative forensic identification: a preliminary study, *Journal of Forensic Sciences* **57**(4): 964–968. Swetswise [Online]. Available at www.swetswise.com (accessed: 16 August 2012).

Muthusubramanian M., Limson K. S. and Julian R. (2005) Analysis of rugae in burn victims and cadavers to simulate rugae identification in cases of incineration and decomposition, *Journal of Forensic Odontostomatology* **23**(1): 26–29.

Myers S. L., Williams J. M. and Hodges J. S. (1999) Effects of extreme heat on teeth with implications for histologic processing, *Journal of Forensic Sciences* **44**(4): 805–809.

Ohtani M., Nishida N., Chiba T., Fukuda M., Miyamoto Y. and Yoshioka N. (2008) Indication and limitations of using palatal rugae for personal identification in edentulous cases, *Forensic Science International* **176**(2): 178–182. ScienceDirect [Online]. Available at www.sciencedirect.com (accessed 20 August 2012).

Olsson T., Thureson P. and Borrman H. (1993) Denture marking: a study of temperature resistance of different metal bands for ID-marking, *Journal of Forensic Odontostomatology* **11**(2): 37–44.

Parsons T. J., Huel R., Davoren J., Katzmarzyk C., Milos A., Selmanović A., Smajlović L., Coble M. D. and Rizvić A. (2007) Application of novel 'mini-amplicon' STR multiplexes to high volume casework on degraded skeletal remains, *Forensic Science International: Genetics*, **1**(2): 175–179. ScienceDirect [Online]. Available at www.sciencedirect.com (accessed 10 September 2012).

Petersen P. E. and Yamamoto T. (2005) Improving the oral health of older people: the approach of the WHO Global Oral Health Programme, *Community Dentistry and Oral Epidemiology* **33**(2): 81–92.

Pretty I. A. and Sweet D. (2001) A look at forensic dentistry. Part 1: The role of teeth in the determination of human identity, *British Dental Journal* **190**(7): 359–366.

Pretty I. A., Pretty R. J., Rothwell B. R. and Sweet D. (2003) The reliability of digitized radiographs for dental identification: a web-based study, *Journal of Forensic Sciences* **48**(6): 1325–1330.

Pye K (2004) Isotope and trace element analysis of human teeth and bones for forensic purposes. In: Pye K and Croft D. J. (eds), *Forensic Geoscience: Principles, Techniques and Applications*. London: Geological Society, pp. 215–236.

Rajan M. and Julian R. (2002) A new method of marking dentures using microchips, *Journal of Forensic Odontostomatology* **20**(1): 1–5.

Ricaut F. X., Keyser-Tracqui C., Crubézy E. and Ludes B. (2005) STR-genotyping from human medieval tooth and bone samples, *Forensic Science International* **151**(1): 31–35. ScienceDirect [Online]. Available at www.sciencedirect.com (accessed 10 September 2012).

Richmond R. and Pretty I. A. (2007) Denture marking: patient preference of various methods, *Journal of Forensic Sciences* **52**(6): 1338–1342. Swetswise [Online]. Available at www.swetswise.com (accessed 10 September 2012).

Richmond R. and Pretty I. A. (2009a) The use of radio-frequency identification tags for labeling dentures: scanning properties, *Journal of Forensic Sciences* **54**(3): 664–668. Swetswise [Online]. Available at www.swetswise.com (accessed: 10 September 2012).

Richmond R. and Pretty I. A. (2009b) A range of postmortem assault experiments conducted on a variety of denture labels used for the purpose of identification of edentulous individuals, *Journal of Forensic Sciences* **54**(2): 411–414. Swetswise [Online]. Available at www.swetswise.com (accessed: 10 September 2012).

Rötzscher K., Bedrich M. R., Jurisch R. and Peitsch P. (1999) Electronic denture marking: an aid for identification, *Journal of Forensic Odontostomatology* **7**(1): 27–29.

Santoro V., Lozito P., Mastrorocco N., DeDonno A. and Introna F. (2009) Personal identification by morphometric analyses of intra-oral radiographs of unrestored teeth, *Journal of Forensic Sciences* **54**(5): 1081–1084. Swetswise [Online]. Available at www.swetswise.com (accessed: 16 August 2012).

Santos C. and Caldas I. M. (2012) Palatal rugae pattern in a Portuguese poplation: a preliminary analysis, *Journal of Forensic Sciences* **57**(3): 86–88. Swetswise [Online]. Available at www.swetswise.com (accessed: 25 August 2012).

Savio C., Merlati G., Danesino P., Fassina G. and Menghini P. (2006) Radiographic evaluation of teeth subjected to high temperatures: experimental study to aid identification processes, *Forensic Science International* **158**(2–3): 108–116. ScienceDirect [Online]. Available at www.sciencedirect.com (accessed 10 September 2012).

Sholl S. A. and Moody G. H. (2001) Evaluation of dental radiographic identification: an experimental study, *Forensic Science International* **115**(3): 165–169.

Shukla D., Chowdhry A., Bablani D., Jain P. and Thapar R. (2011) Establishing the reliability of palatal rugae pattern in individual identification (following orthodontic treatment), *Journal of Forensic Odontostomatology* **29**(1): 20–29. Journal of Forensic Odontostomatology Online [Online]. Available at www.iofos.eu/JFOSOnline2.html (accessed: 3 September 2012).

Sidler M., Jackowski C., Dirnhofer R., Vock P. and Thali M. (2007) Use of multislice computed tomography in disaster victim identification: advantages and limitations, *Forensic Science International* **169**(2–3): 118–128. ScienceDirect [Online]. Available at www.sciencedirect.com (accessed 10 September 2012).

Sosa C., Baeta M., Núñez C., Casalod Y., Luna A. and Martínez-Jarreta B. (2012) Nuclear DNA typing from ancient teeth, *American Journal of Forensic Medical Pathology* **33**(3): 211–214.

Tabak M. (1993) Identification systems for dental prostheses using fluorescence techniques, *Revue Bel ge de Medecin Dentaire*, **48**, 77–84.

Taylor K. T. (2000) A history of forensic art. In: *Forensic Art and Illustration*. New York: CRC Press, pp. 11–43.

Thali M. J., Yen K., Schweitzer W., Vock P., Boesch Ch., Ozdoba Ch., Schroth G., Ith M., Sonnenschein M., Doerhoefer T., Scheuer E., Plattner T. and Dirnhofer R. (2003) Virtopsy, a new imaging horizon in forensic pathology: virtual autopsy by postmortem multislice computed tomography (MSCT) and magnetic resonance imaging (MRI) – a feasibility study, *Journal of Forensic Sciences* **48**(2): 386.

Turner C. G., Nichol C. R. and Richard Scott G. (1991) Scoring procedures for key morphological taits of the permanent dentition: the Arizona State University Dental Anthropology system. In: Kelley M. A. and Larsen C. S. (eds), *Advances in Dental Anthropology*. California: Wiley-Liss, pp. 13–31.

van der Meer D. T., Brumit P. C., Schrader B. A., Dove S. B. and Senn D. R. (2010) Root morphology and anatomical patterns in forensic dental identification: a comparison of computer-aided identification with traditional forensic dental identification, *Journal of Forensic Sciences* **55**(6): 1499–1503. Swetswise [Online]. Available at www.swetswise.com (accessed: 16 August 2012).

Whittaker D. K. and McDonald D. G. (1989) *A Colour Atlas of Forensic Dentistry*. Ipswich:Wolfe.

Winstanley T. D. (1996) Salvaging dark dental radiographs, *Dental Update* **23**(6): 246–249.

Zorba E., Moraitis K., Eliopoulos C. and Spiliopoilou C. (2012) Sex determination in modern Greeks using diagonal measurements of molar teeth, *Forensic Science International* **217**(1–3): 19–26. ScienceDirect [Online]. Available at www.sciencedirect.com (accessed 10 September 2012).

6

Disaster victim identification

Catherine Adams
UKDVI & Powys Teaching Health Board, UK

6.1 Introduction

A disaster is an unexpected, catastrophic event that results in the death or injury of many people. A multiple-fatality incident (MFI) is a catastrophic event that results in the death of many people. Although more correctly these events should be referred to as MFIs, for the purpose of this chapter the author will refer to them as disasters, since forensic dentists are part of an integrated multi-agency team commonly referred to as the Disaster Victim Identification Team (DVIT). Disaster victim identification (DVI) is the process that is undertaken to identify all fatalities that may be the result of a disaster.

A disaster may be due to natural causes (meteorological or geological events) or to technological or man-made causes (structural failures, transportation failures, crowd surges, fire, explosions, war and terrorism).

Disasters may be open or closed, or a combination of both. An *open disaster* is a situation where there is no immediate putative identification of the deceased, so there are likely to be delays obtaining ante-mortem data. A *closed disaster* is a situation where there is a readily available list of possible victims (e.g. a plane crash where there is a passenger list), and generally, ante-mortem comparative data are more quickly available. Combined open/closed disasters may occur when the scenario of the disaster is complicated by, for example, a plane crash into a residential area. This type of situation may also cause some difficulties with ante-mortem data collection.

If the number of fatalities in a disaster exceeds the local resources available, a temporary mortuary facility and holding area need to be established close to the scene and additional mortuary, bereavement and police personnel than are immediately available locally. Thus the response may be a regional, national or international one as required.

It is generally accepted worldwide that deceased human remains should be identified (INTERPOL, 2009). There are many reasons for this:

- providing the dignity of a name to a deceased individual
- to enable the next of kin and loved ones to commence the grieving process

Forensic Odontology: An Essential Guide, First Edition.
Edited by Catherine Adams, Romina Carabott and Sam Evans.

- to allow a funeral to go ahead
- to facilitate the process of a judicial investigation
- to permit the legal process of probate to proceed.

It is essential that all cultural, religious, political and legal issues be taken into consideration within the DVI process. The process is designed to provide the highest possible quality standards to respond to next of kin's requirement for certainty in a prompt, respectful and dignified manner (Lord Justice Clarke, 2000).

The DVI process requires that different expertise areas are integrated and work towards the common goal of identifying all victims. Police, medical and dental specialties all work together. The UK follows the Interpol DVI guidelines, which recommend cooperation with other national DVI teams when different victim nationalities are to be expected.

6.2 Disaster management

The management of any disaster follows the principle of 5 R's:

1. Rescue – immediate medical and humanitarian aid for survivors
2. Recovery – recovery of deceased bodies and body parts
3. Records – ante-mortem and post-mortem data
4. Reconciliation – comparison and matching of post-mortem (PM) with ante-mortem (AM) data
5. Repatriation – return of correctly identified bodies to next of kin for funeral.

The rescue phase of the response begins with emergency measures designed to prevent or minimise further danger. This phase includes medical aid, personal security and property security measures for victims, and personnel deployed for the disaster response operation. The priority is to protect life and prevent further serious harm to life resulting from hazards (chemical, biological, radiological, nuclear, fire, structural failure). The disaster area must be secured so that the response and investigation teams may work without disruption. Once the first medical and humanitarian response to a situation has been completed it will be followed by an investigative (e.g. accident or criminal investigation) phase, if appropriate, and then the deceased bodies will be recovered to an appropriate holding facility so that the process of post-mortem examination may commence. This holding facility is refrigerated and for ease of process should be close to the site of the temporary mortuary. The temporary mortuary itself may be distant from the site of the disaster. This has many advantages – particularly the safe securing of the site – and allows the post-mortem process to continue with minimal disruption and dignity and respect for the victims and the bereaved who may wish to view or be in the same vicinity as their loved ones.

It is important that family assistance and public relations work are integrated from the outset of any incident and that it is recognised that the various agencies, organisations and specialists involved in the response will be initiated and work simultaneously. There is a logical sequence to any DVI response, but there must be flexibility to change the sequence depending on the characteristics of a particular incident – such as terrain, facilities, geographical location, available personnel and state of the deceased bodies.

6.3 DVI planning

The key to an efficient and accurate process is the strategy planning and coordination of a response. To enable this it may be helpful to follow a planning tool, which ensures that all aspects are considered and which may be used by all DVI specialists involved in the response. Senior, experienced members of the various specialist teams are primarily involved in the strategy, coordination and planning phase of a response. The author suggests that any planning includes the following considerations (Chittick, personal communication):

Planning stage 1

1. *Time*. Time to deploy, time to do what is asked of us, time to process bodies. What freedom/constraints are there?
2. *Facilities*. What infrastructure does each speciality need? Space? Body holding?
3. *Environment*. Are there any environmental constraints, such as heat/humidity/geographical issues, that may effect each speciality?
4. *Resources*. Equipment and manpower – what is needed to initiate, sustain and conclude the task? Funding – are there any financial restraints?
5. *Logistics*. Destination, distance, demand and duration – will this impact on each speciality's ability to partake/sustain their input (e.g. specialists who work in the National Health Service)?
6. *Legal* (or religious, depending on locus/scenario). Are there any legal implications that could impact on how the specialists work (e.g. Human Tissue Act, HM Coroner or equivalent considerations)?
7. *Procedures and protocols*. How are the specialities going to conduct their business and how should they be integrated?

Completion of this stage allows discussion of the incident, and three conclusions can be reached:

- Planning guidance – this is what we are going to do; *or*
- Are there any questions to be answered? Is more information needed from other sources before planning guidance can be issued?
- Is there a strategic question to be answered? Do the identification specialities need questions answered by HM Coroner, Senior Investigating Officer (SIO) or Senior Identification Manager (SIM) that is critical to the plan (e.g. what unidentified body parts do we DNA sample)?

Planning stage 2

1. How reliant is the DVI speciality team on external agencies for deployment of equipment/personnel etc.?
2. How is the response going to be initiated and sustained?
3. How will the plan interact with that of police/SIO/SIM/other specialities?
4. Are there any chronological constraints with the plan (e.g. religious festivals)?
5. What is the plan?
6. What are the strengths and weaknesses of the proposed plan?

6.4 DVI and the dentist

Lord Justice Clarke, in his report on the post-mortem process in the Marchioness disaster in 1989 (Thames Safety Inquiry, 2000), clearly stated:

1. Families of victims must always be informed of their rights to attend or elect medical representatives to attend post-mortems. With appropriate counselling, they should be offered the opportunities to view their relative's body. The issue of visual identification must, however, be treated with caution.
2. Removal of hands for the identification of bodies should be done only when all other methods have been exhausted (especially the matching of dental records) and not as a matter of expediency. In such circumstances, mortuary technicians and pathologists must remember that a procedure which may seem standard to them is likely to be deeply distressing and offensive to relatives.
3. We would like to remind all agencies of the importance of keeping detailed and accurate records. Particular attention should be given to the correct documentation of proceedings in the mortuary.

Dental identification of human remains is recognised by INTERPOL as one of the primary methods of DVI. Noteworthy examples where dental identification proved particularly valuable include the Lockerbie air disaster (1988), the Asian tsunami (2004), the London bombings (2005), the Dhow boat disaster (2006) and the Christchurch, New Zealand, earthquake (2011).

Statistics from the Asian tsunami DVI process in Thailand in December 2005 showed the value of dental identification. By May 2005, 1474 bodies had been identified with dental identification being the primary method in 79% of the total; and by December 2001, 3750 bodies had been identified with dental identification contributing to 46.2% of the total as the primary method. This illustrates the value of dental identification as a rapid and efficient identification method where records are available. Forensic dentistry continued to contribute throughout the identification process as a secondary or supportive method where records were either inadequate or missing. Of particular value was dental ageing (Petju *et al.*, 2007).

Forensic dentistry contributes to identification by way of comparison and reconstruction methods (Pretty and Sweet, 2001). Ultimately, identification will rely on comparison between post-mortem dental examinations and ante-mortem dental records. However, when records are not initially available, such as when there is no putative name for an individual, then characteristics of the oro-dental structures may be used to indicate age, sex, medical or dental history etc. Lack of ante-mortem dental records will preclude the possibility of establishing an identification, but information such as ageing of neonatal and child remains may help provide information for fingerprints or DNA experts to establish an identity quicker than may otherwise have been possible when there are a lot of deceased. Ante-mortem records may also be difficult to interpret for a variety of reasons, but especially when they are from foreign dentists as the terminology and charting symbols may be different from what may be used in the UK. A valuable help is a database of foreign dental terminology compiled by and made available by Scheila Manica (www.internationaldentalcharts.com; see also Table 5.4 in Chapter 5).

6.5 The dental DVI team structure

The DVI Commander is a senior police officer experienced in forensic scientific investigation and the Dental Identification Manager (DIM) is directly responsible to him/her. The DIM has overall responsibility for the dental team (Figure 6.1). Each section of the process will have an experienced team leader and team members who are forensic dentists. Working alongside them will be dental team assistants who are dental care professionals (DCPs) with additional training in the DVI process and experience of working within a mortuary environment.

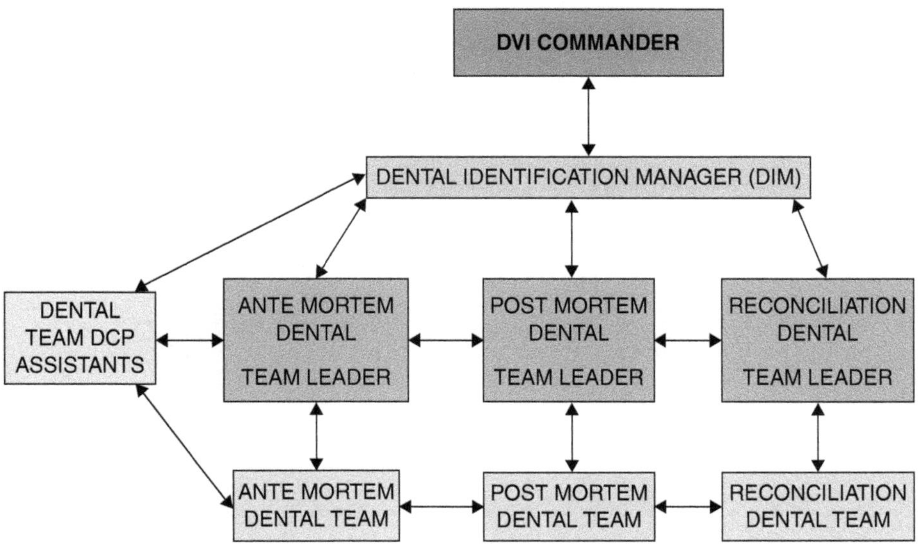

Figure 6.1 DVI odontology team structure in the UK

6.6 Documentation

The accepted international documentation related to DVI is the INTERPOL AM and PM forms, which can be downloaded from the Interpol website. By convention the ante-mortem forms are yellow and the post-mortem forms are pink (Figures 6.2 and 6.3).

There are a number of parts of these forms that refer to dental information, but the main sections for dental information input are the F1 and F2 pages in both AM and PM forms. It is important that ALL parts of these forms are filled in by the examining forensic dentist and then checked and countersigned by another forensic dentist to ensure quality assurance.

Filling in Interpol forms

In section F1, make sure that the reference number is clearly shown, and that the sex is clearly indicated (boxes at the top). Fill in all the details requested further down. Under 'Circumstances of the disappearance', give the shortest possible extract of the police report. Under 'Dental information', list any supplementary information obtained by the police from family members and/or others. Request from the police – and list – exact name, address and telephone number of the dentists/institutions from which records etc. have been obtained; also list the respective periods covered (whole years). Written records should be originals or good photostat copies. Ensure that all record x-rays,

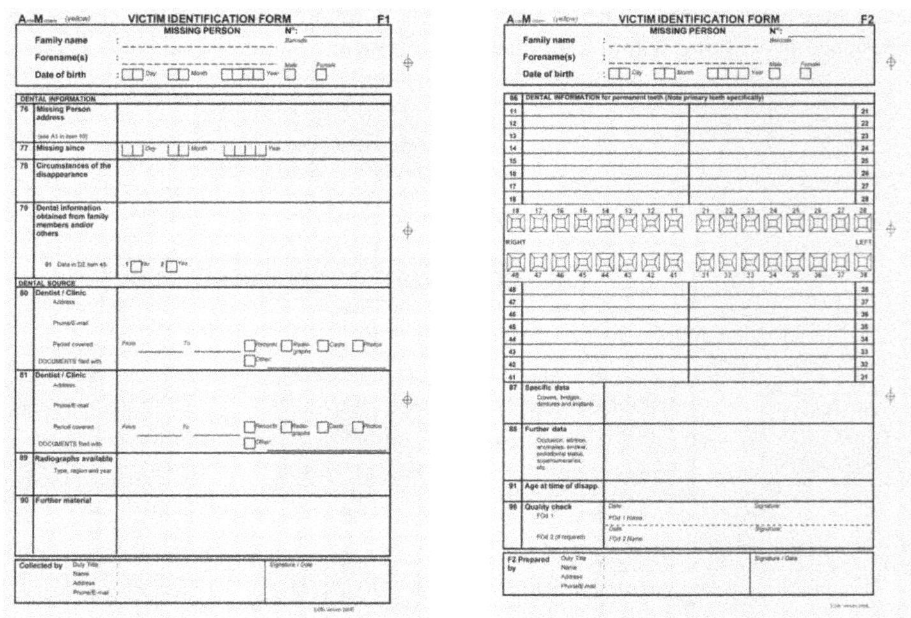

Figure 6.2 F1 and F2 ante-mortem INTERPOL forms (For colour details, please see colour plate section.)

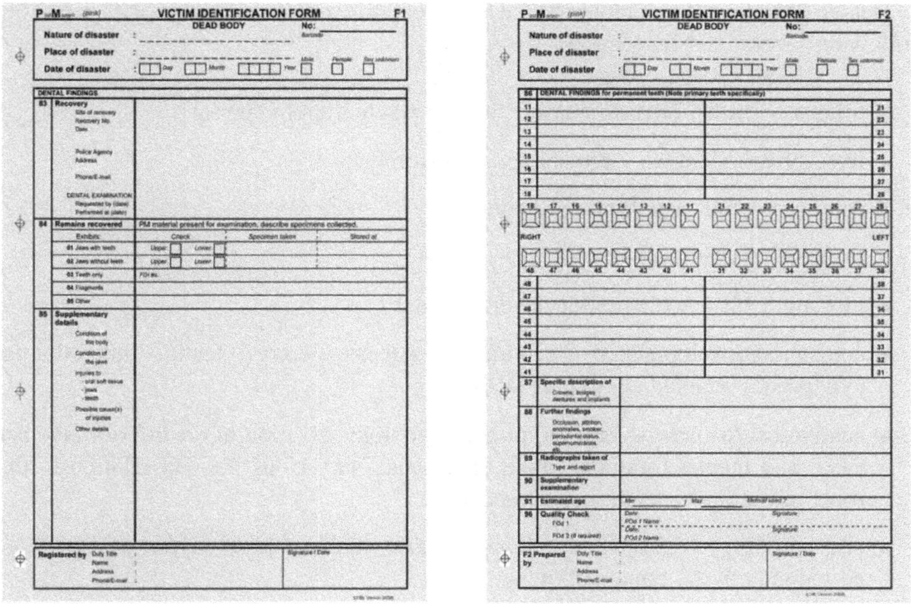

Figure 6.3 F1 and F2 post-mortem INTERPOL forms (For colour details, please see colour plate section.)

models and photographs are clearly marked with the person's name, dentist's name, and date of exposure or production; if they are not, you must do it yourself.

In section F2, the missing person's latest known dental status is to be listed. The status can only be established by extraction from, and rearrangement of, the data listed in one or more dental records – or apparent from x-rays, models, photographs or other material produced. Start with the latest entry in the written record and work your way backwards; in this way, all previous treatment now covered by later treatment can be left out. Indicate surfaces by using the capital-letter system: M = mesial, O = occlusal, D = distal, V = vestibular, L = lingual. If other abbreviations are used, explain them in one of the boxes further down. (Note: there will be a notation only for treatment/conditions actually described or seen in the material.) Next, sketch on the dental chart the location and extent of all fillings and other conditions listed as present according to your rearrangement of data. For colour distinction, use black for amalgam, red for gold, and green for tooth-coloured material. For teeth extracted or not formed, put a large cross (X) over the appropriate tooth square. If the practitioner's record includes a dental chart, compare it with your own and make sure they tally. Do not hesitate to contact the practitioner for clarification of dubious points. If x-rays and/or other material are available, indicate (in the appropriate boxes) type, year of exposure or production, and teeth concerned. Finally, record age at time of disappearance.

Once section F2 has been completed, type your name, address and telephone number (or use your professional stamp) in the box at the bottom of section F1. Finally, enter the date of completion above your personal signature. Remember – this is a legal document, so keep a full copy for your own file. Likewise, make copies of all original record material, before returning them to the practitioner.

Dental PM clinical examination and AM dental record examination will detail the following (Pretty and Sweet, 2001):

- fillings – crown or root, number, shape, position and material
- fixed prosthodontics – crowns, bridges, implants
- dentures – full or partial and material
- orthodontic appliances
- missing teeth – extracted or developmental
- congenital/developmental anomalies – supernumerary teeth, microdontia, hypoplasia, retained deciduous teeth
- anatomical features – root and pulp morphology, position of the inferior alveolar canal and mental foramen, shape of the maxillary sinus floor in relation to the roots of the upper teeth, bony trabeculae
- oral pathology – caries, periodontal disease, retained roots, cysts, periapical or periodontal cysts, bone pathology.

The F2 parts of the forms are normally completed by hand, checked and signed, and then the information may be transferred to a software package, such as Plassdata or Fimag (Rutty *et al.*, 2009). These packages are being upgraded frequently and the Plassdata package has a search facility. There are other software packages available, such as WinID (www.winid.com), but in the author's experience the Plassdata (www.plass.dk/dok/dvi/DVIBrochure.pdf) is the most widely used.

The value of dental radiographs cannot be over-emphasised (Figure 6.4). Dental fillings are now often recorded as covering whole surfaces of the tooth on digital and written records, while in the past it was commonplace for the shape of the filling

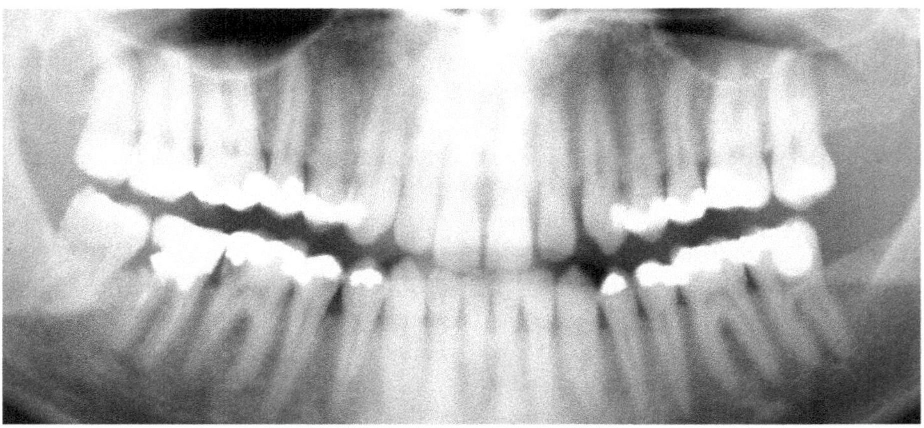

Figure 6.4 Orthopantomogram of an adult human showing the morphology of the permanent dentition, anatomical relationships, dental restorations and endodontic treatment

to be drawn on records. Not all identifying information will be seen on the crown of the tooth, such as root morphology, anatomical relationships, pathology and any iatrogenic features that are not visible to the naked eye (e.g. the shape of the floors of any fillings made by the dentist's drill, pin retainers, root fillings and implants).

Two odontologists are used in each part of the identification process to assure quality and to minimise the possibility of error.

6.7 Retrieval of dental records

AM dental records may contain handwritten and/or digital clinical information, dental and/or facial radiographs, clinical photographs and dental models, and possibly also specific information from relatives and friends. Commonly, it is the handwritten or digitally written clinical information, dental radiographs and an AM smiling photograph that are most readily available.

Features of the dentition may contribute to indentification methods depending on the quality of the AM dental records and photographs available. There are some circumstances where AM smiling photographs may be of tremendous help in comparing PM dental findings, such as discoloration, missing and malformed or misaligned anterior teeth. This information may have been recorded on the dental records, but in the author's experience this is not always the case. However, it is becoming more common, with the advent of digital software for record keeping by dentists, to take images of the dentition. There are often dental images taken if the deceased has had orthodontic treatment, for example, or other aesthetic dentistry procedures, such as crown and bridge work or tooth whitening or dental implants at a specialist practice or as a hospital referral.

Once a putative identification of a victim is obtained it is normally the Coroner's Officer, Family Liaison Officer or police officer who is tasked with obtaining the AM dental records. It is important that the professionals tasked with obtaining them have an understanding of what is required and what should not be accepted. There is a standard operating procedure (SOP) recommended by the British Association for Forensic Odontology DVI team for obtaining these records, as follows:

1. Make immediate contact with the lead odontologist to join the team that is managing and coordinating the procedure.

2. When a dental practice is visited, the Family Liaison Officer should try to speak to the dentist or at least the practice manager rather than the receptionist or nurse.

3. All *original* records should be provided regardless of date. If the records are computerised they should be printed in colour (often computerised records have a colour coding denoting the treatment done) and any x-rays or photographs copied on to CD. If the records have treatment that is colour-coded then the key of explanation should also be printed.

4. Make sure contact details for the dentist providing the records are clearly recorded and provided with the records to the odontologist.

5. Dental records are anything produced by a dental professional (dentist, dental hygienist, dental therapist) or doctor in relation to examination and/or treatment of teeth or jaws; and may be in the form of written examination records, x-rays, photographs, dental models, treatment plans, investigation results. ALL records should be collected even if they are not recent.
6. Dental treatment means anything seen by a dentist:
   - dental examination, scaling (seen by hygienist), fillings, crowns, bridges, dentures, fractured teeth, extractions, bleaching, cosmetic dentistry;
   - includes tooth extraction under a general anaesthetic in a hospital or local specialist practices providing sedation or general anaesthetic;
   - includes dental assessment for patients with medical problems or being treated for medical problems (e.g. heart disease, clotting disorders, complex illnesses, cancer etc.);
   - includes tooth straightening (orthodontics);
   - includes facial and jaw trauma (e.g. in an accident or assault so hospital records may be very helpful).
7. Ask relatives and friends whether the missing person has had any dental treatment, and whether they know who provided it.
8. Ask relatives and schools whether the missing person saw the school dentist or community dental service.
9. Ask colleagues at school, at collage, or at a workplace whether the missing person had been seen by a dentist and/or had any dental treatment.
10. Check on whether the missing person has been seen in a hospital following an accident or facial injury. X-rays may have been taken.
11. If the answer is 'yes', then the following need to be approached:
    - general dental practice (NHS and private) – check if necessary with Dental Practice Board in Eastbourne (NHS patients);
    - dental hospitals – Cardiff, Bristol, Birmingham, King's, Guy's, Royal London (London), Newcastle, Manchester, Sheffield, Liverpool, Glasgow, Edinburgh, Dundee;
    - hospital (non-dental) with dental units – oral and maxillofacial departments, orthodontic departments, restorative departments;
    - community dental services – these treat children, people with physical or mental disorders and provide emergency care;
    - employers who may provide dental care for their employees;
    - army, navy, air force;

- Dental Access units on street corners or any emergency treatment centres.
- Denplan – offices at Winchester (0800 328 3223) – will have a database of patients paying direct debits to Denplan and this should link to date of birth and who the dentist is;
- Practice Plan – similar to above (01691 677966);
- primary healthcare Trusts in each region – will have lists of dentists in the area and will manage primary dental care and emergency dental treatment.

12. It is the responsibility of the forensic odontologist alone to fill in the details in F1 and F2 forms. Resist the temptation to allow the deceased's dentist, dental nurse, practice manager, receptionist, or even yourself to fill in the details.

6.8 Post-mortem dental examination

In single dental identifications, the dental examination of the deceased should be carried out before comparison with ante-mortem dental records is undertaken. In a disaster situation this may not be possible due to delay in getting the ante-mortem records, and there may be circumstances when information from ante-mortem records indicating unusual dental features may be useful to expedite the process of reconciliation in a DVI scenario in a limited number of deceased, for example, fewer than 100 bodies.

The SOP for non-contaminated post-mortem dental examination, as recommended by the British Association for Forensic Odontology DVI team, is as follows:

- two forensic dental examiners working together – 1 clean, 1 dirty
- aim is to get all relevant information in one examination and avoid re-examination.

Dirty forensic dentist

1. Check unique post-mortem numbers on body bag and body.
2. Photograph facial structures – AP and both laterals. Retract lips for comparison with ante-mortem smiling photos. Part the lips slightly so that the incisal edges are visible as the topography may be important.
3. Examine the facial skeleton for gross abnormality prior to examining the teeth.
4. If necessary, do a facial flap to expose mandible, maxilla and associated teeth, avoiding, if possible, direct cuts into facial soft tissues – APT may be very helpful here.
5. If necessary, disarticulate the mandible but always keep with body. If jaws have to be removed for some reason then permission from the Coroner (or equivalent) *must* be sought and granted prior to removal. Jaws *must* be repatriated to the

body as soon as possible. Removal of jaws should be *avoided* unless absolutely necessary.

6. Clean the teeth with toothbrush and alcohol to remove debris.
7. If avulsed teeth are with the body, place them in correct anatomical position. Make a note of this on F2.
8. Photograph jaws and teeth – AP in and out of occlusion, both laterals in and out of occlusion, mandibular and maxillary occlusals. Photograph dentures and orthodontic appliances, in and out of the mouth. Remember to include the unique post-mortem number, time and date.
9. X-ray jaws and teeth of ALL victims. Right and left bitewings and full-mouth periapicals are mandatory for all victims.
10. Take occlusals if there is clinical or radiographic evidence of impacted canines or premolars or pathology – minimum of 2 bitewings (right and left) and periapicals.
11. Check radiographs prior to further examination.
12. Do a full dental examination of the teeth noting teeth present, missing, restorations, occlusion, orthodontic appliances, arch shape, anomalies of tooth position, congenital abnormalities, trauma and pathology.
13. If an orthodontic appliance was worn, take dental impressions in a non-distortable dental impression material. These will need to be disinfected and cast off-site. Photographs of the casts may also be taken off-site with the unique post-mortem identifying number, time and date added.
14. Extract a tooth for DNA – preferably a sound, fully developed (closed apices) second or first molar tooth. If this is not available then extract another molar or premolar tooth. *Avoid* (if possible) extracting anterior teeth and using teeth avulsed post-mortem and found in the bag with the body. If not used the teeth *must* be repatriated to the body as soon as possible.

Clean forensic dentist

1. Process radiographs – wet processing or digital.
2. Mount radiographs in correct orientation. Label with unique post-mortem identifying number, time and date. Both forensic dentists should sign as being correct.
3. Compile a composite dental chart using information from clinical examination and radiographs in consultation with the dirty forensic dentist.
4. Place the tooth extracted for DNA into an appropriate container, secure and label with the unique post-mortem identifying number, date, time and place of examination.
5. Ensure that ALL relevant dental information is entered onto F1 and F2 forms.

6. The odontogram should be filled in with accurate representation of the position, size and shape of any restorations present.
7. Both forensic dentists should check and sign F1 and F2 forms as being correct.

It is becoming more common for the odontologist to work with a forensic dental assistant who is a qualified dental care professional, commonly a dental nurse, dental hygienist or dental therapist, who is registered with the General Dental Council. The use of DCPs is relatively new in the civilian forensic dental world but has been common in the military for many years. The forensic dental team is qualified to do all their own radiography and also raise facial flaps to visualise the dental structures optimally. However, help from the pathologist or Anatomical Pathology Technician (APT) with dissection may be required, as will help from a forensic radiographer.

6.9 Ante-mortem dental records

Forensic dentists are comprehensively involved throughout the identification process. To avoid unnecessary confusion and misinformation, it is advisable that the forensic odontologist be contacted at the initial stages of any identification process where it is thought a dental ID may be possible.

Although it is preferable for the AM dental records to be contemporaneous, this is not necessarily essential, and neither is it essential that obvious dental work be present. A lot of dental fillings are tooth-coloured and quality of restorative work may make it difficult for non-dentists to identify. The presence or absence of dental restorations does not preclude a dental identification, particularly if radiographs are available for comparison.

The SOP recommended by the British Association for Forensic Odontology DVI team for AM dental record inputting is as follows:

1. Check all identifying details on records.
2. If records suggest other records may be available, contact the relevant dentist. Task the Family Liaison Officer to collect them as soon as possible.
3. Make copies of all records and radiographs.
4. Fill in available details on to F1 and F2 forms and compile composite dental records.
5. Check to assure quality with another forensic odontologist, and both sign record copies and F1 and F2 forms ensuring information is accurate and radiographs are correctly orientated.
6. Copies of records should be retained in the exhibits office, stored securely and kept in the missing person's file.
7. Original dental records must be available for dental reconciliation and legal identification (the providing dentist may request them to be returned after the legal ID process has been completed).

6.10 Dental reconciliation

The dental reconciliation process is undertaken by the odontologist and consists of comparing the information obtained in the post-mortem clinical dental examination with that contained in the original ante-mortem dental records. After legal ratification by HM Coroner (or equivalent), the deceased may be repatriated to his/her loved ones.

There is an accepted range of conclusions available to HM Coroner (or equivalent) in human identification, namely:

- *Insufficient information.* There is insufficient information to enable a comparison to be undertaken.
- *Exclusion.* The post-mortem examination and ante-mortem dental records show irreconcilable differences, such that the individual concerned cannot be that person.
- *Possible.* There are features that are comparable between the post-mortem examination and ante-mortem dental records, but either the post-mortem remains are fragmented and incomplete or the ante-mortem dental records lacking in information such that confirmation of ID cannot be established.
- *Probable.* There are no irreconcilable discrepancies between the post-mortem examination and the ante-mortem dental records, but there may only be a fragment of mandible or maxilla with a few teeth or the ante-mortem records are a few years old.
- *Established.* There is complete correlation between the post-mortem examination and ante-mortem dental records, such that identity may be confirmed.

The forensic dentist will compare all the information and determine whether there are any discrepancies. If there are, are they explainable on the grounds of expected dental deterioration if the records are old, expected treatment due to evidence of referral for specialist treatment, or human error in the records?

Young children often will not necessarily have dental records, and if they do the changes due to tooth eruption means that the dentition may change rapidly. However, as mentioned previously, tooth development is sequential and may be extremely helpful in ageing the deceased child and contributing information to other identification specialities as a secondary identifier.

Where there are no AM dental records available, facial mapping techniques may be employed by appropriately trained forensic dentists as a secondary identification method. These techniques compare facial anatomical points and teeth utilising anthropometric measurements and relative proportions or photographic superimposition of an ante-mortem smiling photograph with an equivalently positioned post-mortem facial photograph. Although these techniques have been accepted by the criminal court and used to establish identity (e.g. *R v Rosemary Pauline West* (1996) LTL C0004000), they are generally accepted as more valuable to exclude or provide a possible identification. An additional identification method may then be used to establish an ID – such as fingerprints, DNA, medical or physical information.

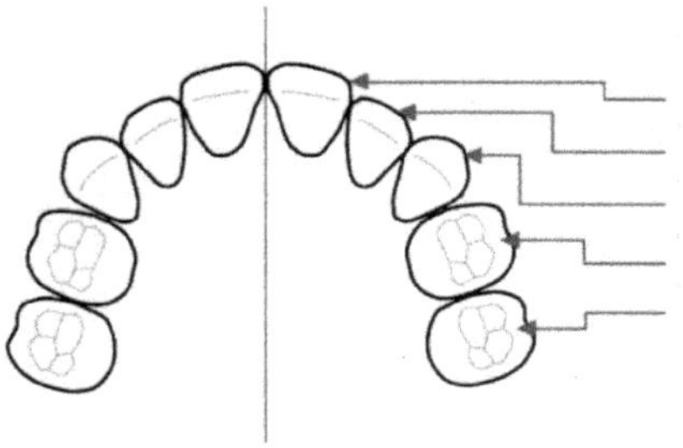

Upper Teeth	Erupt	Exfoliate
Central incisor	8-12 months	6-7 years
Lateral incisor	9-13 months	7-8 years
Canine (cuspid)	16-22 months	10-12 years
First molar	13-19 months	9-11 years
Second molar	25-33 months	10-12 years

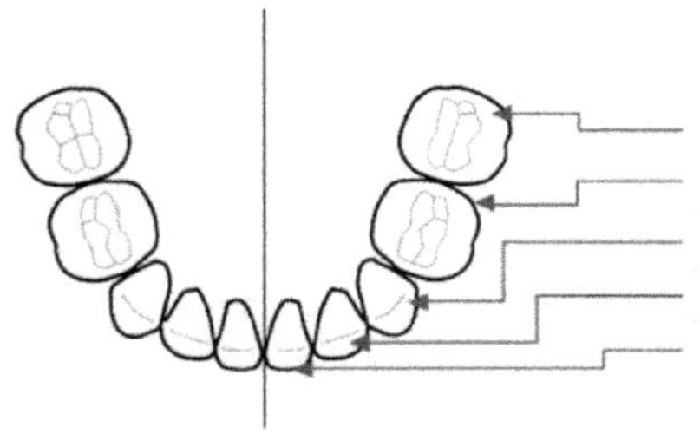

Lower Teeth	Erupt	Exfoliate
Second molar	23-31 months	10-12 years
First molar	14-18 months	9-11 years
Canine (cuspid)	17-23 months	9-12 years
Lateral incisor	10-16 months	7-8 years
Central incisor	6-10 months	6-7 years

Deciduous Mandibular Dental Arch

Figure 6.5 Sequence and timing of human deciduous tooth eruption. Courtesy of Ruth Bowen, Medical Illustrator, Cardiff University

The human dentition develops sequentially (Figures 6.5 and 6.6). The crowns of the deciduous dentition start to mineralise before birth and eruption begins at between 6 months and 3 years of age. Full root development is normally complete approximately 1 year after eruption of the crown of the tooth). At 6 years of age the deciduous dentition begins to exfoliate, beginning with the incisor teeth and then progressively around the mouth until, by the age of 12 years, all the deciduous dentition will have been lost and replaced by the succeeding permanent dentition. Finally, by the age of 18–23 years the third molars will be fully developed and, if there is room, will have erupted into the oral cavity. Complete root development of the permanent teeth normally occurs two to three years after crown eruption.

AlQahtani (2009) has produced an illustrated atlas of tooth development and eruption that may be used in conjunction with radiographs of the developing dentition (see also Figure 7.1 in Chapter 7). It is a clear and very useful aid to determining biological age of neonates and children up to the age of full dental development. Adult dental ageing past the completion of dental development is a complex matter and the variation of results considerably wider than those for younger age groups. For adult ageing the removal of a tooth for histological quantification of age-related deposition of sclerotic dentine, or amino-acid racemisation, biochemical analysis is necessary. This clearly has issues as the removed tooth tissue is often destroyed and so HM Coroner instruction is essential.

The use of imaging is particularly important as dental radiographs show at a glance the whole tooth structure. There is ongoing research investigating the possibility of

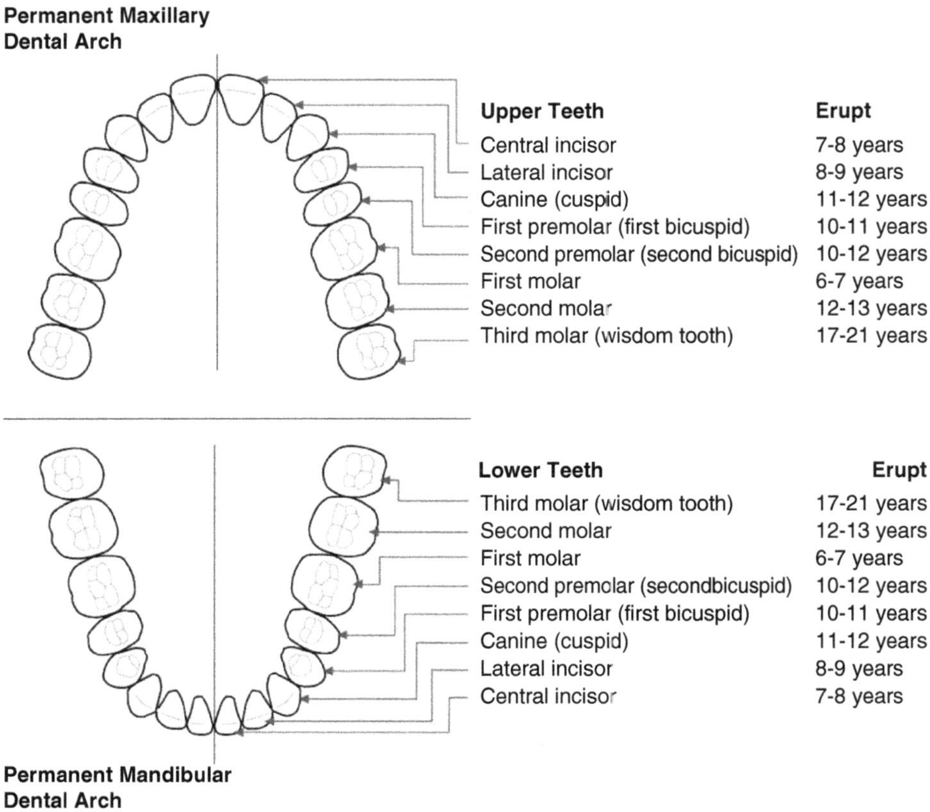

Figure 6.6 Sequence and timing of human permanent tooth eruption. Courtesy of Ruth Bowen, Medical Illustrator, Cardiff University

using multi-detector computed tomography (MDCT) scans as a virtual dental autopsy tool. It has recently been shown to be as effective as conventional dental radiographs when used for dental ageing of neonates and children (Brough *et al.*, 2012) (Figures 6.7 and 6.8). However, currently there are problems to overcome, one being the scatter effect from metal dental restorations.

In a 'chemical, biological, radiological or nuclear' (CBRN) incident, it is essential that the mortuary DVI team be protected from any hazardous materials. Remote methods of visual, x-ray and recording continues to be investigated and improved.

6.11 Equipment for the dental DVI team

The AM and reconciliation dental teams require a variety of standard office equipment including tables, chairs, computers linked to the internet and specialist servers if used, colour printers, colour photocopiers, telephone and fax communication and stationary including Interpol DVI forms, pens, coloured crayons, pencils, erasers, paper clips, staplers, notebooks, printing paper, scissors and sticky tape. The only specialist dental

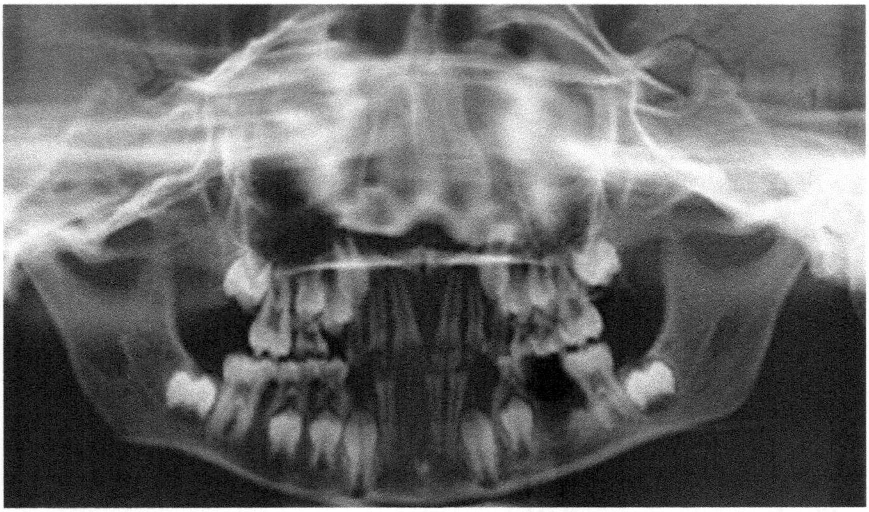

Figure 6.7 Orthopantomogram showing mixed dentition of a 6.5-year-old child. Courtesy of Alison Brough, East Midlands Forensic Pathology Unit, Leicester

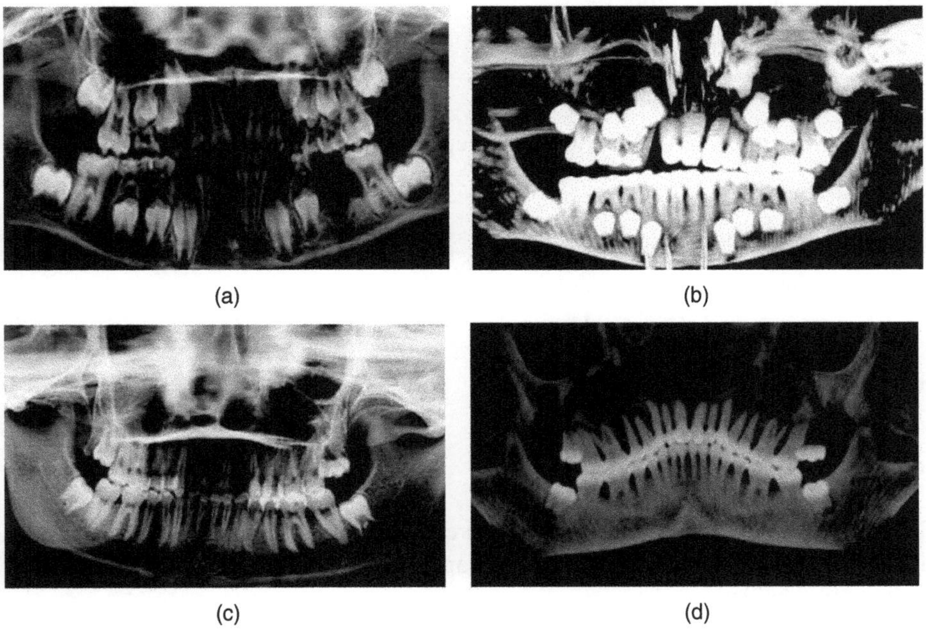

Figure 6.8 Two sets of matched orthopantomogram (OPT) and multi-detector CT (MDCT) 3-dimensional curved multi-planar reconstruction (MPR) images: (a) aged 8–10 years, traditional dental OPT; (b) aged 8–10 years, MDCT 3-dimensional curved MPR (mean intensity projection); (c) aged 18–21 years, traditional dental OPT; (d) aged 18–21 years, MDCT 3-dimensional curved MPR (maximum intensity projection). Research images courtesy of Alison Brough, East Midlands Forensic Pathology Unit, Leicester

equipment are an x-ray viewer and a scanner that allows scanning of non-digital dental radiographs.

The PM team needs equipment that enables them to start their examinations as quickly as possible. A suggested 'grab-bag' based on 20 fatalities is as follows.

General equipment for pathology grab-bag

- Tyvek suits – 20 in total – medium (4), large (12), extra large (4)
- latex-free gloves – 1 pack of each – small, medium, and large
- overshoes – 50 pairs
- face visors – 50 pack
- 10-inch wiper rolls.

Specific dental post-mortem kit

- disposable dental mirrors – 20
- disposable dental probes – 20
- spray container for water/alcohol
- disposable toothbrushes – 20
- lower premolar dental extraction forceps – 4
- self-retaining lip retractors – 10
- disposable pen torches – 20
- dental photographic mirrors – 10
- mouth prop
- mouth gag.

Dental x-ray equipment

Nomad plus sensors and associated software – need both Nomad and rucksack holding other associated equipment. Such as laptop, software, digital sensors and dental radiography holders.

Dental imaging equipment

This may be a simple digital camera that can download images on to the available software as the images will be used for record purposes rather than analysis. If images are required for more advanced purposes (e.g. facial mapping), then specialist equipment and expertise should be sought.

6.12 Maintaining dental team morale

It is extremely important for the dental team to consider the wellbeing of themselves and others in what is going to be a stressful situation. Everyone is responsible for everyone else and there must be an atmosphere of support for one another. The Trauma Risk Management (TRiM) system is a peer support system (Creamer *et al.*, 2012) and aims to identify those who are not coping after potentially traumatising events and ensure they are signposted to professional sources of help. It is used by the police, the military and the Foreign and Commonwealth Office. TRiM practitioners are trained to spot the psychological risk factors that might otherwise go unnoticed in those who are suffering deployment stress, including post-traumatic stress disorder (PTSD). In the author's view it is preferable that there should be members of the team who are TRiM aware and preferably trained as practitioners.

6.13 References

AlQahtani S. J. (2009) *Atlas of Tooth Development and Eruption.* Available at www.atlas.dentistry.qmul.ac.uk (accessed 16 June 2013).

Brough A.L., Rutty G. N., Morgan B., Black S. and Adams C. (2012) 'Anthropological measurement of the juvenile mandible and dental age assessment using multi-detector computed tomography'. Presented at the American Academy of Forensic Sciences, Annual Meeting.

Creamer M. C., Varker T., Bisson J., Darte K., Greenberg N., Lau W., Moreton G., O'Donnell M., Richardson D., Ruzek J., Watson P. and Forbes D. (2012) Guidelines for peer support in high-risk organizations: an international consensus study using the Delphi method, *Journal of Traumatic Stress* **25**: 134–141.

INTERPOL (2009). http://www.interpol.int/INTERPOL-expertise/Forensics/DVI.

Lord Justice Clarke (2000) *Thames Safety Inquiry: Final Report.* January.

Petju M., Suteerayongpraert A., Thongpud R. and Hassiri K. (2007) Importance of dental records for victim identification following the Indian Ocean tsunami disaster in Thailand, *Public Health* **121**(4): 251–257.

Pretty I. A. (2007) Forensic dentistry. 1. Identification of human remains, *Dental Update* **334**(10): 621–622, 624–626, 629–630 passim.

Pretty I. A. and Sweet D. (2001) A look at forensic dentistry. Part1: The role of teeth in the determination of human identity, *British Dental Journal* **190**(7): 359–366 (review).

Rutty G.N., Robinson C., Morgan B., Black S., Adams C. and Webster P. (2009) Fimag: the United Kingdom disaster victim identification imaging system, *Journal of Forensic Sciences* **54**(6): 1438–1442.

7

Dental age assessment

Sakher AlQahtani
King Saud University, Riyadh, Saudi Arabia

7.1 The importance of knowing age

Knowing your age is a basic human right and having it documented is what gives identity to the individual (Unicef, 1989). In the society we live in, one's date of birth is the epitome of one's entity. It is required to enter school, work, get married and get a pension. It also plays a role in unfortunate events pertaining to justice and dealing with offenders rightfully according to their age, and protecting them and the people around them by knowing their appropriate age group. In other words it drives the journey of life from birth to death.

With the importance of knowing one's true age highlighted in every aspect of any society, it is shocking that 30–50% of the 50 million births each year are still unrecorded (Unicef, 2012), violating those babies' human rights and setting up a rocky road for their future life. Moreover, with the increase in armed conflicts around the world, especially in the last two decades up to the recent Arab Spring, more and more people flee their homeland without their documents because they fear for their lives. Their documents are lost or stolen, or are destroyed to avoid the owner being identified. This problem became clear to the developed countries with the surge of asylum seekers who had no documents during the war in Bosnia in the early 1990s. This movement of immigrants seeking shelter in developed countries is on the increase, with people fleeing famine in eastern Africa, ethnic cleansing in middle and western Africa, genocides in the Middle East, and oppressive regimes in the Near and Far East. In 2010, there were 214 million international migrants worldwide, with Europe being their main destination (United Nations, 2011).

The need to know the ages of unidentified asylum seekers, to make sure they are who they claim to be, is not only for the benefit of the hosting country. It is also to protect them from sexual abuse, being taken advantage of, and getting appropriate support. Developed countries also sometimes need to age their own citizens who were not recorded at birth, had their documents stolen or who have been kidnapped at some point. So an easy-to-apply method for age estimation is vital to minimise the time needed for processing cases and training personnel.

Forensic Odontology: An Essential Guide, First Edition.
Edited by Catherine Adams, Romina Carabott and Sam Evans.

Social services that deal with asylum seekers favour the use of social parameters along with physical developmental charts. One problem, however, is that social parameters have never been systematically evaluated, and physical development is affected by the environment. Dental development has been extensively researched and evaluated, but many social workers lobby against taking radiographs, even of the dentition, because of the risks associated with x-ray exposure. They quote advice from the Royal College of Paediatrics and Child Health (RCPCH) that a hand/wrist radiograph to confirm an alleged chronological age is unjustified, because ionising radiation should be used only in cases of clinical need (Levenson and Sharma, 1999). However, Australia, Canada, the UK, the United States and New Zealand all request a chest radiograph as part of their visa application for individuals older than 11 years (IOM, 2012) if they apply through the proper channels, and the risk of radiation exposure when taking a dental radiograph is almost negligible compared to the amount of exposure from a chest radiograph.

Wanting to know the correct age of a person goes beyond the living to the dead. In the past 100 years the world has experienced an upsurge in mass disasters, both natural and man-made. Mass graves from the twentieth century are still being discovered in Bosnia and Africa; new mass graves are being created in the Middle East. Identifying victims of mass murders not only brings closure to relatives but also helps to incriminate people responsible for those atrocities. With the huge numbers in victims of mass murders, which could be thousands in one grave, the need for a simple method of age estimation is crucial because of limited resources and the usual use of volunteers.

7.2 The chronological age

Age is determined by the date of birth and the period of time or number of years elapsed after that to any point of time, which is then called the *chronological age* (Krogman, 1968; Kraemer *et al.*, 1985). It is documented ideally in a birth certificate, hospital records, governmental databases and many more; but in the absence of these documents, other ways to establish age are important.

The age of criminal responsibility can be as young as 7 years (in Switzerland and South Africa) to as old as 18 years (in Belgium and the United States). Currently, the age of criminal responsibility in Scotland is 12 years. In England, Wales and Northern Ireland it is 10 years, and 10- to 12-year-olds can be convicted but not imprisoned, 12- to 15-year-olds can be convicted and incarcerated in special units, 16 years is a milestone for sexual consent and assault, 15- to 17-year-olds will be juvenile offenders, 18- to 21-year-olds will be young offenders, and 21- to 25-year-olds will be young adult offenders (Janes, 2008). Therefore, knowing the right age in the absence of documents can be life-changing for a young person. No finalised government guidelines and/or protocol are in place so far, and no country has got it right.

Age assessment is done when there is a serious doubt. It is a last resort, keeping the best interest of the child as the main priority and giving the benefit of the doubt. Although the law is biased towards a social services assessment using Merton Age Compliance Guidelines published in 2003 (Crawley, 2012), which includes assessing physical appearance, the interaction of the individual during the assessment process, social history, family composition, how the individual responds to authority/instruction, education, independence/self-care skills, health, medical assessment and information from documentation and other sources.

Chronological age can be estimated by determining physiological age, which is the age at which a developing system or organ reaches a specific stage (Braga *et al.*, 2005). Knowledge is needed of the developmental stages of that system or organ, and the time needed for each stage to be achieved, along with population norms or standards. Not all systems or organs can be used for age estimation.

A set of criteria should exist for an system or organ to be an ideal age indicator:

- It has to develop over a long period of time.
- It has to have recognisable and/or measurable stages that can be assessed in the living as well as the dead.
- The stages have to happen over a short period of time.
- It has to be stable, not be affected by environmental or racial factors.
- It has to survive inhumation well.

Many systems and organs have been used to estimate chronological age – starting from the most obvious and least complex (height, weight, secondary sex characteristics), to the less obvious and more complex (molecular methods using biomarkers), and passing through methods of moderate complexity (bone and dental development). What attracted scientists to these is the ability to recognise changes that happen to all people at more or less the same age. These observations led to countless studies in a quest to find the ideal system that will enable the determination of chronological age.

7.3 The dental age

Early records that date back to the first half of the nineteenth century by factories who employed children, and by legal bodies in the UK to impose legal responsibility on children older than 7 years, showed that dental development was used as an age indicator (Saunders, 1837).

The human dentition develops over nearly a third of the average human life, with easily detected and predictable stages. Teeth also survive inhumation very well because of their minimal organic content, which is only 4% in dental enamel. They are very stable and minimally affected by environmental factors, socioeconomic status, nutrition, dietary habits and even by endocrine factors (Garn *et al.*, 1965a,b; Voors, 1973; Demirjian *et al.*, 1985; Krogman and Işcan, 1986; Hillson, 1996; Gutiérrez-Salazara and Reyes-Gasgaa, 2003; Aka *et al.*, 2009).

Ethnic differences do not play a role in tooth development, as research has shown that there are no statistically significant differences between races, and the differences present are merely biological ones (McKenna *et al.*, 2002; Olze *et al.*, 2004; Schmeling *et al.*, 2004; Sisman *et al.*, 2007; Martin-de las Heras *et al.*, 2008; TeMoananui *et al.*, 2008; Ren *et al.*, 2009; Liversidge and Marsden, 2010). The presence of these biological differences necessitates knowing the full range of variations; for a full list refer to AlQahtani *et al.* (2010).

These qualities make the developing dentition the best age indicator compared with other systems. Extensive research has been done on tooth development to provide simple and accurate ways of assessing the physiological dental age.

7.4 Dentition as an age indicator

7.4.1 Dental development

Humans have two sets of teeth: 20 deciduous teeth (four incisors, one canine and four molars in each jaw) and 32 permanent teeth (four incisors, one canine, two premolars and six molars in each jaw).

Dental development can be divided into two main phases: tooth formation and tooth eruption. Tooth formation is the laying down and mineralisation of dental tissues (enamel, dentine and cementum), whereas eruption is the dynamic continuous movement of the developing tooth in an axial direction from the depth to the edge of the alveolar bone, and further to the occlusal level (Demirjian, 1986; Kardos, 1996; Wise *et al.*, 2002; Craddock and Youngson, 2004). Tooth emergence, which is a part of tooth eruption, is the clinical appearance of the cusps of a tooth through the gums.

7.4.2 Dental age assessment

Dental age assessment can be done in an invasive or non-invasive way.

Non-invasive methods

1. *Sequential tooth eruption and/or emergence* (Demirjian, 1973; Carvalho *et al.*, 1989; Nyström *et al.*, 2001; Foti *et al.*, 2003; Moslemi, 2004; Franchi *et al.*, 2008; Olze *et al.*, 2008; Aggarwal 2011; Feraru *et al.*, 2011).
2. *Development by means of calcification and/or root maturation*:
   - developmental schemas (Schour and Massler, 1941; Gustafson and Koch, 1974; Ubelaker, 1978; Kahl and Schwarze, 1988a; AlQahtani *et al.*, 2010);
   - dental developmental stages (Kronfeld, 1935; Gleiser and Hunt, 1955; Garn *et al.*, 1958; Garn *et al.*, 1959; Nolla, 1960; Moorrees *et al.*, 1963b; Haataja, 1965; Nanda and Chawla, 1966; Wolanski, 1966; Fass, 1969; Haavikko, 1970, 1974; Fanning and Brown, 1971; Liliequist and Lundberg, 1971; Demirjian *et al.*, 1973; Anderson *et al.*, 1976; Demirjian and Goldstein, 1976; Nyström *et al.*, 1977; Van der Linden *et al.*, 1985a,b,c,d; Nyström *et al.*, 1986; Carels *et al.*, 1991; Smith, 1991; Mincer *et al.*, 1993; Köhler *et al.*, 1994; Mörnstad *et al.*, 1994; Mesotten *et al.*, 2002);
   - root developmental stages (Harris and Nortjé, 1984; Kullman *et al.*, 1992; Gunst *et al.*, 2003; Rai *et al.*, 2008).

3. *Morphological tooth parameters* (Gustafson, 1950; Dalitz, 1962; Johanson, 1971; Moore and Corbett, 1971, 1973; Miles, 1978; Brothwell, 1981; Lovejoy, 1985; Solheim, 1993; Kvaal and Solheim, 1994; Constandse-Westermann, 1997).
4. *Tooth measurements* (Stack, 1960, 1967; Liversidge *et al.*, 1993; Kullman *et al.*, 1995; Kvaal *et al.*, 1995; Liversidge and Molleson, 1999a,b; Aka *et al.*, 2009).

Invasive methods

1. *Biomarkers* (Wehner *et al.*, 2007; Alkass *et al.*, 2009; Griffin *et al.*, 2009).
2. *Root dentine translucency* (Dalitz, 1962; Bang and Ramm, 1970; Solheim, 1993; Prince and Konigsberg, 2008).
3. *Incremental lines* (Solheim, 1990, 1993; FitzGerald, 1998; Jankauskas *et al.*, 2001; Bojarun *et al.*, 2003; Smith and Avishai, 2005; Czermak *et al.*, 2006; Aggarwal *et al.*, 2008; Antoine *et al.*, 2009).

One of the easiest and comprehensive tooth formation stages used is the one adopted by (AlQahtani *et al.*, 2010) that has written description added to the 13 formation stages from cusp initiation to full root maturation; deciduous teeth have an extra three resorption stages (Tables 7.1–7.3). Eruption through the alveolar bone is a good reference point, which makes it more favourable than gingival emergence; and allowance should be made for clinical gingival emergence when using alveolar eruption in the presence of oral soft tissues (AlQahtani *et al.*, 2010) (Table 7.4).

7.4.3 Techniques using dental development

Several techniques have been developed to utilise dental development to estimate chronological age, from charts of tooth formation and eruption to mathematical formulae that calculate dental age. Many studies testing each and every method have also been done in the quest to find the method with the best performance measures. What performs well in one population doesn't appear to perform well in another; what is simple to one scientist is complicated to another. Methods have been modified, re-modified, tested and re-tested. Diagrams have been redrawn and adopted, yet there are still problems associated with most of these methods. Lack of evidence behind the technique is the most profound problem (Smith, 1991; Braga *et al.*, 2005), even with the most widely used techniques. The lack of documented details of the studied sample (Fass, 1969), the restriction to a small age range (Gustafson and Koch, 1974), an insufficient sample size, or the absence of samples all together are just examples (Schour and Massler, 1941). Some of these methods were even based on estimates (Ubelaker, 1978).

7.4.4 Accuracy of dental age estimation techniques

The accuracy of dental age estimation is defined by how closely the difference between real age and estimated age is to zero and how closely that can be predicted and reproduced (Cardoso, 2007a; Butti *et al.*, 2008; Cameriere *et al.*, 2008b).

Table 7.1 Description of modified Moorrees' stages used to identify tooth developmental stages of single-rooted teeth (Moorrees *et al.*, 1963a,b). PDL, periodontal ligament space

	Ci: initial cusp formation	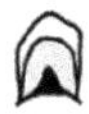	**Ri**: initial root formation with diverging edges
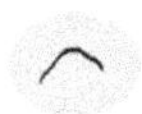	**Cco**: coalescence of cusps	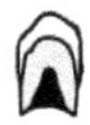	**R 1/4**: root length less than crown length
	**Coc**: cusp outline complete	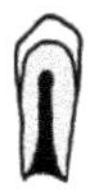	**R 1/2**: root length equals crown length
	**Cr 1/2**: crown half completed with dentine formation	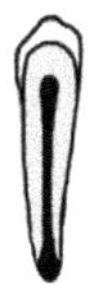	**R 3/4**: three-quarters of root length developed with diverging ends
	**Cr 3/4**: crown three-quarters completed	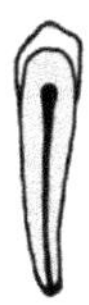	**Rc**: root length completed with parallel ends
	**Crc**: crown completed with defined pulp roof	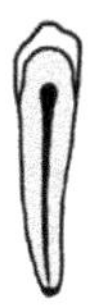	**A 1/2**: apex closed (root ends converge) with wide PDL
		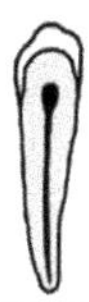	**Ac**: apex closed with normal PDL width

Table 7.2 Description of modified Moorrees' stages used to identify tooth developmental stages of multi-rooted teeth (Moorrees *et al.*, 1963a,b). PDL, periodontal ligament space

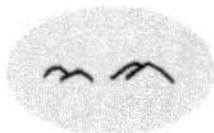	**Ci**: initial cusp formation		
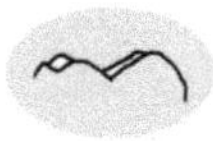	**Cco**: coalescence of cusps	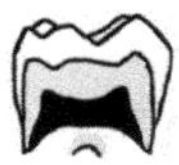	**R 1/4**: root length less than crown length with visible bifurcation area
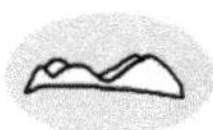	**Coc**: cusp outline complete	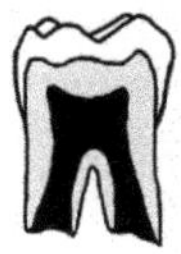	**R 1/2**: root length equals crown length
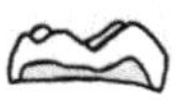	**Cr 1/2**: crown half completed with dentine formation	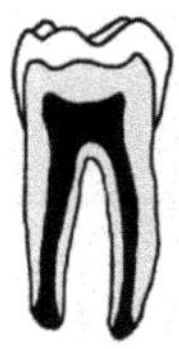	**R 3/4**: three-quarters of root length developed with diverging ends
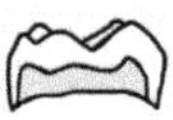	**Cr 3/4**: crown three-quarters completed	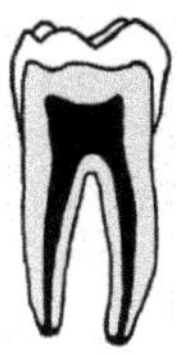	**Rc**: root length completed with parallel ends
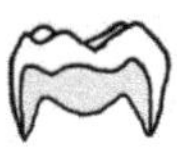	**Crc**: crown completed with defined pulp roof	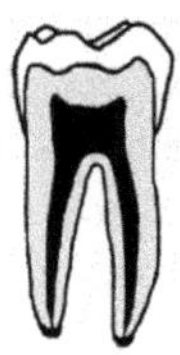	**A 1/2**: apex closed (root ends converge) with wide PDL
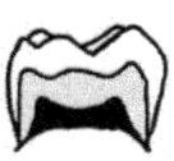	**Ri**: initial root formation with diverging edges	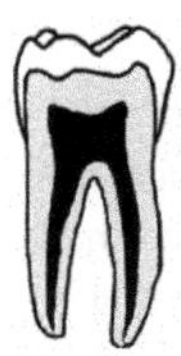	**Ac**: apex closed with normal PDL width

Table 7.3 Description of modified Moorrees' stages used to identify root resorption in single- and multi-rooted teeth (Moorrees *et al*., 1963b)

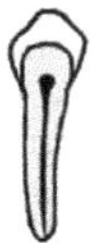	**Ac**: apex closed with normal PDL width	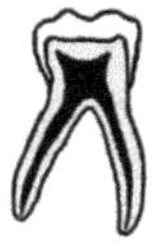
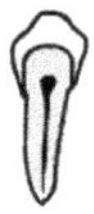	**Res 1/4**: resorption of apical quarter of the root	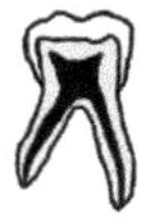
	**Res 1/2**: resorption of half the root	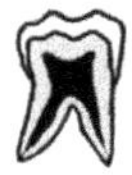
	**Res 3/4**: resorption of three-quarters of the root	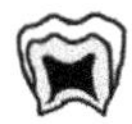

Table 7.4 Description of modified Bengston's stages used to identify tooth eruption (Bengston, 1935)

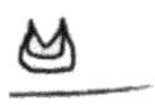	**Position 1**: when the occlusal or incisal surface is covered entirely by bone	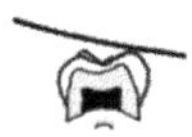
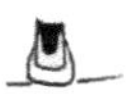	**Position 2**: when the occlusal or incisal surface breaks through the crest of the alveolar bone	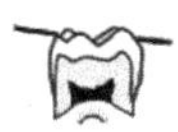
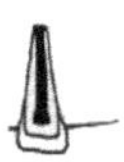	**Position 3**: when the occlusal or incisal surface is midway between the alveolar bone and the occlusal plane	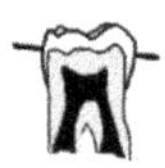
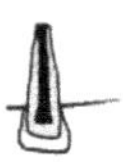	**Position 4**: when the occlusal or incisal surface is in the occlusal plane	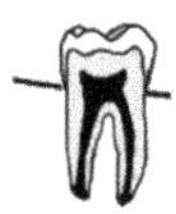

Many studies have tested the accuracy of different age estimation methods based on dental development, with varying results. In general the methods are more accurate in children because of the number of developing teeth; as the number of developing teeth decreases, so does the accuracy (Hägg and Matsson, 1985; Hägg and Hägg, 1986; Staaf *et al.*, 1991; Thorson and Hägg, 1991; Saunders *et al.*, 1993; Davis and Hagg, 1994; Liversidge, 1994; Kullman, 1995; Willems, 2001; Solari and Abramovitch, 2002; Liversidge *et al.*, 2003; Chaillet and Demirjian, 2004; Chaillet *et al.*, 2004a,b; Smith, 2005; Brkic *et al.*, 2006; Cameriere *et al.*, 2006; Maber *et al.*, 2006b; Smith *et al.*, 2006; Bhat and Kamath, 2007; Cardoso, 2007a,b; Halcrow *et al.*, 2007; Tao *et al.*, 2007; Cardoso, 2009; Griffin *et al.*, 2009; Shi *et al.*, 2009; Cruz-Landeira *et al.*, 2010).

The common drawbacks of the earlier methods are the lack of uniform age distribution and/or the limited age range that fails to cover the entire developing dentition. A uniform age distribution with similar numbers for each year of age improves variance across the age range (Bocquet-Appel and Masset, 1982; Konigsberg and Frankenberg, 2002); whereas a normal age distribution has high precision around the mean value but low precision at the age extremes.

7.4.5 Schemas of dental development

There are several methods of age estimation based on dental age, but most of them are based on formulae and lengthy techniques only a specialist can deliver (Demirjian *et al.*, 1973; Roberts *et al.*, 2008), sometimes using special equipment (Bauer, 2007; Heinrich *et al.*, 2007). In mass disaster situations, the need for an accurate, reliable, cheap, fast and easy-to-use method is imperative for the victim identification process, especially when the lack of personnel or resources dictates the help of untrained volunteers. In these cases, using a comparison method in the form of a diagram or computer software with the radiograph of developing teeth that would give an estimate of chronological age would be ideal.

Various schemas have been compiled throughout the last century to show dental development. One of the first schemas to be used widely is Schour and Massler's *Atlas* (1941) and it has been the benchmark for the past 70 years. Gustafson and Koch (1974) used data from 20 sources combining anatomical, radiographic and gingival eruption to construct a schematic representation of tooth formation and eruption from prenatal to the age of 16 years. It illustrates the range of tooth development and the peak age for each stage. Ubelaker's chart (1978) was loosely based on Schour and Massler's *Atlas* using additional North American Indian population data. Brown *et al.* (1985) demonstrated permanent tooth development using anatomical tooth illustrations tabulated for the ages 3 to 12 years based on Schour and Massler's *Atlas*. Kahl and Schwarze (1988b) updated the *Atlas* using 993 radiographs of children aged 5 to 24 years and produced anatomical charts for the sexes.

All the past schemas cover a limited age range, except for Schour and Massler's and Ubelaker's schemas that cover dental development from prenatal to early adulthood, which made them the most wildly used ones. The limitations of these schemas, however, are the lack of clarity in identifying crown and root developmental stages, as almost all of these schemas were based on dental radiographical description of tooth development directly or indirectly, yet they presented anatomical drawings, concealing the internal tooth developmental stages.

When assessing tooth development from dental radiographs, one can distinguish between consecutive developmental stages more easily using internal hard tissues, such as the shape of the pulp chamber or root canal, improving sensitivity and performance measures (Moorrees *et al.*, 1963a,b; Demirjian, 1973; Haavikko, 1974), yet no schematic method delivers that. All the previously mentioned schemas used anatomical representations of teeth that mask internal tooth structures and with no information regarding eruption reference, with the exception of Ubelaker (1978), who used gingival emergence as a reference.

Publication of the 'London atlas' (AlQahtani *et al.*, 2010) (Figure 7.1) brought a new comprehensive evidence-based method of dental age estimation to forensics. It is based on tooth development covering all ages between 28 weeks *in utero* to 23 years. Each age group in this represents the median stages of tooth development from 24 individuals. It has been used in many workshops, incorporated into several universities' curricula around the world and adopted by several forensic societies. It is available as a free download from the website of the Institute of Dentistry at Queen Mary, University of London (www.atlas.dentistry.qmul.ac.uk) in 17 languages – Arabic, traditional Chinese, simplified Chinese, Croatian, Dutch, English, Farsi, French, German, Greek, Hindi, Japanese, Malay, Portuguese, Russian, Spanish and Urdu.

7.5 Age estimation methods in children and young adults

7.5.1 Essentials

Choosing the right age assessment method relies heavily on the individual in question, according to the presence or absence of teeth in the oral cavity, and whether the subject is alive. With living children, the guidelines for dealing with cases of age dispute according to the United Nations Convention on the Rights of the Child (UNCRC) and the United Kingdom Border Agency (UKBA) are as follows:

- There should be no discrimination based on race, colour, sex, language, religion, political or other opinion, national, ethnic or social origin, property, disability, birth or other status.
- Consider the best interests of the child in all actions, whether undertaken by public or private social welfare institutions, courts of law, administrative authorities or legislative bodies.
- Ensure that the child has protection and care as is necessary for his/her wellbeing, taking into account the rights and duties of the parents, legal guardians, or other individuals legally responsible for him/her. To this end, take all appropriate legislative and administrative measures.
- Every child matters, even if he/she is someone subject to immigration control.

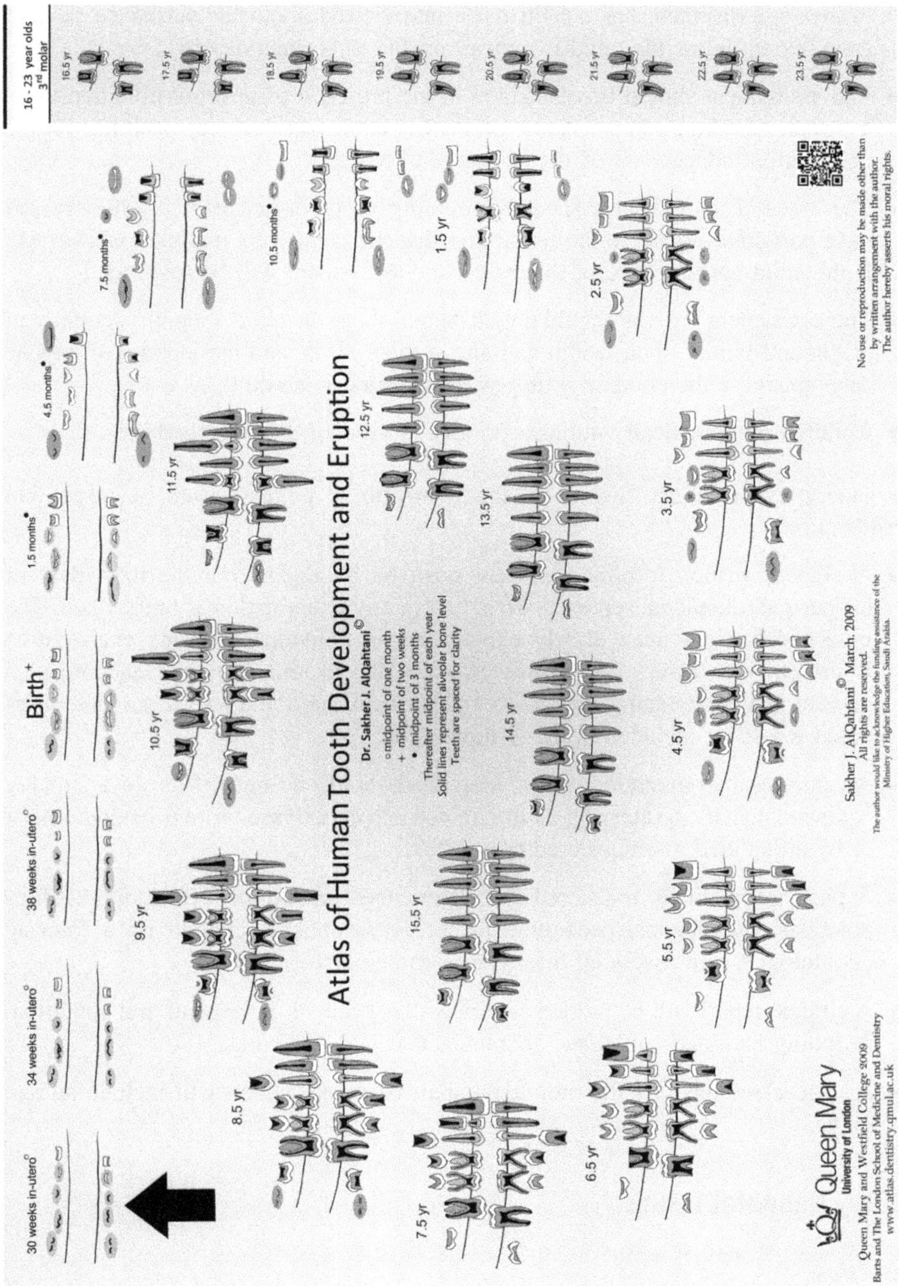

Figure 7.1 Human tooth development and eruption. © 2009: all rights reserved (For colour details, please see colour plate section.)

- Children should have their cases dealt with in a way that minimises the uncertainty that they may experience.
- An accompanied or unaccompanied child (over the age of 12 years), who has his/her age disputed, has a right to be interviewed about the substance of their assessment, unless the child is unfit or unable to be interviewed.
- The assessment should be conducted in the presence of a responsible adult (i.e. a parent, guardian, representative or another adult who has responsibility for the child but is independent of the Secretary of State).
- The assessor should have specialist training in age assessment of children and have particular regard to the possibility that the child feels inhibited or alarmed. If the child appears tired or distressed, the assessment will be suspended.
- The assessment process should obtain details about the child's identity, country of origin and family, their health and any special needs, and the identity of anyone accompanying the child or acting as their responsible adult.
- Children must be dealt with as a priority in view of their vulnerability.

For general cases of age dispute in the living, these points should be taken into consideration:

- A signed, written informed consent must be obtained from the individual or his/her guardian/legal representative, before any examination is undertaken. The informed consent must clearly explain to the individual that the examination is primarily to assess age. However, since the examination will encompass a general health screening, any abnormal medical, hard and soft tissue pathology noted would be included in the written report.
- An intra-oral examination of the individual should be undertaken in a suitably equipped dental operatory by a fully trained and experienced forensic odontologist or by a qualified and registered radiologist.
- A panel of qualified, registered and experienced practitioners (including anthropologists, radiologists, paediatricians, or orthodontists), chaired by a forensic odontologist, will assess all information gathered.
- A clinical report will be written covering all aspects of the general oral condition, including hard and soft tissue anomalies that may be found.
- An age assessment of the individual shall be given, which will include an age range.

7.5.2 Neonatal issues

Cusp tips

Histological tooth development starts from the 6th week *in utero*. Mineralisation that allows teeth to be visible on a radiograph will not happen until the second trimester, in the form of cusp tips of the deciduous teeth at around 12 weeks after histological tooth development. These cusp tips are very small and are held in their crypt by soft tissues. The challenge in dealing with neonates in this age group is to preserve and find these cusp tips and incisal edges that could be easily misplaced or lost after soft tissue decomposition.

The loss of the supporting soft tissues within the crypt and the porosity of the jaw bone at this age can lead to these cusp tips falling off and being misplaced in the surrounding soil if the neonate was buried, or within the cloth or garment if the neonate was wrapped. Therefore, it is important that the forensic odontologist examines the body of the neonate before it is moved from its place to locate the cusp tips and incisal edges necessary for age estimation.

In crime scenes, usually the forensic pathologist starts the body examination, but the only one who knows what to look for and where in regard to teeth is the forensic odontologist. If a body of a neonate is found, the area around it should be secured and the body covered from weather elements and a forensic odontologist called to the scene. Great care should be exercised not to lose or overlook any cusp tips or break the fragile occlusal cusps that started to coalesce.

If no mineralised tooth tissue is present, a radiograph should be taken of the jaw. Then histological examination is carried out by dissecting the jaw and looking into the crypts of the teeth.

If isolated cusp tips are recovered, they can be examined with the naked eye. Age estimation can be done by either dry weighing (Stack, 1960), or by comparing them to the diagrams supplied in Figure 7.1. The performance measure of the London atlas for this age group in 95% confidence intervals is: bias (difference between real age and estimated age) = 0.0847 months with ±0.22 months standard deviation. In cases of skeletal remains, radiographs should be taken of the skull and dental development compared to diagrams of the London atlas.

The neonatal line

When ageing a neonate using tooth developmental stages, corrected gestation age should be followed (40 gestational weeks) (AlQahtani *et al.*, 2010) keeping in mind that birth is an event that doesn't affect dental development. The neonatal line forms a clear demarcation between the prenatal and postnatal enamel deposition and it is independent of gestational age or size at birth (Smith and Avishai, 2005).

Finding the neonatal line will reveal that the infant was in fact born alive and lived for at least 7–10 days, which is the time necessary for visualisation of the neonatal line as a band between pre- and postnatal enamel. The amount of enamel formed after birth can then be measured to evaluate the duration of postnatal survival in skeletal remains (Whittaker and Richards, 1978; Eli *et al.*, 1989; Skinner and Dupras, 1993; Kodaka *et al.*, 1996; Sabel *et al.*, 2008).

7.5.3 Infants from birth to 2 years

This age group starts with no teeth in the oral cavity. Within months, deciduous teeth start to emerge through the gums. The sequence of eruption and tooth count may be the only way to estimate the age of the living infant, as radiographs are *contraindicated* in this age group and the difficulty of obtaining a radiograph from an infant is predictable. Also, tooth eruption is highly affected by nutrition, infection, pathology, trauma, tooth agenesis, tooth loss and crowding, so the assessor should be familiar with these limitations and with the anatomy and anomalies of teeth (Demirjian, 1973; Brown, 1978; Lauzier and Demirjian, 1981; Hägg and Matsson, 1985; Tanguay *et al.*, Buschang and Demirjian, 1986; Carvalho *et al.*, 1989; Holman and Jones, 1991, 1998, 2003; Choi and Yang, 2001; Nyström *et al.*, 2001; Foti *et al.*, 2003; Psoter *et al.*, 2003; Liversidge and Molleson, 2004; Moslemi, 2004; Holman and Yamaguchi, 2005; Bastos *et al.*, 2007; Folayan *et al.*, 2007; Franchi *et al.*, 2008; Olze *et al.*, 2008; AlQahtani *et al.*, 2010; Blenkin and Evans, 2010; Aggarwal *et al.*, 2011; Feraru *et al.*, 2011).

In cases of skeletal remains or crime scenes, a radiograph will be appropriate to examine the tooth development and compare it to the London atlas (AlQahtani *et al.*, 2010). There is a bias of 0.059 years and a standard deviation of ±0.343 at 95% confidence interval for this age group. A lateral oblique radiograph and/or an anterior radiograph would be optimal to show all the developing dentition.

7.5.4 Children and adolescents from 2 to 18 years

This age group displays the full deciduous dentition in the oral cavity at age 2 years and the beginning of permanent tooth eruption at 5 years. This eruption of the permanent dentition could be utilised for age assessment between the ages of 5 and 14 years, keeping in mind the limitations of relying on tooth eruption mentioned earlier. Extra studies that evaluated the eruption of permanent teeth in different populations can be referred to as well (Perreault *et al.*, 1974, 1975; Kochhar and Richardson, 1998; Nyström *et al.*, 2001; Mugonzibwa *et al.*, 2002; Diamanti and Townsend, 2003; Nizam *et al.*, 2003; Rousset *et al.*, 2003; Friedrich *et al.*, 2008, 2009; AlQahtani *et al.*, 2010).

Radiographic analysis of the developing dentition as well as the clinical tooth emergence in various phases will help in age determination. A good-quality radiograph is invaluable, be it a panoramic or peri-apical radiograph, a CT scan or even a lateral oblique. The London atlas (Figure 7.1) shows a bias of 0.0279 years with standard deviation ±0.908 at 95% confidence interval for this age group.

Demirjian's method

Many studies have tested measurement techniques, but the most widely used with good results is Demirjian's method (Demirjian *et al.*, 1973; Demirjian and Goldstein, 1976). Using it with self-weighted maturity scores and modified regression models to reflect local samples gives better results (Chen *et al.* 2010; Nyström *et al.*, 1977; Hägg and Matsson, 1985; Gaethofs *et al.*, 1999; Lehtinen *et al.*, 2000; Krailassiri *et al.*, Anuwongnukroh and Dechkunakorn, 2002; McKenna *et al.*, 2002; Solari and Abramovitch, 2002; Olze *et al.*, 2003; Leurs *et al.*, 2005; Neves *et al.*, 2005; Liversidge *et al.*, 2006; Maber *et al.*, 2006a; Jamroz *et al.*, 2006; Başaran *et al.*, 2007; Heuzé and

Cardoso, 2008; Introna *et al.*, 2008; Mani *et al.*, 2008; Martin *et al.*, 2008; Moananui *et al.*, 2008; Tunc and Koyuturk, 2008; Mitchell *et al.*, 2009; Peiris 2009; Cruz-Landeira *et al.*, 2010; Liversidge *et al.*, 2010; Bagherian and Sadeghi, 2011; Jayaraman *et al.*, 2011; Nik-Hussein *et al.*, 2011; Nur 2012).

In Demirjian's method, each stage of dental development is given a score that provides an estimate of dental maturity on a scale 0 to 100. There are eight stages of dental development in this method. The assessor can use either seven mandibular teeth (Demirjian, 1978) or four mandibular teeth (Demirjian and Goldstein, 1976), missing teeth from one side can be substituted by the same tooth type from the other side of the jaw and a missing first molar can be substituted with a central incisor. The limitations of this method, however, are that it can only be applied on mandibular teeth and it has no scores for third molars.

7.5.5 Adults aged 18 years and above

In the UK, 'turning eighteen' is the step that defines an individual as now being an adult. In age dispute cases, this is therefore a sensitive age because of the impact it has on life, not only on the individual but also on those around him/her.

At the age of 15 years, all permanent teeth have reached maturation except for the third molars, which provide the only possibility to use dental development for age assessment. There is, however, controversy surrounding the reliability of third molar development, with it being the tooth with the most variation in size, time of formation and time of eruption (Thorson and Hägg, 1991; Kullman *et al.*, 1992; Mincer *et al.*, 1993). Recent studies have suggested that the age of attainment of complete closure of the apices of the third molars is an indication that the living individual is over the age of 18 years and thus, by definition, an adult (Mincer *et al.*, 1993), but some studies showed differences with regard to race and gender (Cameriere *et al.*, 2008a). Many studies have revealed some regional differences with regard to third molar development, so referring to the applicable population standards in the case under study is advisable (Staaf *et al.*, 1991; Mincer *et al.*, 1993; Krailassiri *et al.*, 2002; McKenna *et al.*, 2002; Solari and Abramovitch, 2002; Olze *et al.*, 2003, 2004, 2008; De Salvia *et al.*, 2004; Prieto *et al.*, 2005; Dhanjal *et al.*, 2006; Maber *et al.*, 2006a; Başaran *et al.*, 2007; Orhan *et al.*, 2007; Sisman *et al.*, 2007; Bai *et al.*, 2008; Cameriere *et al.*, 2008a; Introna *et al.*, 2008; Martin-de las Heras *et al.*, 2008; Moananui *et al.*, 2008).

The London atlas showed no bias when tested on 18-year-olds, with an absolute mean difference of 1.07 years and a standard deviation of ± 1.25 years at 95% confidence interval. The positive likelihood ratio was 12.11 and the positive predictive value was 31.75%.

7.6 Age assessment after tooth development

With living individuals in age-disputed cases, obtaining radiographs is the non-invasive method of choice. Good-quality radiographs should be attained for age assessment based on one of the following methods:

7.6.1 Pulp ratio

Kvaal *et al.* (1995) developed a regression analysis formula, with age as the dependent variable and gender as an independent variable. Pulp size measurements are taken from a peri-apical radiograph. Six teeth should be examined:

- maxilla – central incisor, lateral incisor and second premolar
- mandible – lateral incisor, canine and first premolar.

The regression formula appears to be most reliable if only one jaw is included, and weakest if only the mandibular canine is measured (Kvaal *et al.*, 1995; Willems, 2001).

7.6.2 Other markers

Teeth go through many changes throughout adult life. Regressive changes such as attrition, secondary dentine formation, loss of periodontal attachment, apposition of apical root cementum, apical resorption and the translucency of root dentine can be utilised to assess the age of an adult.

A method for age estimation based on the length of the apical translucent zone in millimetres of a given tooth was published by Bang and Ramm (1970). They differentiated for tooth position, side and whether an intact tooth was being assessed or a tooth section.

A method based on all tooth morphologic parameters was published by Gustafson (1950). He assigned scores on a scale from 0 to 3 and, by adding these, an overall score can be obtained and used in a regression formula for age estimation.

Johanson (1971) published an improvement to Gustafson's technique, and this became the most widely accepted among forensic odontologists. Seven different stages are assigned instead of the original four, but the same six parameters are evaluated: attrition (A), secondary dentine formation (S), periodontal attachment loss (P), cementum apposition (C), root resorption (R) and apical translucency (T). Johanson's regression formula is then:

$$\text{age} = 11.02 + 5.14^*A + 2.3^*S + 4.14^*P + 3.71^*C + 5.57^*R + 8.98^*T.$$

In cases where tooth preservation is necessary, the use of a method developed by Solheim is advisable, because some of its calculations are based on unsectioned tooth measurements – which makes this technique of particular interest (Solheim, 1993; Willems, 2001). Kvaal and Solhiem (1994) published a method that takes into account the tooth type assessed, along with both radiographical and morphological tooth parameters.

The results from methods of age determination after dental development are used only as an indication, as they are based on multiple regressions which tend to overestimate the age in young individuals (Solheim and Vonen, 2006).

7.6.3 Biomarkers

Biomarkers, which are biochemical features, can be used to examine the ageing process. They measure the degeneration of the RNA ends that happens every time the cell divides (Ritz-Timme *et al.*, 2000; Bauer, 2007; Heinrich *et al.*, 2007; Jiang *et al.*, 2008; Griffin *et al.*, 2009; Ren *et al.*, 2009). Racemisation of aspartic acid in dentine or tooth enamel can determine the date of death, and radiocarbon dating of postnatal tooth enamel can determine the date of birth (Alkass *et al.*, 2009). Combination of these two techniques can provide chronological age estimation up to an accuracy of ±1.6 years (Alkass *et al.*, 2009). The drawback, however, is that it requires a sample from the tooth, which is an invasive procedure in living individuals. It is also expensive and time-consuming.

7.7 Writing a dental age report

Age estimation will always be within a range rather than an exact age because of the biological differences between individuals. This fact should always be emphasised when writing a dental age report. In preparing a legal deposition, the exact choice of words and conclusions depend on the circumstances. The conclusion may be that the findings were 'consistent with an individual of that age', or the degree of dental certainty or probability of the findings may be specified.

Two forensic odontologists should work together in age assessment. The second examiner need only to examine the radiographs or the prepared tooth. Both examiners should agree to the exact conclusion and their signatures be on the report, but if deemed necessary, the second examiner should re-examine the case. The second examiner should also read the report and suggest corrections.

The International Organization for Forensic Odonto-Stomatology (IOFOS, 2008) gave recommendations for quality assurance in age estimation, and these are summarised below.

General

The purpose of the age estimation is to:

- estimate the most likely age of the individual.
- express the likelihood of an official age, if it exists (optional).
- express the likelihood of an alternative age, if it exists (optional).

All available information should be used for the final estimate (optional), including:

- the expert's own assessment.
- information from the person on living conditions and diseases.
- results from scientific statistical methods.

Background information (optional)

The assessor should ask (if the individual in question is alive) questions relevant for tooth development and maintenance, such as:

- family economy.
- food and water supply.
- current or prior systemic diseases.
- previous dental problems and treatment.
- dental hygiene.

Methods

- Use as many appropriate parameters as possible.
- Make reference to the methods used.
- Use methods as originally described in the literature.
- Use as many teeth as possible.
- Use, if possible, at least two independent statistical methods (optional).

Clinical examination (in both living and dead individuals)

- Establish the identity of the person.
- Examine the oral mucosa (optional).
- Describe the dentition (optional): teeth present in the mouth; individual characteristics of the teeth; the degree of attrition; occlusion; colour of the teeth; staining and calculus; periodontal condition.
- Assess the age visually, based solely on the teeth (optional).

Radiographic examination

- Take radiographs appropriate to the methods you have decided to use.
- Describe the dentition and individual characteristics of the development of the teeth.

Evaluation

- Make an assessment of the most likely chronological age.
- Assess whether the methods are appropriate in relation to the individual (optional).

- Assess factors that may have influenced tooth development or ageing (optional).
- Assess especially whether pathological factors or other may have influenced the findings (optional).

7.8 Final comments

Dental age assessment can be very subjective, so testing inter- and intra-observer variations and their extent is crucial. When selecting a new method, it is useful to calibrate oneself by testing the method on individuals of known age, thereby gauging the likely margin of over- or under-estimation (Willems, 2001).

Different teeth erupt at different ages, in a relatively constant chronological order; therefore using them for age assessment can be safe, and child- and gender-sensitive. It is the non-invasive technique of choice for individuals still in the process of tooth eruption and exfoliation of deciduous teeth up to the age of 2 years, and in mixed dentition from the age of 5 years until the final stages of second permanent molar eruption at the age of 10 years.

Schemas of dental development show diagrammatic representations of the developing dentition from prenatal onwards and are based on current data. Since any age assessment derived from an atlas comparison will be reported as an age range, this allows for a determination of age based on 'the balance of probabilities'. This addresses concerns noted in the Convention of the Rights of the Child (CRC). Atlas comparisons are the technique of choice for age assessment of individuals who, on intra-oral examination, have all deciduous teeth erupted – which makes them over the age of 2 years because of the need to take a radiograph.

From the age of 15 years to the early twenties, there are few reliable dental methods of age estimation other than the tooth development. Third molar statistics are often presented as evidence of the likelihood of the age of attainment (complete closure of the apex of the root), or as a percentage of the population who would be aged 18 years when the third molar has completed development. This method of age assessment, of necessity, involves the capture of radiographic images of the third molars as they lie within the mandible and maxilla, and ethical issues need to be addressed before images are captured.

The forensic academy recommendation for using teeth in age estimation is that the method has to give results within 6 months of the actual age for it to be legally acceptable (Schmeling *et al.*, 2006; Rösing *et al.*, 2007; Peiris *et al.*, 2009). One should keep in mind that the standard deviation for adults is in general 10–12 years (Willems, 2001).

7.9 References

Aggarwal P., Saxena S. and Bansal P. (2008) Incremental lines in root cementum of human teeth: an approach to their role in age estimation using polarizing microscopy, *Indian Journal of Dental Research* **19**(3): 326–330.

Aggarwal K. K., Kaur A. and Kumar R. (2011) Chronological pattern of eruption of permanent teeth in the adolescent age group in patiala district, Punjab, *Journal of Punjab Academy of Forensic Medicine & Toxicology* **11**(1): 12–19.

Aka P. S., Canturk N., Dagalp R. and Yagan M. (2009) Age determination from central incisors of fetuses and infants, *Forensic Science International* **184**(1–3): 15–20.

Alkass K., Buchholz B. A., Ohtani S., Yamamoto T., Druid H. and Spalding K. L. (2009) Age estimation in forensic sciences: application of combined aspartic acid racemization and radiocarbon analysis, *Molecular & Cellular Proteomics* **9**(5): 1022–1030.

AlQahtani S. J., Hector M. P. and Liversidge H. M. (2010) Brief communication: the London atlas of human tooth development and eruption, *American Journal of Physical Anthropology* **142**(3): 481–490.

Anderson D., Anderson G. and Popovich F. (1976) Age of attainment of mineralization stages of the permanent dentition, *Journal of Forensic Sciences* **21**: 191–200.

Antoine D., Hillson S. and Dean M. C. (2009) The developmental clock of dental enamel: a test for the periodicity of prism cross-striations in modern humans and an evaluation of the most likely sources of error in histological studies of this kind, *Journal of Anatomy* **214**(1): 45–55.

Bagherian A. and Sadeghi M. (2011) Assessment of dental maturity of children aged 3.5 to 13.5 years using the Demirjian method in an Iranian population, *Journal of Oral Science* **53**(1): 37-42.

Bai Y., Mao J., Zhu S. and Wei W. (2008) Third-molar development in relation to chronologic age in young adults of central China, *Journal of Huazhong University of Science and Technology – Medical Sciences* **28**(4).

Bang G. and Ramm E. (1970) Determination of age in humans from root dentin transparency, *Acta Odontologica Scandinavica* **28**(1): 3–35.

Başaran G., Özer T. and Hamamc N. (2007) Cervical vertebral and dental maturity in Turkish subjects, *American Journal of Orthodontics and Dentofacial Orthopedics* –(4): 447.e13–447.e20.

Bastos J. L., Peres M. A., Peres K. G. and Barros A. J. D. (2007) Infant growth, development and tooth emergence patterns: a longitudinal study from birth to 6 years of age, *Archives of Oral Biology* **52**(6): 598–606.

Bauer M. (2007) RNA in forensic science, *Forensic Science International: Genetics* **1**(1): 69–74.

Bhat V. J. M. D. and Kamath G. P. M. D. S. (2007) Age estimation from root development of mandibular third molars in comparison with skeletal age of wrist joint, *American Journal of Forensic Medicine and Pathology* **28**(3): 238–241.

Blenkin M. R. B. and Evans W. (2010) Age estimation from the teeth using a modified Demirjian system, *Journal of Forensic Sciences* **55**(6): 1504–1508.

Bocquet-Appel J. and Masset C. (1982) Farewell to paleodemography, *Journal of Human Evolution* (11): 321–333.

Bojarun, R., Garmus A. and Jankauskas R. (2003) Microstructure of dental cementum and individual biological age estimation, *Medicina (Kaunas)* **39**(10): 960–964.

Braga J., Heuze Y., Chabadel O., Sonan N. K. and Gueramy A. (2005) Non-adult dental age assessment: correspondence analysis and linear regression versus Bayesian predictions, *International Journal of Legal Medicine* **119**(5): 260–274.

Brkic H., Milicevic M. and Petrovecki M. (2006) Age estimation methods using anthropological parameters on human teeth, *Forensic Science International* **162**(1–3): 13–16.

Brothwell D. R. (1981) *Digging up Bones: The Excavation, Treatment, and Study of Human Skeletal Remains*. Ithaca, New York: Cornell University Press.

Brown A. C., Beeler W. J., Kloka A. C. and Fields R. W. (1985) Spatial summation of pre-pain and pain in human teeth, *Pain* **21**(1): 1–16.

Brown T. (1978) Tooth emergence in Australian aboriginals, *Annals of Human Biology* **5**(1): 41–54.

Butti A. C., Clivio A., Ferraroni M., Spada E., Testa A. and Salvato A. (2008) Haavikko's method to assess dental age in Italian children, *European Journal of Orthodontics*: cjn081.

Cameriere R., Ferrante L. and Cingolani M. (2006) Age estimation in children by measurement of open apices in teeth, *International Journal of Legal Medicine* **120**(1): 49–52.

Cameriere R., Ferrante L., Angelis D. D., Scarpino F. and Galli F. (2008a) The comparison between measurement of open apices of third molars and Demirjian stages to test chronological age of over 18-year-olds in living subjects, *International Journal of Legal Medicine* **122**(6).

Cameriere R., Ferrante L., Liversidge H. M., Prieto J. L. and Brkic H. (2008b) Accuracy of age estimation in children using radiograph of developing teeth, *Forensic Science International* **176**(2–3): 173–177.

Cardoso H. F. V. (2007a) Accuracy of developing tooth length as an estimate of age in human skeletal remains: the deciduous dentition, *Forensic Science International* **172**(1): 17–22.

Cardoso H. F. V. (2007b) A test of the differential accuracy of the maxillary versus the mandibular dentition in age estimations of immature skeletal remains based on developing tooth length, *Journal of Forensic Sciences* **52**(2): 434–437.

Cardoso H. F. V. P. (2009) Accuracy of developing tooth length as an estimate of age in human skeletal remains: the permanent dentition, *American Journal of Forensic Medicine and Pathology* **30**(2): 127–133.

Carels C. E., Kuijpers-Jagtman A. M., Van Der Linden F. P. and Van't Hof M. A. (1991) Age reference charts of tooth length in Dutch children, *Journal de Biologiel Buccale* **19**(4): 297–303.

Carvalho J. C., Ekstrand K. R. and Thylstrup A. (1989) Dental plaque and caries on occlusal surfaces of first permanent molars in relation to stage of eruption, *Journal of Dental Research* **68**(5): 773–779.

Chaillet N. and Demirjian A. (2004) Dental maturity in south France: a comparison between Demirjian's method and polynomial functions, *Journal of Forensic Sciences* **49**(5): 1059–1066.

Chaillet N., Nystrom M., Kataja M. and Demirjian A. (2004a) Dental maturity curves in Finnish children: Demirjian's method revisited and polynomial functions for age estimation, *Journal of Forensic Sciences* **49**(6): 1324–1331.

Chaillet N., Willems G. and Demirjian A. (2004b) Dental maturity in Belgian children using Demirjian's method and polynomial functions: new standard curves for forensic and clinical use, *Journal of Forensic Odonto-Stomatology* **22**(2): 18–27.

Chen J. W., Guo J., Zhou J., Liu R. K., Chen T. T. and Zou S. J. (2010) Assessment of dental maturity of western Chinese children using Demirjian's method, *Forensic Science International* **197**(1–3): 119.e1–119.e4.

Choi N. K. and Yang K. H. (2001) A study on the eruption timing of primary teeth in Korean children, *ASDC Journal of Dentistry for Children* **68**(4): 244–249, 228.

Constandse-Westermann T. S. (1997) Age estimation by dental attrition in an independently controlled early 19th century sample from Zwolle, the Netherlands, *Human Evolution* **12**(4).

Craddock H. L. and Youngson C. C. (2004) Eruptive tooth movement: the current state of knowledge, *British Dental Journal* **197**(7): 385–391.

Crawley H. (2012) Asylum age disputes and the process of age assessment. In: Kelly E. and Bokhari F. (eds), *Safeguarding Children from Abroad: Refugee, Asylum-seeking and Trafficked Children in the UK*. London, Jessica Kingsley Publishers, pp. 55–68.

Cruz-Landeira A., Linares-Argote J., Martínez-Rodríguez M., Rodríguez-Calvo M. S., Otero X. L. and Concheiro L. (2010) Dental age estimation in Spanish and Venezuelan children: comparison of Demirjian and Chaillet's scores, *International Journal of Legal Medicine* **124**(2): 105–112.

Czermak A., Czermak A., Ernst H. and Grupe G. (2006) A new method for the automated age-at-death evaluation by tooth-cementum annulation, *Anthropologischer Anzeiger* **64**(1): 25–40.

Dalitz G. D. (1962) Age determination of adult human remain by teeth examination, *Journal of Forensic Sciences Society* **3**: 11–21.

Davis P. J. and Hägg U. (1994) The accuracy and precision of the Demirjian system when used for age determination in Chinese children, *Swedish Dental Journal* **18**(3): 113–116.

De Salvia A., Calzetta C., Orrico M. and De Leo D. (2004) Third mandibular molar radiological development as an indicator of chronological age in a European population, *Forensic Science International* **146** (Suppl. 1): S9–S12.

Demirjian A. (1973) Tooth eruption in the French Canadian child, *Journal Dentaire du Quebec* **10**(10): 9.

Demirjian A. (1978) [Dental development: index of physiologic maturation], *Medecine et Hygiene* **36**(1302): 3154–3159.

Demirjian A. (1986) Dentition. In: Falkner F. and Tanner J. (eds), *Human Growth: A Comprehensive Treatise*, vol. 2. New York: Plenum Press, pp. 269–298.

Demirjian A. and Goldstein H. (1976) New systems for dental maturity based on seven and four teeth, *Annals of Human Biology* **3**(5): 411–421.

Demirjian A., Goldstein H. and Tanner J. M. (1973) A new system of dental age assessment, *Human Biology* **45**(2): 211–227.

Demirjian A., Buschang P. H., Tanguay R. and Patterson D. K. (1985) Interrelationships among measures of somatic, skeletal, dental, and sexual maturity, *American Journal of Orthodontics* **88**(5): 433–438.

Dhanjal K. S., Bhardwaj M. K. and Liversidge H. M. (2006) Reproducibility of radiographic stage assessment of third molars, *Forensic Science International* **159** (Suppl. 1): S74–S77.

Diamanti J. and Townsend G. C. (2003) New standards for permanent tooth emergence in Australian children, *Australian Dental Journal* **48**(1): 39–42.

Eli I., Sarnat H. and Talmi E. (1989) Effect of the birth process on the neonatal line in primary tooth enamel, *Pediatric Dentistry* **11**(3): 220–223.

Fanning E. and Brown T. (1971) Primary and permanent tooth development, *Australian Dental Journal* **16**: 41–43.

Fass E. (1969) A chronology of growth of the human dentition, *ASDC Journal of Dentistry for Children* **36**(6): 391–401.

Feraru I.-V., Rãducanu A. M., Feraru S. E. and Herpeliu C. (2011) The sequence and chronology of the eruption of permanent canines and premolars in a group of Romanian children in Bucharest, *Oral Health and Dental Management* **10**(4).

FitzGerald C. M. (1998) Do enamel microstructures have regular time dependency? Conclusions from the literature and a large-scale study, *Journal of Human Evolution* **35**(4–5): 371–386.

Folayan M., Owotade F., Adejuyigbe E., Sen S., Lawal B. and Ndukwe K. (2007) The timing of eruption of the primary dentition in Nigerian children, *American Journal of Physical Anthropology* **134**(4): 443–448.

Foti B., Lalys L., Adalian P., Giustiniani J., Maczel M., Signoli M., Dutour O. and Leonetti G. (2003) New forensic approach to age determination in children based on tooth eruption, *Forensic Science International* **132**(1): 49–56.

Franchi L., Baccetti T., De Toffol L., Polimeni A. and Cozza P. (2008) Phases of the dentition for the assessment of skeletal maturity: a diagnostic performance study, *American Journal of Orthodontics and Dentofacial Orthopedics* **133**(3): 395–400.

Friedrich R. E., Leist A. and Scheuer H. A. (2008) Eruption times of permanent teeth in children and adolescents in the German state of Saarland, *Archiv fur Kriminologie* **222**(3–4): 73–104.

Friedrich R. E., Habib S. and Scheuer H. A. (2009) Eruption times of permanent teeth in children and adolescents in Latakia (Syria), *Archiv fur Kriminologie* **223**(3–4): 84–97.

Gaethofs M., Verdonck A., Carels C. and de Zegher F. (1999) Delayed dental age in boys with constitutionally delayed puberty, *European Journal of Orthodontics* **21**(6): 711–715.

Garn S. M., Lewis A. B., Koski . and Polacheck D. L. (1958) The sex difference in tooth calcification, *Journal of Dental Research* **37**(3): 561–567.

Garn S. M., Lewis A. B. and Polacheck D. L. (1959) Variability of tooth formation, *Journal of Dental Research* **38**(1): 135–148.

Garn S. M., Lewis A. B. and Blizzard R. M. (1965a) Endocrine factors in dental development, *Journal of Dental Research* **44** (Suppl.): 243–258.

Garn S. M., Lewis A. B. and Kerewsky R. S. (1965) Genetic, nutritional, and maturational correlates of dental development, *Journal of Dental Research* **44** (Suppl.): 228–242.

Gleiser I. and Hunt E. E. (1955) The permanent mandibular first molar: its calcification, eruption and decay, *American Journal of Physical Anthropology* **13**(2): 253–283.

Griffin R. C., Chamberlain A. T., Hotz G., Penkman K. E. H. and Collins M. J. (2009) Age estimation of archaeological remains using amino acid racemization in dental enamel: a comparison of morphological, biochemical, and known ages-at-death, *American Journal of Physical Anthropology* **140**(2): 244–252.

Gunst K., Mesotten K., Carbonez A. and Willems G. (2003) Third molar root development in relation to chronological age: a large-sample-sized retrospective study, *Forensic Science International* **136**(1–3): 52–57.

Gustafson G. (1950) Age determination on teeth, *Journal of American Dental Association* **41**(1): 45–54.

Gustafson G. and Koch G. (1974) Age estimation up to 16 years of age based on dental development, *Odontologisk Revy* **25**(3): 297–306.

Gutiérrez-Salazara M. d. P. and Reyes-Gasgaa J. (2003) Microhardness and chemical composition of human tooth, *Materials Research* **6**(3): 367–373.

Haataja J. (1965) Development of the mandibular permanent teeth of Helsinki children, *Proceedings of the Finnish Dental Society* **61**: 43–53.

Haavikko K. (1970) The formation and the alveolar and clinical eruption of the permanent teeth: an orthopantomographic study, *Suom hammaslääk toim* **66**(3): 103–170.

Haavikko K. (1974) Tooth formation age estimated on a few selected teeth: a simple method for clinical use, *Proceedings of the Finnish Dental Society* **70**(1): 15–19.

Hägg U. and Hägg E. (1986) The accuracy and precision of assessment of chronological age by analysis of tooth emergence, *Journal of International Association of Dentistry for Children* **17**(2): 45–52.

Hägg U. and Matsson L. (1985) Dental maturity as an indicator of chronological age: the accuracy and precision of three methods, *European Journal of Orthodontics* **7**(1): 25–34.

Halcrow S. E., Tayles N. and Buckley H. R. (2007) Age estimation of children from prehistoric southeast asia: are the dental formation methods used appropriate? *Journal of Archaeological Science* **34**(7): 1158–1168.

Harris M. J. and Nortjé C. J. (1984) The mesial root of the third mandibular molar: a possible indicator of age, *Journal of Forensic Odontostomatology* **2**(2): 39–43.

Heinrich M., Matt K., Lutz-Bonengel S. and Schmidt U. (2007) Successful RNA extraction from various human postmortem tissues, *International Journal of Legal Medicine* **121**(2): 136–142.

Heuzé Y. and Cardoso H. F. V. (2008) Testing the quality of nonadult bayesian dental age assessment methods to juvenile skeletal remains: the Lisbon collection of children and secular trend effects, *American Journal of Physical Anthropology* **135**(3): 275–283.

Hillson S. (1996) *Dental Anthropology*. Cambridge:Cambridge University Press.

Holman D. J. and Jones R. E. (1991) Longitudinal analysis of deciduous tooth emergence in indonesian children. I: Life table methodology, *American Journal of Human Biology* **3**(4): 389–403.

Holman D. J. and Jones R. E. (1998) Longitudinal analysis of deciduous tooth emergence. Ii: Parametric survival analysis in Bangladeshi, Guatemalan, Japanese, and Javanese children, *American Journal of Physical Anthropology* **105**(2): 209–230.

Holman D. J. and Jones R. E. (2003) Longitudinal analysis of deciduous tooth emergence. Iii: Sexual dimorphism in Bangladeshi, Guatemalan, Japanese, and Javanese children, *American Journal of Physical Anthropology* **122**(3): 269–278.

Holman D. J. and Yamaguchi K. (2005) Longitudinal analysis of deciduous tooth emergence. Iv: Covariate effects in Japanese children, *American Journal of Physical Anthropology* **126**(3): 352–358.

Introna F. M. D. P., Santoro V. D. D. S., De Donno A. M. D. and Belviso M. P. (2008) Morphologic analysis of third-molar maturity by digital orthopantomographic assessment, *American Journal of Forensic Medicine and Pathology* **29**(1): 55–61.

IOFOS (2008) Dental age estimation, quality assurance. Available from http://iofos.eu/Quality-Ass/Age-IOFOS.htm (accessed: July 2012).

IOM (2012) Global health assessment programmes (2005 to present). Available from www.iom.int/jahia/Jahia/projects-assessments/cache/offonce (accessed: July 2012).

Jamroz G., Kuijpers-Jagtman A., van't Hof M. and Katsaros C. (2006) Dental maturation in short and long facial types. Is there a difference? *Angle Orthodontist* **76**(5): 768–772.

Janes L. (2008) Criminal liability of minors and severity of penalties: European trends and developments. *The Howard League for Penal Reform*, E. rights. England and Wales, www.europeanrights.eu.

Jankauskas R., Barakauskas S. and Bojarun R. (2001) Incremental lines of dental cementum in biological age estimation, *Homo Gottingen* **52**(1): 59–71.

Jayaraman J., King N. M., Roberts G. J. and Wong H. M. (2011) Dental age assessment: are Demirjian's standards appropriate for southern Chinese children? *Journal of Forensic Odontostomatology* **2**(29): 22–28.

Jiang H., Schiffer E., Song Z. *et al.,* (2008) Proteins induced by telomere dysfunction and DNA damage represent biomarkers of human aging and disease, *Proceedings of the National Academy of Sciences* **105**(32): 11299–11304.

Johanson G. (1971) Age determination from human teeth: a critical evaluation with special consideration of changes after fourteen years of age, *Odontologisk Revy* **22** (Suppl. 21): 1–126.

Kahl B. and Schwarze C. (1988a) Updating of the dentition tables of I. Schour and M. Massler of 1941, *Fortschr Kieferorthop* **49**(5): 432–443.

Kahl B. and Schwarze C. W. (1988b). [Updating of the dentition tables of I. Schour and M. Massler of 1941], *Fortschritte der Kieferorthopadie* **49**(5): 432–443.

Kardos T. B. (1996) The mechanism of tooth eruption, *British Dental Journal* **181**(3): 91–95.

Kochhar R. and Richardson A. (1998) The chronology and sequence of eruption of human permanent teeth in Northern Ireland, *International Journal of Paediatric Dentistry* **8**(4): 243–252.

Kodaka T., Sano T. and Higashi S. (1996) Structural and calcification patterns of the neonatal line in the enamel of human deciduous teeth, *Scanning Microscopy* **10**(3): 737–743; discussion 743–744.

Köhler S., Schmelzle R., Loitz C. and Püschel K. (1994) Die entwicklung des weisheitszahnes als kriterium der lebensalterbestimmung, *Annals of Anatomy* **176**: 339–345.

Konigsberg L. W. and Frankenberg S. R. (2002) Deconstructing death in paleodemography, *American Journal of Physical Anthropology* **117**(4): 297–309.

Kraemer H., Korner A. and Horwitz S. (1985) A model for assessing the development of preterm infants as a function of gestational, conceptual, or chronological age, *Developmental Psychology* **21**: 806–812.

Krailassiri S., Anuwongnukroh N. and Dechkunakorn S. (2002) Relationships between dental calcification stages and skeletal maturity indicators in thai individuals, *Angle Orthodontist* **72**(2): 155–166.

Krogman W. M. (1968) Biological timing and the dento-facial complex. 3, *ASDC Journal of Dentistry for Children* **35**(5): 377–381.

Krogman W. M. and Işcan M. Y. (1986) The human skeleton. In: Charles C. (ed.), *Forensic Medicine*. Springfield, IL, Thomas Pub.

Kronfeld R. (1935) Postnatal development and calcification of the anterior permanent teeth, *Journal of American Dental Association* **22**: 1521–1536.

Kullman L. (1995) Accuracy of two dental and one skeletal age estimation method in Swedish adolescents, *Forensic Science International* **30**(75): 225–236.

Kullman L., Johanson G. and Akesson L. (1992) Root development of the lower third molar and its relation to chronological age, *Swedish Dental Journal* **16**(4): 161–167.

Kullman L., Martinsson T., Zimmerman M. and Welander U. (1995) Computerized measurements of the lower third molar related to chronologic age in young adults, *Acta Odontologica Scandinavica* **53**(4): 211–216.

Kvaal S. I. and Solheim T. (1994) A non-destructive dental method for age estimation, *Journal of Forensic Odontostomatology* **12**(1): 6–11.

Kvaal S. I., Kolltveit K. M., Thomsen I. O. and Solheim T. (1995) Age estimation of adults from dental radiographs, *Forensic Science International* **74**: 175–185.

Lauzier C. and Demirjian A. (1981) [Emergence of primary teeth in French-Canadian children], *Union Medicale du Canada* **110**(12): 1061–1064.

Lehtinen A., Oksa T., Helenius H. and Rönning O. (2000) Advanced dental maturity in children with juvenile rheumatoid arthritis, *European Journal of Oral Sciences* **108**(3): 184–188.

Leurs I. H., Wattel E., Aartman I. H. A., Etty E. and Prahl-Andersen B. (2005) Dental age in Dutch children, *European Journal of Orthodontics* **27**: 309–314.

Levenson R. and Sharma A. (1999) *The Health of Refugee Children: Guidelines for Paediatricians*. London: Royal College of Paediatrics and Child Health.

Liliequist B. and Lundberg M. (1971) Skeletal and tooth development: a methodologic investigation, *Acta Radiologica Diagnosis (Stockh)* **11**(2): 97–112.

Liversidge H. M. (1994) Accuracy of age estimation from developing teeth of a population of known age (0–5.4 years), *International Journal of Osteoarchaeology* **4**(1): 37–45.

Liversidge H. M. and Marsden P. H. (2010) Estimating age and the likelihood of having attained 18 years of age using mandibular third molars, *British Dental Journal* **209**(8): E13.

Liversidge H. M. and Molleson T. I. (1999a) Deciduous tooth size and morphogenetic fields in children from Christ Church, Spitalfields, *Archives of Oral Biology* **44**(1): 7–13.

Liversidge H. M. and Molleson T. I. (1999b) Developing permanent tooth length as an estimate of age, *Journal of Forensic Sciences* **44**(5): 917–920.

Liversidge H. M. and Molleson T. I. (2004) Variation in crown and root formation and eruption of human deciduous teeth, *American Journal of Physical Anthropology* **123**(2): 172–180.

Liversidge H. M., Dean M. C. and Molleson T. I. (1993) Increasing human tooth length between birth and 5.4 years, *American Journal of Physical Anthropology* **90**(3): 307–313.

Liversidge H. M., Lyons F. and Hector M. P. (2003) The accuracy of three methods of age estimation using radiographic measurements of developing teeth, *Forensic Science International* **131**(1): 22–29.

Liversidge H. M., Chaillet N., Mornstad H., Nystrom M., Rowlings K., Taylor J. and Willems G. (2006) Timing of Demirjian's tooth formation stages, *Annals of Human Biology* **33**(4): 454–470.

Liversidge H. M., Smith B. H. and Maber M. (2010) Bias and accuracy of age estimation using developing teeth in 946 children, *American Journal of Physical Anthropology* **143**(4): 545–554.

Lovejoy C. O. (1985) Dental wear in the Libben population: its functional pattern and role in the determination of adult skeletal age at death, *American Journal of Physical Anthropology* **68**(1): 47–56.

Maber M., Liversidge H. M. and Hector M. P. (2006) Accuracy of age estimation of radiographic methods using developing teeth, *Forensic Science International* **159** (Suppl. 1): S68–S73.

Mani, S. A., L. I. N. Naing, J. John and A. R. Samsudin (2008). "Comparison of two methods of dental age estimation in 7–15-year-old malays." International Journal of Paediatric Dentistry **18**(5): 380-388.

Martin-de las Heras S., GarcÃa-Fortea P., Ortega A., Zodocovich S. and Valenzuela A. (2008) Third molar development according to chronological age in populations from Spanish and Magrebian origin, *Forensic Science International* **174**(1): 47–53.

Martin M. B., Li C.-S., Rowland C. C., Howard S. C. and Kaste S. C. (2008) Correlation of bone age, dental age, and chronological age in survivors of childhood acute lymphoblastic leukaemia, *International Journal of Paediatric Dentistry* **18**(3): 217–223.

McKenna C., James H, Taylor J. and Townsend G. (2002) Tooth development standards for South Australia, *Australian Dental Journal* **47**(3): 223–227.

Mesotten K., K. Gunst, A. Carbonez and G. Willems (2002). "Dental age estimation and third molars: A preliminary study." Forensic Science International **129**(2): 110–115.

Miles A. (1978) Teeth as an indicator of age in man. In: Butler P. M. and Joysey K. A. (eds), *Development, Function and Evolution of Teeth*. London: Academic Press.

Mincer H., Harris E. and Berryman H. (1993) The a.BFO study of third molar development and its use as an estimator of chronological age, *Journal of Forensic Science* **38**(2): 379–390.

Mitchell J. C., Roberts G. J., Donaldson A. N. A. and Lucas V. S. (2009) Dental age assessment: reference data for British caucasians at the 16-year threshold, *Forensic Science International* **189**(1–3): 19–23.

Moananui R. T., Kieser J. A., Herbison P. and Liversidge H. M. (2008) Advanced dental maturation in New Zealand Maori and Pacific Island children, *American Journal of Human Biology* **20**(1): 43–50.

Moore W. J. and Corbett M. E. (1971) The distribution of dental caries in ancient British populations. I: Anglo-saxon period, *Caries Research* **5**: 151–168.

Moore W. J. and Corbett M. E. (1973) The distribution of dental caries in ancient British populations. It: Iron Age, Romano-British and mediaeval periods, *Caries Research* **7**: 139–153.

Moorrees C., Fanning E. and Hunt E. (1963a) Formation and resorption of three deciduous teeth in children, *American Journal of Physical Anthropology* **21**: 205–213.

Moorrees C., Fanning E. and Hunt E. (1963b) Age variation of formation stages for ten permanent teeth, *Journal of Dental Research* **42**: 1490–1502.

Mörnstad H., Staaf V. and Welander U. (1994) Age estimation with the aid of tooth development: a new method based on objective measurements, *European Journal of Oral Sciences* **102**(3): 137–143.

Moslemi M. (2004) An epidemiological survey of the time and sequence of eruption of permanent teeth in 4- to 15-year-olds in Tehran, Iran, *International Journal of Paediatric Dentistry* **14**(6): 432–438.

Mugonzibwa E. A., Kuijpers-Jagtman A. M., Laine-Alava M. T. and Van't Hof M. A. (2002) Emergence of permanent teeth in Tanzanian children, *Community Dentistry and Oral Epidemiology* **30**(6): 455–462.

Nanda R. and Chawla T. (1966) Growth and development of dentitions in Indian children. I: Development of permanent teeth, *American Journal of Orthodontics and Dentofacial Orthopedics* **52**: 837.

Neves L. S., Pinzan A., Janson G., Canuto C. E., de Freitas M. R. and Cançado R. H. (2005) Comparative study of the maturation of permanent teeth in subjects with vertical and horizontal growth patterns, *American Journal of Orthodontics and Dentofacial Orthopedics* **128**(5): 619–623.

Nik-Hussein N. N., Kee K. M., Gan P. *et al.,* (2011) Validity of Demirjian and Willems methods for dental age estimation for Malaysian children aged 5–15 years, *Forensic Science International* **204**(1–3): 208.e1–208.e6.

Nizam A., Naing L. and Mokhta N. (2003) Age and sequence of eruption of permanent teeth in Kelantan, north-eastern Malaysia, *Clinical Oral Investigations* **7**(4): 222–225.

Nolla C. (1960) The development of the permanent teeth, *Journal of Dentistry for Children* **27**: 254–266.

Nur B., Kusgoz A., Bayram M., Celikoglu M., Nur M., Kayipmaz S. and Yildirim S. (2012) Validity of Demirjian and Nolla methods for dental age estimation for north-eastern Turkish children aged 5–16 years, *Medicina Oral, Patologia Oral y Cirugia Bucal* **17**(5): e871–e877.

Nyström M., Kilpinen E. and Kleemola-Kujala E. (1977) A radiographic study of the formation of some teeth from 0.5 to 3.0 years of age, *Proceedings of the Finnish Dental Society* **73**(4): 167–172.

Nyström M., Haataja J., Kataja M., Evälahti M., Peck L. and Kleemola-Kujala E. (1986) Dental maturity in Finnish children, estimated from the development of seven permanent mandibular teeth, *Acta Odontologica Scandinavica* **44**(4): 193–208.

Nyström M., Kleemola-Kujala E., Evälahti M., Peck L. and Kataja M. (2001) Emergence of permanent teeth and dental age in a series of Finns, *Acta Odontologica Scandinavica* **59**(2): 49–56.

Olze A., Taniguchi M., Schmeling A., Zhu B.-L., Yamada Y., Maeda H. and Geserick G. (2003) Comparative study on the chronology of third molar mineralization in a Japanese and a German population, *Legal Medicine* **5** (Suppl. 1): S256–S260.

Olze A., Schmeling A., Taniguchi M., Maeda H., Niekerk P. V., Wernecke K. –D. and Geserick G. (2004) Forensic age estimation in living subjects: the ethnic factor in wisdom tooth mineralization, *International Journal of Legal Medicine* **118**(3): 170–173.

Olze A., Peschke C., Schulz R. and Schmeling A. (2008) Studies of the chronological course of wisdom tooth eruption in a German population, *Journal of Forensic and Legal Medicine* **15**(7): 426–429.

Orhan K., Ozer L., Orhan A. I., Dogan S. and Paksoy C. S. (2007) Radiographic evaluation of third molar development in relation to chronological age among Turkish children and youth, *Forensic Science International* **165**(1): 46–51.

Peiris T. S., Roberts G. J. and Prabhu N. (2009) Dental age assessment: a comparison of 4- to 24-year-olds in the United Kingdom and an Australian population, *International Journal of Paediatric Dentistry* **19**(5): 367–376.

Perreault J. G., Demirjian A. and Jenicek M. (1974) [Eruption of permanent teeth in French-Canadian children], *Journal Dentaire* **40**(4): 306–313.

Perreault J. G., Chaumont A, Jenicek M. and Demirjian A. (1975) [Eruption of permanent teeth in Canadian children of French origin. 2: Development from the piercing of the gingiva to the complete clinical crown], *Journal Dentaire* **41**(10): 572–577.

Prieto J. L., Barbería E., Ortega R. and Magaña C. (2005) Evaluation of chronological age based on third molar development in the Spanish population, *International Journal of Legal Medicine* **119**(6).

Prince D. A. and Konigsberg L. W. (2008) New formulae for estimating age-at-death in the Balkans utilizing Lamendin's dental technique and Bayesian analysis, *Journal of Forensic Sciences* **53**(3): 578–587.

Psoter W. J., Morse D. E., Pendrys D. G., Zhang H. and Mayne S. T. (2003) Median ages of eruption of the primary teeth in White and Hispanic children from Arizona, *Pediatric Dentistry* **25**(3): 257–261.

Rai B., Krishan K., Kaur J.and Anand S. (2008) Age estimation from mandible by lateral cephalogram: a preliminary study. *Journal of Forensic Odonto-Stomatology* **26**(1) 24–28.

Ren F., Li C., Xi H., Wen Y. and Huang K. (2009) Estimation of human age according to telomere shortening in peripheral blood leukocytes of Tibetans, *American Journal of Forensic Medicine and Pathology* **30**(3): 252–255.

Ritz-Timme S., Cattaneo C., Collins M., Waite E., Schütz H. W., Kaatsch H. and Borrman H. (2000) Age estimation: the state of the art in relation to the specific demands of forensic practice, *International Journal of Legal Medicine* **113**(3): 129–136.

Roberts G. J., Parekh S., Petrie A. and Lucas V. S. (2008) Dental age assessment: a simple method for children and emerging adults, *British Dental Journal* **204**(4): E7.

Rösing F., Graw M., Marré B., Ritz-Timme S., Rothschild M., Rötzscher K., Schmeling A., Schröder I. and Geserick G. (2007) Recommendations for the forensic diagnosis of sex and age from skeletons, *Homo Gottingen* **58**(1): 75–89.

Rousset M.-M., Boualam N., Delfosse C. and Roberts W. E. (2003) Emergence of permanent teeth: secular trends and variance in a modern sample, *Journal of Dentistry for Children* **70**(3): 208–214.

Sabel N., Johansson C., Kühnisch J., Robertson A., Steiniger F., Norén J. G., Klingberg G. and Nietzsche S. (2008) Neonatal lines in the enamel of primary teeth: a morphological and scanning electron microscopic investigation, *Archives of Oral Biology* **53**(10): 954–963.

Saunders E. (1837) The teeth, a test of age, considered with reference to the factory children. Addressed to the members of both Houses of Parliament. Renshaw, London.

Saunders S., DeVito C., Herring A., Southern R. and Hoppa R. (1993) Accuracy tests of tooth formation age estimations for human skeletal remains, *American Journal of Physical Anthropology* **92**(2): 173–188.

Schmeling A., Olze A., Reisinger W. and Geserick G. (2004) Forensic age diagnostics of living people undergoing criminal proceedings, *Forensic Science International* **144**(2–3): 243–245.

Schmeling A., Reisinger W., Geserick G. and Olze A. (2006) Age estimation of unaccompanied minors. Part i: General considerations, *Forensic Science International* **159** (Suppl. 1): S61–S64.

Schour L. and Massler M. (1941) The development of the human dentition, *Journal of American Dental Association* **28**.

Shi G., Lie R., Tao J., Fan L. and Zhu G. (2009) Application of Demirjian's method for chronological age estimation in teenagers of Shanghai Han population, *Fa Yi Xue Za Zhi* **3**(25): 168–171.

Sisman Y., Uysal T., Yagmur F. and Ramoglu S. I. (2007) Third-molar development in relation to chronologic age in Turkish children and young adults, *Angle Orthodontist* **77**(6): 1040–1045.

Skinner M. and Dupras T. (1993) Variation in birth timing and location of the neonatal line in human enamel, *Journal of Forensic Sciences* **38**(6): 1383–1390.

Smith B. H. (1991). Standards of human tooth formation and dental age assessment. In: Kelley M. A. and Larsen C. S. (eds), *Advances in Dental Anthropology*. New York: Wiley-Liss, pp. 143–168.

Smith E. L. (2005) A test of Ubelaker's method of estimating subadult age from the dentition, *Human Biology*. University of Indianapolis, Indianapolis. Master's thesis.

Smith P. and Avishai G. (2005) The use of dental criteria for estimating postnatal survival in skeletal remains of infants, *Journal of Archaeological Science* **32**(1): 83–89.

Smith T. M., Reid D. J. and Sirianni J. E. (2006) The accuracy of histological assessments of dental development and age at death, *Journal of Anatomy* **208**(1): 125–138.

Solari A. and Abramovitch K. (2002) The accuracy and precision of third molar development as an indicator of chronological age in Hispanics, *Journal of Forensic Sciences* **47**(3): 531–535.

Solheim T. (1990) Dental cementum apposition as an indicator of age, *Scandinavian Journal of Dental Research* **98**: 510–519.

Solheim T. (1993) A new method for dental age estimation in adults, *Forensic Science International* **59**: 137–147.

Solheim T. and Vonen A. (2006) Dental age estimation, quality assurance and age estimation of asylum seekers in Norway, *Forensic Science International* **159** (Suppl. 1): S56–S60.

Staaf V., Mörnstad H. and Welander U. (1991) Age estimation based on tooth development: a test of reliability and validity, *Scandinavian Journal of Dental Research* **99**(4): 281–286.

Stack M. V. (1960) Forensic estimation of age in infancy by gravimetric observations on the developing dentition, *Journal of the Forensic Science Society* **1**(1): 49–59.

Stack M. V. (1967) Vertical growth rates of the deciduous teeth, *Journal of Dental Research* **46**(5): 879–882.

Tanguay R., Buschang P. H. and Demirjian A. (1986) Sexual dimorphism in the emergence of deciduous teeth: its relationship with growth components in height, *American Journal of Physical Anthropology* **69**(4): 511–515.

Tao J., Wang Y., Liu R., Xu X. and Li X. (2007) Accuracy of age estimation from orthopantomograph using Demirjian's method, *Fa Yi Xue Za Zhi* **23**(4): 258–260.

TeMoananui R., Kieser J. A., Herbison G. P. and Liversidge H. M. (2008) Estimating age in Maori, Pacific Island, and European children from New Zealand, *Journal of Forensic Sciences* **53**(2): 401–404.

Thorson J. and Hägg U. (1991) The accuracy and precision of the third mandibular molar as an indicator of chronological age, *Swedish Dental Journal* **15**(1): 15–22.

Tunc E. S. and Koyuturk A. E. (2008) Dental age assessment using Demirjian's method on northern Turkish children, *Forensic Science International* **175**(1): 23–26.

Ubelaker D. H. (1978) *Human Skeletal Remains: Excavation, Analysis, and Interpretation*. Chicago:Aldine Publishing.

Unicef (1989) Convention on the rights of the child. Available from www.unicef.org/crc (accessed: 1 May 2012).

Unicef (2012) Fact sheets: birth registration. Available from www.unicef.org/newsline/2003/03fsbirthregistration.htm (accessed 1 May 2012).

United Nations (2011) International migration in a globalizing world: the role of youth. Technical paper, Department of Economic and Social Affairs: Population Division, New York. 2011/1.

Van der Linden F. P., Wassenberg H. J. and Bakker P. J. (1985a) [Development of the human dentition. I], *Dental Cadmos* **53**(6): 17, 19–29, 31–45.

Van der Linden F. P., Wasenberg H. J. and Bakker P. J. (1985b) [Development of the human dentition. Ii], *Dental Cadmos* **53**(7): 19, 21–22, 25–30.

Van der Linden F. P., Wasenberg H. J. and Bakker P. J. (1985c) [Development of the human dentition. Iii], *Dental Cadmos* **53**(9): 17, 19–36, 39–40.

Van der Linden F. P., Wassenberg H. J. and Bakker P. J. (1985d) [Development of the human dentition. Iv], *Dental Cadmos* **53**(11): 15, 17–18, 23–30.

Voors A. (1973) Can dental development be used for assessing age in underdeveloped communities? *Journal of Tropical Pediatrics & Environmental Child Health* **19**: 242.

Wehner F., Secker K., Wehner H., Gehring K. and Schulz M. (2007) Immunohistochemical proof of amelogenin in teeth: a contribution to the evaluation of the age in the identification of unknown corpses, *Arch Kriminol* **220**(1–2): 44–50.

Whittaker D. K. and Richards D. (1978) Scanning electron microscopy of the neonatal line in human enamel, *Archives of Oral Biology* **23**(1): 45–50.

Willems G. (2001) A review of the most commonly used dental age estimation techniques, *J Forensic Odontostomatology* **19**(1): 9–17.

Wise G. E., Frazier-Bowers S. and D'Souza R. N. (2002) Cellular, molecular, and genetic determinants of tooth eruption, *Critical Reviews in Oral Biology & Medicine* **13**(4): 323–335.

Wolanski N. (1966) A new method for the evaluation of tooth formation, *Acta Genetica (Basel)* **16**: 186–197.

8

Bite marks – I

Douglas R. Sheasby
University of Glasgow, UK

8.1 Introduction

Human bite marks occur in a minority of forensic medico-legal investigations, usually as a result of human beings biting one another. Forensic bite marks occur in a variety of violent crimes, assault, rape, murder and child abuse. Occasionally, forensic bite marks have been reported in food and a miscellaneous group of inanimate materials.

MacDonald (1974) defined a bite mark as 'a mark caused by the teeth either alone or in combination with other mouth parts'. Clearly, a bite mark in skin is evidence of contact between the teeth, either alone or in combination with other mouth parts, and the skin. Consequently, a human bite mark is produced by three contributory components – dentition and/or mouth parts, skin and the episode of contact. The components are variable, as are the inter-relationships between the components of a particular bite mark. In effect, a bite mark is the result of a potentially unique episode of contact between the dentition and/or mouth parts and the skin. The nature of the contact between the biter and the victim can have a major influence on the appearance of the resultant bite mark.

Human bite marks in skin are complex injuries and consequently the main challenge in forensic odontology is the analysis of bite marks in skin. Bite mark analysis is the interpretation and comparison of two pieces of evidence, namely, the photographic record of the bite mark and the dental casts of the suspect biter. The interpretation of the representation of the dentition and/or mouth parts in skin is a complex cerebral process that constitutes the focal point of bite mark analysis.

8.2 Bite mark components

8.2.1 Dentition and mouth parts

A human bite mark in skin is a representation of certain features of the dental anatomy of the biter. The relevant anatomical features are the dental arches, teeth, interproximal

Forensic Odontology: An Essential Guide, First Edition.
Edited by Catherine Adams, Romina Carabott and Sam Evans.

embrasures, tongue, lips, gingivae and palatal rugae. Bite marks are normally produced by the maxillary and mandibular arches and teeth anterior to the second premolars; bite marks are most commonly caused by the biting edges/cusps of teeth.

Dental arches

The dental arch features recorded in a bite mark normally provide the information required to orientate the bite mark. The initial orientation of a bite mark comprising two opposing arcs of marks is determined comparatively by which arc was caused by the maxillary arch and which by the mandibular arch. The maxillary arch is normally larger and is composed of larger incisors and canines compared to the mandibular arch. However, a class III malocclusion may demonstrate a larger mandibular arch than the maxillary arch, although the size of the teeth remains characteristic for each arch. The orientation of a bite mark comprising one arc of marks is determined solely by the size and shape of the arc and the individual tooth elements. Clearly, the maxillary and mandibular arch centre points are important orienting features in bite mark analysis.

Arch size is usually expressed as the *inter-canine distance*. The average adult male maxillary and mandibular inter-canine distances are approximately 34 mm and 27 mm respectively; the average values in adult females are approximately 1 mm less. Rawson *et al.* (1984b) recorded an average maxillary arch width of 32.3 mm in 397 adults.

Arch shape is normally described as a *catenary curve*, which may vary to either a square or V-shape.

Teeth

There are many individual tooth features that are important in bite mark analysis. The presence or absence of a tooth is important; although the apparent absence of a tooth in a bite mark may be false, the tooth could be present but not produce a mark. The location of the mesial and distal incisal angles of incisors determines their width and centre point; similarly, the locations of the cusps of canines are also important individual tooth features. The cusps of first premolars are features that are rarely recorded in a bite mark.

The character of the incisal edges and cusps may be affected by a variety of factors. The functional aspects of occlusion and malocclusion produce incisal and cuspal characteristics. The edges of newly erupted upper and lower permanent incisors show three small tubercles that are worn level with occlusion (Scott and Symons, 1972). However, anterior teeth that are out of occlusion may retain the notches indefinitely; for example, in a class II division I malocclusion. Attrition of incisors and canines has usually been associated with age; however, it is common in much younger groups of both modern and primitive societies (Dahlberg, 1960). Fracture of incisors or canines may result in a deficiency in the incisal/cuspal level that may be represented as either a false absence or a faint element in the bite mark. Alternatively, a fracture may result in an angulation of the incisal edge or cusp that may be represented as a variation in the density of an element in the bite mark. Class IV restorations with a defective incisal cavo-surface angle, crowns with a wider labio/palatal or lingual dimension, prostheses, caries and developmental peg-shaped lateral incisors are further examples of variation in the character of the incisal edges and cusps.

The position or status of a tooth may be expressed as displacement and/or rotation. The interproximal embrasures are important distinguishing features between adjacent teeth. The petechial haemorrhages often seen in bite marks that are associated with the interproximal embrasures provide incisor width information and a representation of the spacing between individual teeth. Duguid and McKay (1981) concluded that tooth position was the most constant feature relative to an ideal dental arch and that embrasure intervals were more variable relative to an ideal dental arch. Consequently, variation in tooth position is of greater statistical significance and variation in embrasure interval is of less statistical significance.

Tongue and other mouth parts

The action of sucking produces a reduced intra-oral pressure that can traumatise the capillaries in the embouched tissue. The occurrence of sucking during biting may introduce a dimensional change in the dental arch components due to obvious ‘tenting’ of the bitten tissue. The presence of a diffuse ovoid zone of bruising within the centre of a bite mark is indicative of sucking activity (Sopher, 1976).

Sucking may be accompanied by tongue thrusting, in which case the appropriate descriptive term is ‘suckling’ (Harvey, 1976; Harvey *et al.*, 1976). The tongue is a muscular organ that can produce pressure marks in the tissue held in the mouth. Tongue pressure marks are caused by a tongue thrusting action forcing the embouched tissue against the palatal and lingual surfaces of the anterior dentition and the anterior palate. The relevant anatomical features are the palatal/lingual tooth surfaces, gingival margins, interproximal embrasures and rugae. The resultant tongue pressure marks may demonstrate patterns of bruising attributable to specific anatomical features (MacDonald, 1974). The marks may be extremely accurate and detailed. The presence of a prosthesis may also be reflected in tongue pressure marks; patterns of diffuse bruising may be due to pressure against a smooth acrylic baseplate; by contrast, patterns of specific bruising may be due to pressure against a chrome cobalt skeleton or a fixed bridge.

Tongue pressure marks due to either sucking or suckling usually occur in cases of an assailant biting a victim.

8.2.2 Skin

The different skin areas of the body surface vary widely in structure and in the degree of development of certain features. Adaptations to varying external conditions take place and considerable change occurs with age (Garven, 1965). Skin, when fully developed, consists of an epidermis, a dermis and a hypodermis.

- The *epidermis* is a highly developed compound epithelium; this is a layer of keratinising stratified squamous epithelium that is avascular, so minor injuries are relatively harmless.

- The *dermis* is a connective tissue layer with many special features; the blood vessels, lymphatic vessels and nerves of the skin are present in the dermis. Skin is visco-elastic owing to the interaction of elastic fibres, collagen fibres and ground substance in the dermis. Langer's lines represent the directional differences of the pre-existing tension lines in skin; these result from the principal axis of orientation of collagen fibres in the dermis. Skin tension is increased along Langer's lines that vary in direction with the region of the body.
- The *hypodermis* or subcutaneous layer extends from the lower surface of the dermis to the underlying structure, muscle, fascia, ligament or bone. In many areas the hypodermis is a layer of adipose tissue.

Skin is considered to be a poor impression medium because it is not dimensionally stable and is not capable of reproducing detail. There are a number of histological and physiological features that have a contributory influence; in particular, these relate to age and anatomical location.

Age

Babies bruise easily, but bruises in babies are sometimes difficult to see because of abundant subcutaneous fat.

According to Gresham (1986), bite marks in children are often faint and difficult to see. An interesting feature of such bite marks is that the initial lesion may fade away only to become visible a few months after injury. The likely explanation for this is that melanocytes tend to migrate slowly to the edges of wounds and they indicate their presence by absorbing ultraviolet light. The wounds may be demonstrated only by ultraviolet photography when a sufficient quantity of melanocytes has collected at the wound edges.

Important changes take place in the skin with ageing. In old age, the epidermis is very much thinned. The elastic fibre content of the dermis decreases with age; in old age, the dermis is relatively avascular and elastic fibres have almost disappeared. The aged person bruises easily owing to poor collagen support of blood vessels, so slight pressure can produce an extensive bruise.

In contrast to infants and old people, teenagers and adults bruise less easily (Harvey, 1976; Gresham, 1986).

Anatomical location

In certain anatomical locations the hypodermis binds the tissues above tightly to those below, so little movement between the two is possible. Examples are the nose, scalp, pinna of the ear, finger pads, palms, sole and plantar surface of toes. In other locations the two parts, skin and underlying tissues, slide on one another freely; for example, eyelids, penis and scrotum. Bruising develops more easily in soft, vascular, lax tissues such as the eyelids than in tough and less vascular ones such as the palm of the hand or the sole of the foot (Simpson and Knight, 1985). Laceration occurs more readily in sites where the skin is relatively fixed to unyielding bone, such as the scalp (Gresham, 1986).

The contour or shape of the body varies depending on the anatomical location. In effect the quantity of tissue available for biting varies in different locations. The scalp is an example of minimal available tissue whereas the female breast is usually an example of maximum available tissue. Obesity increases the available tissue. The quantity of tissue available for biting is important because soft tissue absorbs and dissipates the kinetic energy of biting to a greater extent than hard tissue. Consequently, skin overlying soft tissue will be subjected to significantly lower levels of pressure than skin overlying hard tissue. The ability to absorb kinetic energy is directly proportional to the quantity of soft tissue.

Bite marks usually occur in skin that is not covered by clothing. The presence of clothing at the time of biting reduces the degree of tooth pressure on the skin. The effect can mask the details in the resultant bite mark and may even be responsible for the absence of particular tooth injuries; for example, maxillary lateral incisor injuries may be absent, but this finding should not necessarily be interpreted as indicative of absent lateral incisors (Sopher, 1976). Clearly, the thickness of clothing is important; the thicker the clothing, the greater is the reduction in the degree of tooth pressure on the skin.

8.2.3 Episode of contact

The dynamics of the action of human beings biting one another are produced by an extensive number of component factors – force, pressure, time, relationship of mandible to maxilla, movement of assailant and victim, nature of bite and mental status of victim and assailant. The factors are variable, as are the inter-relationships and consequently, the dynamics of the action of humans biting one another are complex.

The degree of force and pressure exerted by the dentition on the skin can range from a minimal contact, to a degree of holding of the tissue, to incision and avulsion of the tissue.

The dynamics of movement involve variations in speed, acceleration and angle of contact. The movement of the assailant and/or victim can range from static to extreme movement. The mental status of the victim and the assailant are the conditioning factors of movement. The range in movement is exemplified in certain cases; bite marks that are clearly defined and appear to have been inflicted slowly and deliberately with little movement, probably as part of a sexual act; by contrast, bite marks that are poorly defined as a result of extreme movement during a violent attack and/or defence.

The nature of biting can range from amorous to aggressive with concomitant bite mark severity (MacDonald, 1974). An amorous bite mark, 'love bite', occurs during the sexual arousal of lovers. The mark is usually bruising caused by sucking and perhaps by gentle nibbling with the anterior teeth. The mark is characterised by diffuse bruising in the centre; individual tooth marks are not a feature. By contrast, an aggressive bite mark is inflicted with the intention of causing pain. The marks relate mostly to teeth; the teeth marks usually form an ellipse leaving a central area relatively unmarked; alternatively, the teeth marks constitute scrape marks due to movement between the teeth and skin.

Bites are painful injuries and consequently the mental status of the victim is relevant to the episode of contact. When the victim is conscious and cerebral function is unaffected by other factors, the response to pain is either fight or flight; the resultant movement has an influence on the appearance of the bite mark. Alternatively, the victim's mental status may be affected by sexual arousal, alcohol and/or drug intoxication; in these cerebral conditions, the pain threshold is elevated and consequently a greater degree of injury may be tolerated by the victim. When the victim is unconscious or dead, response is non-existent and consequently more extensive injury is possible. Similarly, the assailant's mental status may be affected by anger, sexual arousal, alcohol and/or drug intoxication and these cerebral conditions may further potentiate the assailant's actions.

The variable and complex nature of the dynamics of human beings biting one another indicates that every episode of contact between the dentition and/or mouth parts and the skin is potentially a unique event. Variation in the episode of contact is illustrated in multiple bite marks that vary in appearance and are caused by a single biter in one victim (Whittaker and MacDonald, 1989). The ability to reproduce a bite mark would depend on an identical episode of contact which in practical terms is difficult to conceive. The view that a bite mark is not reproducible was expressed by Levine (1977). The indication that every episode of contact is a unique event would mean that every bite mark is unique for a particular episode of contact; this raises another hypothetical possibility, that different dentitions could produce similar bite marks.

8.3 Nature of the injury

The shape of a single bite mark is usually oval or almost circular. Occasionally, multiple bite marks are superimposed on one another which results in variations in the shape of the overall mark. The occurrence of a variety of other injuries superimposed on a bite mark is a rare complicating factor.

The injuries in skin are caused by the surface anatomy of the teeth – the biting edge or cusp produces crush injuries. The angle between the biting surface and the long axial surface causes damage due to marked flexion and extension of the skin as it is sharply deformed round the angle. The interproximal embrasure produces petechial haemorrhages due to skin stretching across the embrasure or skin being forced into the embrasure. In these various ways, teeth impress their shape and surface markings in skin. Owing to its elastic nature, skin is capable of absorbing considerable kinetic energy prior to the level of pressure required to produce visible injury (Sopher, 1976). At the time of injury, particular tooth mark indentations will be present; however, the passage of time results in a smoothing out of the tooth indentations owing to the visco-elastic nature of skin and its ability to reconstitute to its original contour.

The degree and type of tissue injury is determined by the severity of the bite, which can range from a minor contact to extreme clenching of the tissue. Consequently, the bite mark can demonstrate considerable variation in the degree and type of injury ranging from mild bruising to avulsion of the bitten tissue (MacDonald, 1974; Sopher, 1976; Whittaker and MacDonald, 1989). The degree and type of injury may be related to the nature of the crime. In addition, there are a number of general factors that influence the response of skin to injury – age, anatomical location, sex (females bruise more readily than males), systemic disease, and certain conditions and medications increase the bleeding tendency (Sopher, 1976). Variation in the severity of the bite and the influence of general factors result in bite marks that may vary markedly in appearance and duration.

At the microscopic level, the tissue response to biting is characterised by evidence of polymorphonuclear leucocytes within a few hours; evidence of granulation tissue occurs within 24–48 hours (D. G. MacDonald, personal communication,1992). These findings are dependent on a circulation and blood pressure and consequently the histological findings have a contributory value when considering the time of injury relative to the time of death.

Bite marks in skin are composed of one or more of the following injuries: bruise, abrasion, laceration (Sopher, 1976; Gresham, 1986).

Bruise

A bruise or contusion in skin is usually caused by contact with a blunt object (Gresham, 1986). The pressure of the contact disrupts capillaries, allowing extravasation of blood into the dermis; the surface may or may not be intact. Blood will spread along normal tissue planes from the injury and a coloured area develops. Owing to the breakdown of haemoglobin, the colour changes through a spectrum of red, brown, purple, green and yellow in the first week after injury. Gravity may cause the bruise to change position. According to Sopher (1976), due to the diffusion of haemorrhage, a phenomenon that may persist post-mortem, the area of a bruise related to a particular tooth or portion thereof will be slightly larger than the surface area that caused the injury. Indeed, the shape of a bruise may or may not bear a good relation to the contour of the tooth. This process of diffusion is responsible for the fading or haziness of the bite mark with time and the subsequent loss of what otherwise may represent an individual characteristic.

Abrasion

An abrasion is a superficial injury of the skin where the surface layer of epidermis is rubbed off either by a sliding force or by direct pressure (Gresham, 1986). According to Gresham, abrasions can be subdivided into scratches, grazes and imprint abrasions due to pressure. Scratches demonstrate heaping of the epidermis at the finishing edge of the scratch. Similarly, when a sharp incisal edge or cusp scrapes across the surface of skin, the movement may produce heaping of the epidermis at the point where the tooth movement stops. Grazes are a form of scratch produced by injury from a rough surface and the pattern of grazing will depend on the nature of the surface. Imprint or pressure abrasions are produced by localised pressure to the skin.

Laceration

A laceration involves the splitting of the full thickness of the skin by a blunt injury (Gresham, 1986). According to Gresham, lacerations are often accompanied by bruising and abrasion of the wound edges.

8.4 Bite mark incidence

Bite marks occur in a variety of violent crimes, assault, rape, murder and child abuse. The crimes involve varying degrees of violence; assault and murder may also be sex-related. Bite marks are found on all anatomical sites. Over 40% of victims have more than one bite mark and many have bite marks on more than one part of the body (Vale and Noguchi, 1983). Consequently, when one bite mark is discovered, a complete body examination of the victim should be conducted. According to Vale and Noguchi, in female victims, bite marks are most common on the breasts, arms and legs; in male victims, the arms and shoulders are the most common sites. The morbidity associated with significant bites is well recognised (Mann, 1977; Burton *et al.*, 1981).

The circumstances of biting are variable in adults. The usual occurrence is the assailant biting the victim; the victim biting the assailant occurs infrequently. Rarely the victim has a self-inflicted bite mark, for example, when the victim's hand is forced into the victim's mouth to stifle screaming. Bite marks are not usually observed in cases of natural death; however, self-inflicted bite marks can occur extremely rarely in two ways. Self-biting may be an emotional response to pain or a type of counter-irritation to alleviate pain, for example, during myocardial ischaemia (Warnick *et al.*, 1987). Self-biting is a type of self-destructive behaviour that has been described in individuals who are mentally retarded or psychologically disturbed (Altmeyer *et al.*, 1985; Sobel and Perper, 1985). Most bite marks noted in a medico-legal death investigation are associated with violent death; consequently, self-inflicted bite marks are rarely seen in cases referred for medico-legal death investigation.

The circumstances of biting are less variable in children. Usually there are a very limited number of people who have the opportunity to abuse the child; the abuser is usually the biter (Levine, 1977; Sopher, 1977). The occurrence of children biting other children during play has to be recognised as an innocent bite mark. Similarly, self-inflicted bite marks in mentally retarded children are innocent and are related to attention-seeking behaviour. Rawson *et al.* (1984a) reported an epidemic of biting activity in a selected group of children in care. There is a perception that the incidence of non-accidental injury to children is increasing either in real terms or in increased reporting.

Bite marks on the victim and/or the assailant have been caused by either the other party, self or a third party. Consequently, the practical application is to examine all suspect dentitions in the relevant time-line of a bite mark case. In the case of a suspected self-inflicted bite mark, the anatomical location is the significant consideration – is it physically possible for the bite mark to have been self-inflicted?

8.5 Principles of bite mark analysis

8.5.1 Distortion

A recurring difficulty in analysis arises from the distortion which is a variable feature of bite marks. The term 'distortion' is defined as 'a twisting awry; deformation without breaking; crookedness' (Chambers, 1989). In the context of a bite mark, distortion may modify the appearance or the photographs of a bite, such that it is not an exact image of the features of the dentition and/or mouth parts of the biter. Distortion may complicate or even preclude the valid comparison of a bite mark with a suspect biter's dentition. A review of trial transcripts reveals that distortion and the interpretation of distortion are the main factors in contentious cases (Rawson *et al.*, 1986a).

Distortion can occur at different stages in the causation and investigation of bite marks. *Primary distortion* may occur at the time of biting. *Secondary distortion* may occur subsequent to a bite mark being made or be introduced at the stage when a bite mark is being examined or recorded (Sheasby and MacDonald, 2001).

Primary distortion

The two main components of primary distortion are dynamic distortion due to the dynamics of the biting process and tissue distortion due to the nature of skin (Sheasby and MacDonald, 2001). Dynamic and tissue distortion are complex and unpredictable phenomena that are closely related because of their simultaneous occurrence during the episode of contact between the dentition and skin.

Dynamic distortion may be produced by the dynamics of the action of biting (Rawson, 1982). The degree of movement between the teeth and skin can range from essentially nil in static bite marks to extreme in tooth scrape marks. Dynamic distortion is directly proportional to the degree of movement. The dynamic event is composed of multiple component movements by the assailant and/or the victim during the episode of contact between the teeth and skin. Consequently, every episode of contact is potentially a unique event; accordingly, a dentition can produce bite marks that exhibit variations in appearance. This phenomenon is illustrated in cases of multiple bite marks produced by a single biter in the same anatomical location in one victim; the bite marks vary in appearance due to variation in the episode of contact between the teeth and skin (Whittaker and MacDonald, 1989).

Tissue distortion is due to the nature of skin (Barbanel and Evans, 1974; Rawson and Brooks, 1984). Skin is an elastic medium capable of distortion due to pressure and reconstituting to its original contour when the pressure is removed. Skin elasticity, due to elastic fibres in the dermis, varies depending on age and anatomical location. Langer's lines represent the directional differences of the pre-existing tension lines in the skin. Skin tension, due to collagen fibres in the dermis, is increased along Langer's lines. Skin is visco-elastic owing to the interaction of elastic fibres, collagen fibres and ground substance in the dermis. The phenomenon of stretching and relaxing produces a variable degree of tissue distortion in all bite marks. Tissue distortion can also arise due to oedema produced in response to biting (Barbanel and Evans, 1974).

The quantity of tissue available for biting is another contributory factor in tissue distortion. When a quantity of tissue is taken into the mouth, this may produce 'tenting' of the tissue which results in dimensional changes in the skin. Clearly, the quantity of tissue taken into the mouth is subject to variation.

Secondary distortion

According to Sheasby and MacDonald (2001), there are three categories of secondary distortion:

- Time-related distortion occurs when a bite mark changes in appearance with the time elapsed subsequent to the bite being made.
- Posture distortion and photographic distortion occur during the examination and evidence recording of a bite mark.

Time-related distortion in living victims can take different forms. Where there is a laceration or where a segment of tissue has been bitten off, the subsequent healing can involve changes, particularly tissue contraction, which can modify the dimensions and detail of a bite mark. In a bruise, the changes with time can result in migration of part of the bruise to a slightly different anatomical location. The bruise may also diffuse variably, giving an altered shape.

Posture distortion occurs when a bite mark is viewed or recorded in a position that is different from the position of the anatomical location at the time of biting. The degree of posture distortion depends on the variation in body position and anatomical location. The greater the variation in body positions between the time of biting and evidence recording, the greater the likely degree of posture distortion. Different anatomical locations potentially demonstrate varying degrees of posture distortion. Marked posture distortion can be observed in a limb depending on the degree of flexion and extension and in the female breast depending on the body position and arm position (Figures 8.1 and 8.2). Posture distortion occurs, to a lesser extent, in the torso related to limb position and in the neck related to head position.

In order to minimise posture distortion during photography, it is necessary to attempt to reconstruct a victim's body position at the time of biting (DeVore, 1971). Clearly this ideal is not always possible and, if not, it is suggested that bite marks are photographed in a range of positional possibilities (Bernstein, 1985). Reconstruction of a victim's known body position at the time of biting or the reconstruction of a range of positional possibilities is most applicable to a live victim. In cases involving a dead victim, the body position at the time of biting is unknown and the reconstruction of a range of possible body positions is not so readily achieved. Therefore, the possible occurrence of posture distortion may be more difficult to account for in dead victims.

The morphology of the female breast can be altered by body position and also by wearing a brassière. In bite mark cases involving a bitten female breast, it is important to establish whether the victim was wearing a brassière. In cases where a brassière was worn, the reconstruction of the known body position of the victim at the time of biting will also require the actual brassière to be worn. When a bite mark occurs in the skin beyond the edge of the brassière, it is possible to reconstruct the body position wearing the actual brassière and photograph the bite mark, thereby minimising any potential posture distortion in the photographs. When a bite mark occurs through the brassière, it is still possible to reconstruct the body position and photograph the bite mark; however, the photographs of the bite mark will record an unknown degree of posture distortion due to the absence of the brassière.

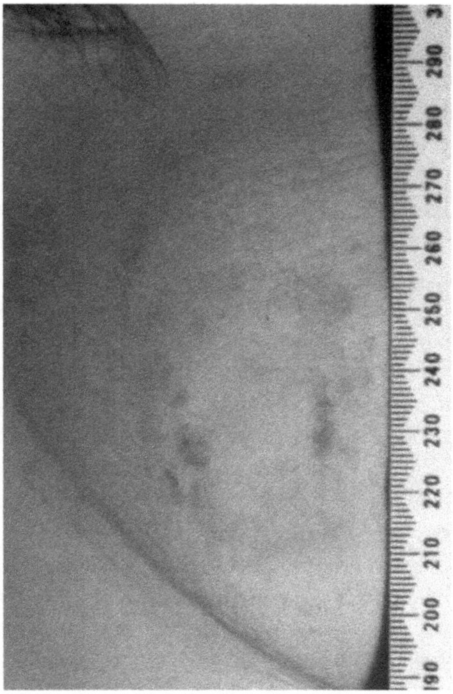

Figure 8.1

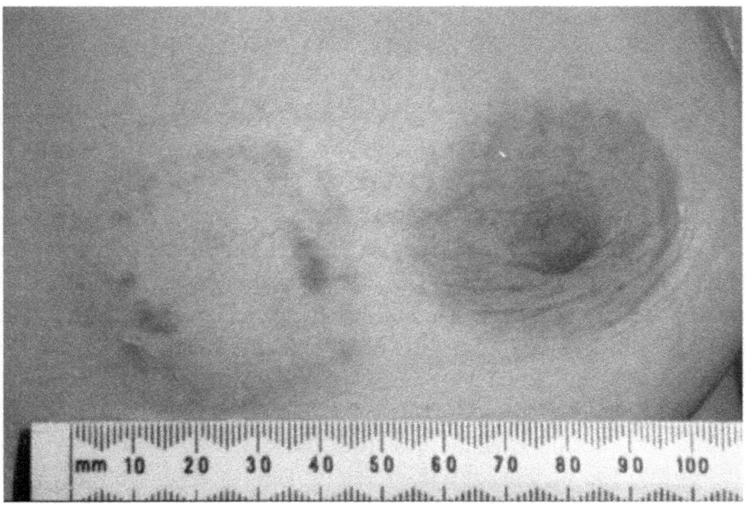

Figure 8.2

Posture distortion in a bite mark on the right breast photographed on successive days with the right arm raised to an unknown position on day 1 (Fig. 8.1) and the arm down by the victim's right side on day 2 (Fig. 8.2). The police photographer was not supervised by an odontologist. The photographs demonstrate posture distortion that produced a significant variation in the size and shape of the bite mark. The variation measures approximately 25% in the vertical axis and 12.5% in the horizontal axis (For colour details, please see colour plate section.)

Photographic distortion may be produced by the photographic method of recording a bite mark (Stimson, 1982). Photographic distortion arises as a result of the influence of the angle of the film to the bite mark and body curvature. The ideal photographic angle is 90 degrees, the camera being perpendicular to the centre of the bite mark (Rawson *et al.*, 1986a). This angle produces parallelism between the film/digital plane and the bite mark plane and consequently photographic distortion is minimised. Variation from the perpendicular will produce photographic distortion in proportion to the extent of the variation. In effect, moving the camera to one side or the other of the bite mark creates photographic parallax. The American Board of Forensic Odontology Bite Mark Guidelines Committee (Rawson *et al.*, 1986a) suggested that a circular scale should be included in photographs, to permit accurate calculations of the photographic angle and to allow correction for any distortion caused by improper angulation. If the roundness of the circular scale is re-established in the superimposition process, then the photographic distortion in the bite mark is also corrected. This suggestion resulted in the development of the bite mark standard reference scale – ABFO no. 2 (Hyzer and Krauss, 1988). The plane of the scale must be parallel to the bite mark plane and on the same level.

According to Rawson *et al.* (1986a), a curved body surface that allows visualisation of the entire bite mark has a surface angle too small to produce significant photographic distortion. This statement can only be made if the entire bite mark can be viewed from one direction. If the body curvature is so great as to obscure part of the bite mark, then the surface angle is large enough to cause significant photographic distortion and multiple photographs would have to be taken of the various parts of the bite mark.

Discussion of distortion

A bite mark may demonstrate more than one type of distortion. Some degree of distortion is probably present in all bite marks and may be produced by a variety of factors (Barbanel and Evans, 1974; DeVore, 1971; Levine, 1977; Rawson *et al.*, 1986a). Consequently, an exact match in arch size is fortuitous and unpredictable, questioning the significance of this criterion. Clearly, exact superimposition is possible only in bite marks exhibiting minimal distortion. The objective of accurate reproduction of a bite mark must be considered in perspective. The intention is not to produce exact superimposition, but rather to preserve maximum visual information and reduce secondary distortion in an already unpredictably distorted finding.

The degree of distortion present in a bite mark is variable and affects arch size and shape. Clearly, size-matching techniques are applicable only to bite marks exhibiting minimal distortion. The incidence of discrete morphological points of comparison and distinctive features in a bite mark are the most significant criteria in bite mark analysis. This is partly due to their relative immunity to distortion. As the degree of distortion increases, bite mark analysis relies progressively more on distinctive features. The role of superimposition-based analysis is to demonstrate comparability/incomparability between the size, shape and position of the features identified in the photographs of the bite mark and the teeth of the suspect biter, taking account of all possible types of distortion.

8.5.2 Uniqueness of the human dentition

Bite mark analysis is based on two postulates (Hale, 1978):

1. The characteristics of the anterior teeth that caused the bite mark are unique.
2. This asserted uniqueness of the anterior teeth is accurately recorded in the bite mark.

Initial statistical research into the uniqueness of the human dentition was conducted by MacFarlane *et al.* (1974). The authors studied certain characteristics of the maxillary and mandibular incisors and canines in 200 dental casts of adults. The authors noted the number and shape of each tooth, the presence of incisal restorations, the relationship of teeth to arch form and four categories of tooth rotation. The study demonstrated that certain characteristics were not inter-related, and consequently, the products of their incidences could be used to indicate an overall frequency. However, certain features, such as the mesiopalatal rotation of the maxillary central incisors, were inter-related. This finding, that certain features were not independent, provided significant evidence that the product rule could not be applied to the statistical assessment of the uniqueness of the human dentition. The authors concluded that the study had not confirmed the uniqueness of the human anterior teeth.

Historically, the generally accepted view had been that the human dentition was unique, except perhaps in identical twins. However, Sognnaes *et al.* (1982) concluded that, in terms of dental arch form and individual tooth position, the dentitions of five pairs of young adult male monozygotic twins were not dentally identical.

Rawson *et al.* (1984b) aimed to confirm the unique nature of the anterior segment of the human dentition statistically. The study examined the maxillary and mandibular incisors and canines; each of the 12 teeth had six selected positions – buccal, lingual, mesial, distal, mesial rotation and distal rotation. The objective of the research was to determine the statistical probability of different individuals having these 12 teeth in matching positions. The study sample consisted of 397 bites selected from 1200 bites from various locations in the United States. The sample bites were selected to be representative of the general population. Each bite was recorded in wax 1 mm thick which was coated on each side of hard cardboard also 1 mm thick. The bite was registered in protrusion such that the incisal edges of the six maxillary and six mandibular teeth were recorded in the wax to a depth of 1 mm. A calibrated 1 cm scale was also impressed in the wax. The bite mark indentations were filled with zinc powder, radiographed and hand-traced on to gridded computer paper. The position of each tooth was recorded to allow for a ± 1 mm variation in the centre point and for a ± 5 degree variation in the angle of rotation. A number of possible positions were determined for each tooth; the individual probabilities were multiplied to establish an overall probability for the study sample. The authors concluded that the probability of finding two dentitions with all six anterior teeth in the same position was 1.4×10^{13}. With an assumed world population of 4×10^{9}, Rawson stated that a match of five teeth in a bite mark would be sufficient evidence to positively identify an individual as the biter to the exclusion of all others. Unfortunately, the authors incorrectly assumed that the position of each tooth was independent of the positions of the other anterior teeth.

Consequently, the calculation of the overall probability was based on the inappropriate application of the product rule to multiple the individual probabilities. Pretty (2006) concluded that Rawson had proved the uniqueness of the human dentition, although perhaps not to the statistical certainty expressed in the paper.

Clearly, further research was required to determine the uniqueness of the human dentition. Kieser *et al.* (2007) used geometric morphometric techniques to study the individuality of the human dentition. The incisor and canine occlusal surfaces of 50 randomly selected, post-operative orthodontic casts of 17 to 20 year olds of both sexes formed the material for the study. Only individuals with post-orthodontic normal occlusion and unrestored teeth were selected because the authors expected this group to display a lower level of individuality than the general population. The orthodontic casts were scanned and the images were saved in JPEG format. Two landmarks and two semi-landmarks located on each occlusal surface of the incisors and canines were used to describe the maxillary and mandibular anterior dentition. The geometry of the morphology of the occlusal surfaces was captured by a new family of geometric morphometric methods. These recorded subtle differences about the morphological variation and the relative spatial location of the individual occlusal surfaces; in addition, these methods recorded a good description of overall arch form. The study demonstrated that there were clear differences in the shape and form of the anterior dental arcade. The main shape variation seemed to be related to general changes in the depth and width of the arcades. These differences were greater than those due to the relative position of teeth or their individual morphology. However, when individuals with a very similar arcade shape were superimposed, differences in tooth orientation were still evident. The authors noted that in the present sample, selected to have lower levels of individuality than the general population, there were no two individuals with identical tooth morphology. Kieser concluded that the study supported the postulate of the uniqueness of the human anterior dentition.

Bowers and Pretty (2009) stated that there was general acceptance that the teeth of an individual were unique, although the degree to which a particular individual's dentition was unique would vary.

8.5.3 Representation of uniqueness

The second postulate that bite mark analysis is based on is that the uniqueness of the anterior dentition is accurately recorded in the bite mark (Hale, 1978). The recording medium for a human bite mark is skin and the recording process occurs during a potentially unique episode of contact between the teeth and skin. Clearly, these factors are not conducive to the accurate recording of the unique features of the dentition and/or mouth parts in skin.

The experimental bite marks which Rawson *et al.* (1984b) analysed were recorded statically in wax. The position of each tooth was recorded to allow for a ± 1 mm variation in the centre point and for a ± 5 degree variation in the angle of rotation. These tolerances were relevant to the statistical confirmation of the unique nature of the human anterior dentition. Rawson stated that a match of five teeth in a bite mark would be sufficient evidence to positively identify an individual as the biter to the exclusion of all others. The validity of this statement depends on three factors:

- the accurate representation of the teeth in skin to Rawson's tolerances
- the assumption that the odontologist correctly interprets the representation
- Rawson's statistics.

The unique features of the anterior dentition are rarely represented accurately and completely in human bite marks in skin to satisfy Rawson's tolerances. The interpretation of the representation of uniqueness is dependent on the evidential value of the bite mark and the competence of the odontologist. Pretty (2006) concluded that Rawson had proved the uniqueness of the human dentition, although perhaps not to the statistical certainty expressed in the paper. Clearly, statements regarding uniqueness are not transferable to the representation of uniqueness of the teeth in skin. Kieser *et al.* (2007) suggested that the unique features of the anterior incisal surfaces would not necessarily be transferred to a bitten substrate.

One of the questions posed in bite mark analysis is: how accurate or distorted is the representation of the uniqueness of the dentition in the skin? The representation of uniqueness is influenced by primary and secondary distortion. Primary distortion may occur during the episode of contact between the teeth and skin. The effects of dynamic and tissue distortion are complex, unpredictable and difficult to recognise and interpret. Primary distortion is, to an unknown and variable degree, intrinsic in a bite mark. Consequently, it is not possible to prevent or limit the effects of dynamic and tissue distortion. Secondary distortion may occur subsequent to a bite mark being made and/or during evidence recording. Time-related distortion is usually easily recognised, but interpretation may be complex. Posture and photographic distortion may occur during the photographic recording of the appearance of a bite mark. It is the responsibility of the odontologist to recognise and manage potential posture and photographic distortion. Consequently, it may be possible to limit the effects of posture and photographic distortion during evidence recording by the odontologist supervising the photographer. However, an important distinction exists in cases where the photographs were taken without supervision and these may have recorded an unknown degree of these types of distortion.

Bite marks demonstrate considerable variation in appearance, ranging from a mild bruise without identifiable features to an accurate and complete representation of the dentition and/or mouth parts. Clearly, the recognition and assessment of the evidential value of a bite mark is important in bite mark analysis. Pretty (2007) produced a bite mark severity and significance scale to demonstrate and simplify the relationship between bite mark severity and the forensic significance of a bite mark. The scale describes six categories of bite mark severity ranging from very mild bruising to complete avulsion of tissue. The scale is linear with respect to bite mark severity: level 1 is the lowest and level 6 is the highest level of severity. However, the scale is not linear in respect of the forensic significance of a bite mark: levels 3 and 4 represent marks of high forensic significance and levels 1, 2, 5 and 6 represent marks of low forensic significance. In effect, the forensic significance of a bite mark increases from the extremes of severity to the two middle categories which are positively identified as human bite marks. The forensic significance in the scale is related to the gross, class and unique characteristics of a dentition that are observed in a bite mark: marks that demonstrate either gross characteristics or a few class characteristics are of low forensic significance; marks that show numerous unique characteristics are of high forensic significance. Clement and Blackwell (2010) commented on the value of this scale in determining the forensic significance of a bite mark, and thus in selecting a mark that was amenable to bite mark analysis. Avon *et al.* (2010) suggested research to evaluate the evidentiary value of bite marks using a standard reference scale such as the one developed by Pretty.

Pretty and Sweet (2010) also commented on the selection of bite marks that were amenable to analysis; accordingly, they referred to bite marks that had a high forensic significance and that exhibited minimal distortion. The authors expressed the view that these conditions were essential for meaningful bite mark analysis; the converse view was also expressed that a level of forensic significance be determined, below which bite marks should not be analysed. Bowers and Pretty (2009) examined 49 bite marks in cases that had been the subject of an appellate proceeding in the United States; the bite mark evidence was part of the appeal hearing in each case. The bite marks were allocated a forensic significance score; the mean bite mark significance scores were evaluated against crime type, experts' opinion and judicial outcome. The authors reported that the study sample consisted of bite marks with low forensic significance scores; this was related to the contentious nature of the cases which introduced a degree of bias in the sample. This metric assessment demonstrated a clear relationship between the forensic significance of a bite mark and the experts' opinion. Marks that were assessed of low forensic significance were more likely to result in disagreement between experts; conversely, marks of higher forensic significance were more likely to result in agreement. The study provided statistical evidence to support the hypothesis that, below a certain level of forensic significance, a bite mark cannot be analysed reliably. Further research is required to determine the threshold level of the forensic significance score that would justify proceeding with bite mark analysis.

8.5.4 Interpretation of representation of uniqueness

Interpretation of the representation of the uniqueness of the human dentition in a bite mark in skin is the focal point of bite mark analysis. The key question is whether the degree of correlation between a bite mark and a dentition can be determined reliably (Rawson *et al.*, 1986b). Experimental research of bite marks in human skin is, by its nature, difficult to conduct. Consequently, previous studies have mainly used experimental bite marks in animal skin or artificial media. One study demonstrated that the dentition that produced test bites in wax was recognised with a high degree of reliability by examiners; however, experimental bite marks produced in non-vital pig skin demonstrated a much lower degree of reliability by the examiners determining the causal dentition (Whittaker, 1975). Similarly, experimental bite marks produced without movement in vital dog skin demonstrated a low degree of reliability by examiners determining the dentition that caused the mark (Rawson *et al.*, 1986b).

Ström (1963) considered details more important than the numbers of teeth in a bite mark and emphasised the importance of identifying characteristic details of the biter's teeth that may be recorded in the bite mark. The importance of distinctive features was also emphasised by Keiser-Nielson (1967). Dinkel (1974) stated that there was no specific number of points of comparison required to identify the biter. Subsequently, the Bite Mark Guidelines Committee of the American Board of Forensic Odontology (1986) formulated a system of scoring each bite mark according to overall arch size and shape, tooth positions and morphology. The scoring system was developed with the basic premise that unusual features were weighted compared to usual features in a bite mark. Consequently, the scoring system produced a high score for an unusual tooth in an unusual position; in effect, the scoring system was designed to reflect the evidential value of a bite mark in numerical terms. Rawson *et al.* (1986b) concluded that the American Board of Forensic Odontology scoring system demonstrated a method of evaluation that produced a high degree of reliability between odontologists. Additionally, it demonstrated the ability to differentiate between different degrees of comparability between a bite mark and teeth, high scores supporting a high confidence level in the identification of the biter. Furthermore, Rawson stated that, if a bite mark was analysed by a group of odontologists independently and there was a high level of agreement between the examiners, this provided further evidence in support of the confidence level expressed in the conclusions of the analyses. Similarly, Ström (1963) and Ligthelm and de Wet (1983) stated that there was greater certainty if a positive identification of a biter was confirmed by more than one odontologist analysing a bite mark independently.

Research has continued into the interpretation of the representation of the uniqueness of the dentition in skin. Pretty and Sweet (2001) assessed the ability of experienced odontologists to use computer-generated overlays on artificial bite marks in pig skin; the authors reported reasonable results, although the intra- and inter-examiner reliability scores were not strong. Miller *et al.* (2009) investigated the possibility of identifying the biter from a group of similar dentitions. Groups of similar dental models were impressed in various anatomical locations in human cadaver skin; the indentations were photographed. The authors noted that it was not possible to identify the actual biter from the group of biters with similar dentitions. The paper indicated that human skin as a bitten medium prevents the differentiation of bite marks caused by similar dentitions. Bush *et al.* (2009) assessed the effect of posture distortion on a bite mark produced by a single biter. A single dental model was impressed in various anatomical locations in human cadaver skin; the indentations were photographed with the body position unaltered and re-photographed with the body in a different position. The authors stated that not one of the bite marks made by the same dentition was measurably identical. The paper demonstrated that posture distortion alters the dimensions and shape of a bite mark significantly.

Stols and Bernitz (2010) applied the mathematical concept of affine transformations to a bite mark case. This showed that mathematically calculable affine transformation had occurred during biting and that the bite mark was a distorted representation of the biter's dentition. The technique depended on the selection of three points on the biter's dentition that corresponded with three points in the bite mark; this selection demonstrated an interpretation of the representation of the biter's dentition in the bite mark by the odontologist. The paper showed that the interpretation of the representation of the biter's dentition in a minimally distorted bite mark could also be confirmed mathematically.

Clement and Blackwell (2010) commented on the natural human tendency of seeing what one wants to see, thereby tempting examiners to over-interpret bite marks.

8.6 Bite mark evidence recording

8.6.1 Initial examination of the alleged/suspected bite mark

The aim of the initial examination of the alleged/suspected bite mark is to determine whether it can be identified as a human bite mark. In order to do this, it is preferable that it be viewed directly. Marks that are identified as human bite marks are double swabbed for DNA analysis if possible. The collection of forensic biological specimens is undertaken by forensic scientists to satisfy forensic and legal considerations in the UK.

The details of the case are recorded in contemporaneous notes, which subsequently provide important case information for the bite mark analysis report. The time of biting is confirmed and the time of the initial examination is also noted. The chronology of events from the time of biting through the various stages of evidence recording is important in two respects:

1. The appearance of the bite mark will alter with the time elapsed from the time of biting. Consequently, it is preferable that the initial examination and the photography of the bite mark are conducted at the earliest stage of the investigation. Clearly, the appearance of the mark between the time of biting and the commencement of photography will remain unknown.
2. The potential for change to the anatomy of the suspect biter's anterior teeth will increase with the time elapsed between biting and the dental examination. This time lapse may extend by many months.

The clinical examination of the bite mark records its anatomical location and determines the number of bite marks present. The location may raise the possibility of self-infliction. In living subjects, it may be possible to record the body position of the victim and the orientation of the assailant to the victim at the time of biting. The presence and thickness of clothing covering the skin at the time of biting is noted. Bite marks occasionally exhibit indentations that may be recorded by an impression. The impression is obtained by the odontologist and transferred to the dental technician who pours master and duplicate dental stone casts. The casts are signed and dated by the technician and odontologist.

There are significant differences in the evidence recording of bite marks in living and dead victims. In general terms, information is more limited in cases where the victim is dead. The time of biting, the victim's body position and assailant's orientation at the time of biting, and the presence of clothing may all be unknown in dead victims.

The contemporaneous notes detail relevant information known to the odontologist and refer to relevant information that is unknown.

8.6.2 Photography of the bite mark

The next stage of evidence recording is photography of the bite mark. These photographs constitute evidence and are subject to the legal rules governing the admissibility of evidence in the UK. One aspect of admissibility depends on proof of the continuity of evidence recording; this is satisfied by the police photographing the bite mark, thereby ensuring that the photographs are accepted as admissible evidence by the court. The appropriate photography of the bite mark depends on the recognition and management of the distortion that occurs in bite marks; this is the responsibility of the odontologist who supervises the police photographer. This combination of personnel satisfies the legal and forensic considerations implicit in the photography of bite marks.

The initial photograph is a facial view of the victim for identification and evidential purposes; this is followed by a general view showing the location of the bite mark. A number of photographs will be required in cases of multiple bite marks in various anatomical locations. The next photograph is a view of the bite mark without the presence of a scale; this demonstrates that the scale in subsequent views is not obscuring any evidence.

Bite mark analysis requires life-size, scaled photographs of the bite mark for comparison with the dental casts of the suspect biter. A bite mark standard reference scale, similar to the ABFO no. 2 scale, is used to produce these scaled photographs. The odontologist holds the rigid, right-angled scale adjacent to the bite mark; the plane of the scale must be parallel to the bite mark plane and the two planes must be coincident (Figure 8.3). The police photographer holds the camera perpendicular to the centre of the bite mark; this angle produces parallelism between the film/digital plane and the bite mark plane. This technique minimises photographic distortion in the photographs of the bite mark.

In living victims where the body position at the time of biting is known, the bite mark is photographed with the body in the same position. This technique minimises posture distortion. Where the body position at the time of biting is unknown, the bite mark is also photographed in a range of positional possibilities (Figures 8.4, 8.5 and 8.6); this procedure records the potential occurrence of posture distortion in the photographs. Different anatomical locations may predispose to varying degrees of posture distortion. When a bite mark occurs in an anatomical location, which is susceptible to posture distortion, it is essential that the bite mark is also photographed in a range of possible positions. This procedure records the occurrence of an unknown degree of posture distortion in the photographs of the bite mark.

In dead victims the body position at the time of biting is unknown and the reconstruction of a range of body positions is limited. Therefore, the possible occurrence of posture distortion in a bite mark may be more difficult to record and demonstrate in photographs of a bite mark in dead victims. Similarly, when a bite mark occurs in an anatomical location which is susceptible to posture distortion, the occurrence and degree of posture distortion may be more difficult to record.

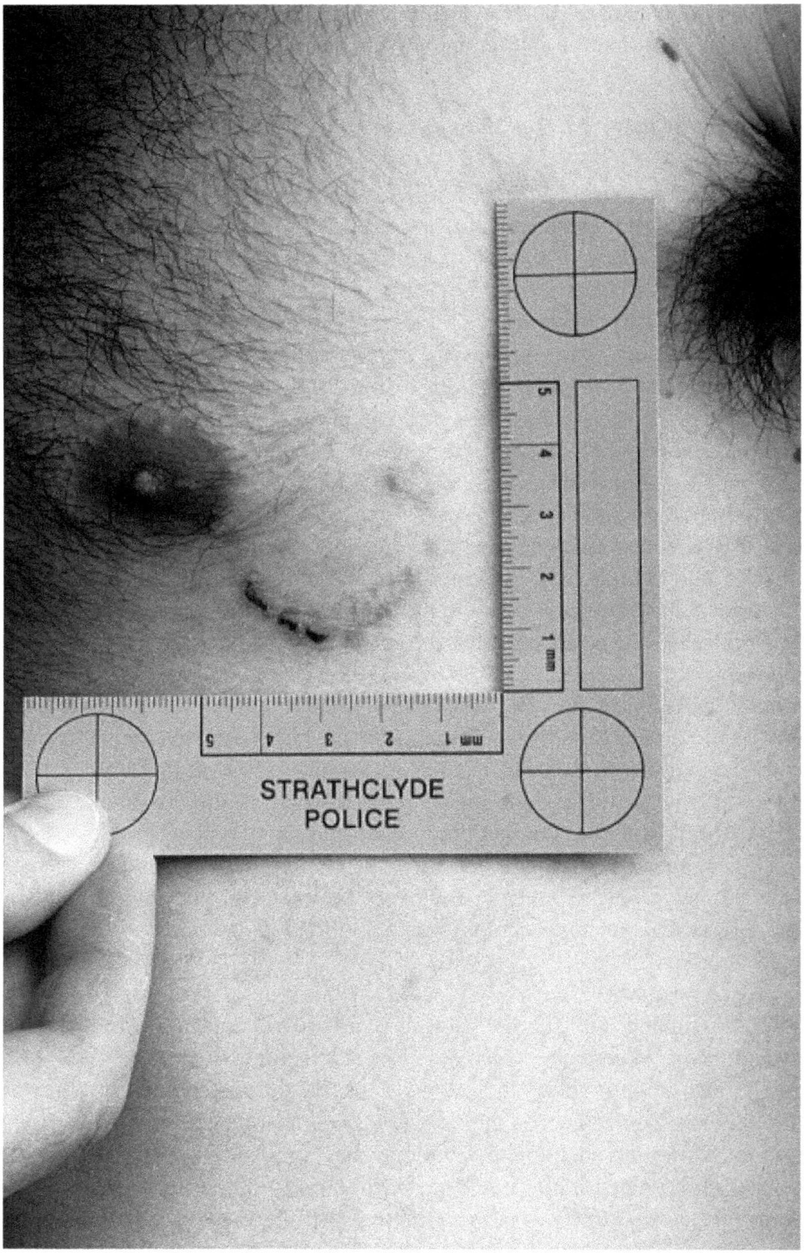

Figure 8.3 The odontologist holds the ABFO no. 2 type scale adjacent to the bite mark. The planes of the scale and bite mark must be parallel and coincident (For colour details, please see colour plate section.)

In cases where the curvature of the anatomical location prevents a single view of the entire bite mark, multiple scaled photographs taken perpendicularly to the centre of the various parts of the overall mark are required. This technique minimises photographic distortion in each of the photographs of the bite mark (Figures 8.7, 8.8 and 8.9).

The appearance of marks in both living and dead victims alters with time. It is not possible to predict the point in time when a bite mark will demonstrate maximum evidential value; consequently the photographic sequence should be repeated, which could be daily, until the mark fades. The dates of all photography are noted in the contemporaneous notes.

The photographs are routinely taken in colour and printed in colour and in black and white. The photographs are printed life-size in order that they can be compared with the dental casts of the suspect biter. The dimensional accuracy of the photographs of the bite mark is confirmed by placing a metric scale against each axis of the scale in the photograph. The coincidence of the scales in each axis also verifies that the scale in the photograph is parallel to the film plane.

The photographs taken by police photographers are likely to be produced digitally without a filter. Specialist photographic filters may be used with infrared or ultraviolet or other methods of illumination in exceptional circumstances. These techniques sometimes reveal the presence of earlier injuries that may not be visible to the naked eye.

The photography of bite marks in live victims is preferably conducted in a photographic studio. Bite marks in dead victims are photographed in the mortuary.

8.6.3 Dental examination of the suspect biter

The final stage of evidence recording is the dental examination of the suspect biter. This is usually conducted in a dental surgery in the presence of an appropriate chaperone. The dental examination is part of a criminal investigation, so it has legal authorisation and instruction. The odontologist confirms the suspect's name, informs the suspect of what the examination involves and requests a signed acceptance to the examination. The suspect has the legal right to refuse to undergo the dental examination; refusal is binding on the odontologist and, clearly, has adverse legal consequences for the suspect.

The contemporaneous notes record the date, location and names of the persons in attendance at the dental examination. The odontologist confirms the date and details of the suspect's latest dental treatment with particular reference to the maxillary and mandibular anterior teeth. The suspect is questioned about accidental or non-accidental damage/alteration to the front teeth from the time of biting and the details are recorded. It is important to note that any change to the anatomy of the anterior teeth between the time of biting and the dental examination may limit valid bite mark analysis.

The clinical dental examination records the teeth present, restorations present, tooth mobility and the presence of a removable prosthesis. The incisal edges of the upper and lower incisors and the cusps of the upper and lower canines and premolars are examined in detail and the findings recorded. Upper and lower complete arch dental impressions are obtained; where a removable prosthesis is worn, the impressions are obtained with and without the denture *in situ*. The occlusion is recorded.

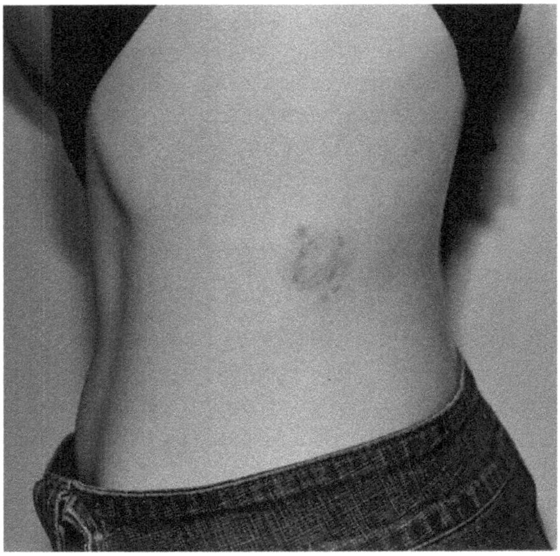

Figure 8.4 General photograph showing the location of a bite mark on the left side of the torso

The upper and lower impressions are identified by the odontologist and transferred to the dental technician who pours master and duplicate, upper and lower, dental stone casts. The casts are signed and dated by the technician and odontologist, thereby demonstrating the continuity of evidence recording. This procedure ensures that the dental casts are accepted as admissible evidence by the court.

8.7 Bite mark analysis techniques

8.7.1 Biological comparison

Sweet *et al.* (1997) pioneered the work on the recovery of salivary DNA from bite marks. The techniques are objective and offer a scientifically validated method of bite mark analysis. However, the techniques are expensive and require extensive laboratory equipment and expertise. It should also be noted that DNA can become degraded and is susceptible to environmental factors. According to Pretty (2003) there is an increasing use of DNA technology by odontologists in bite mark cases. The use of DNA technology in bite mark analysis satisfies the rules on the admissibility of expert witness testimony in the United States because of the large number of peer-reviewed publications supporting its use, including data on error rates and reliability.

Borgula *et al.* (2003) and Rahimi *et al.* (2005) researched the genotyping of oral bacteria, mostly oral streptococci. With over 2000 species in an individual's mouth it may be possible to develop a bacterial identity for each individual.

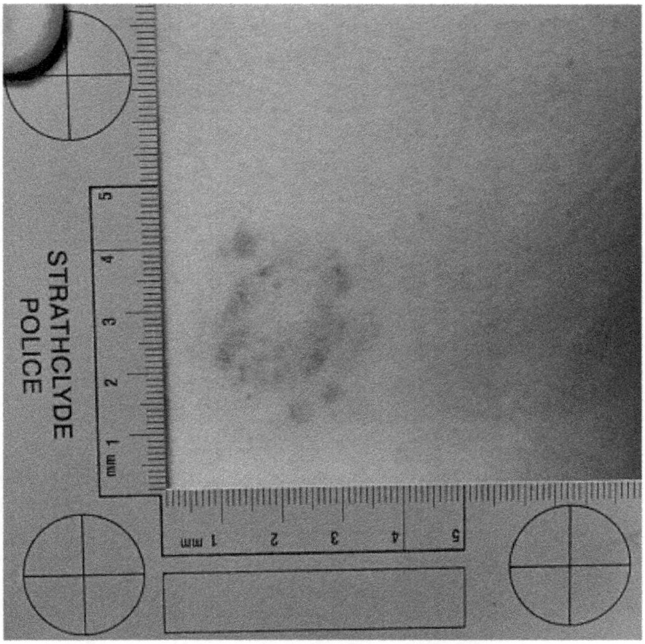

Figure 8.5

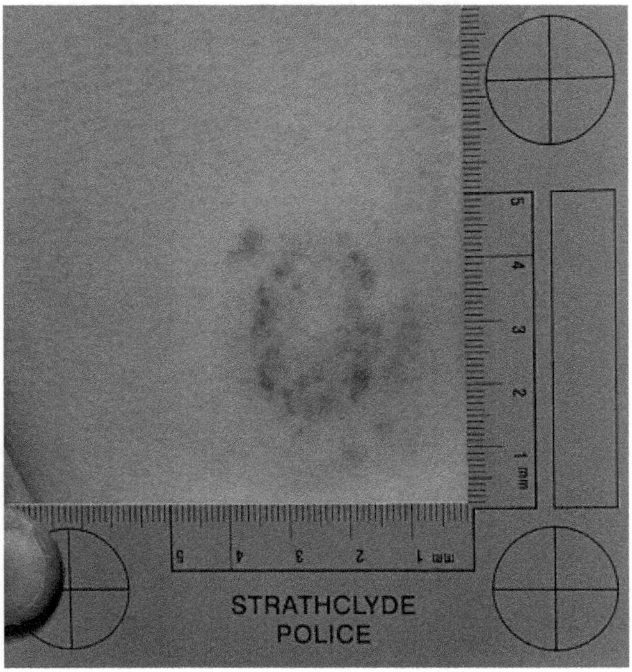

Figure 8.6

Scaled photographs of the bite mark on the torso with the victim standing vertically (Fig. 8.5) and standing and bending from the waist forwards (Fig. 8.6), taken under the supervision of an odontologist. The photographs demonstrate posture distortion that produced a variation in the shape of the bite mark

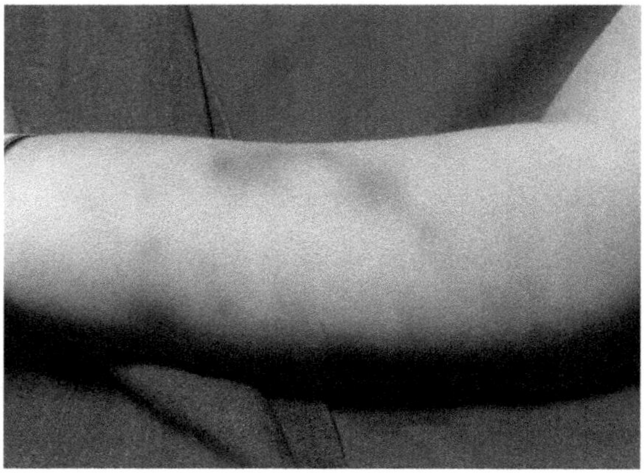

Figure 8.7 General photograph showing the location of a bite mark on the opposing surfaces of the child's left forearm. The entire bite mark cannot be viewed from a single direction; to minimise photographic distortion, the opposing surfaces of the forearm are photographed separately

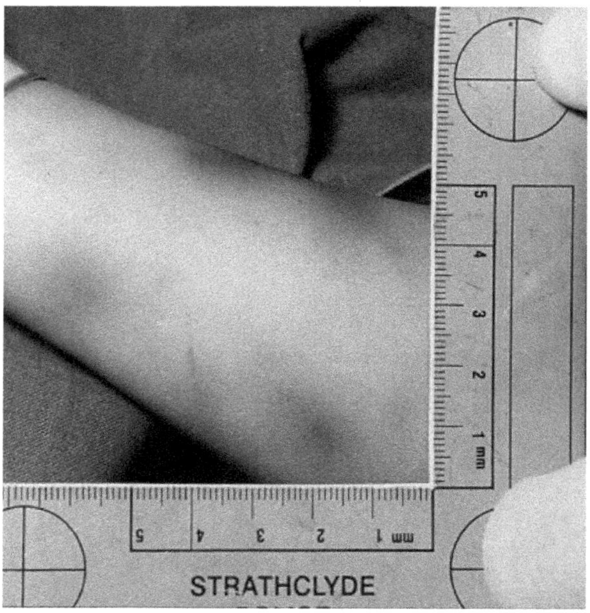

Figure 8.8 Scaled photograph of the arc of marks on the posterior surface of the left forearm taken under the supervision of an odontologist

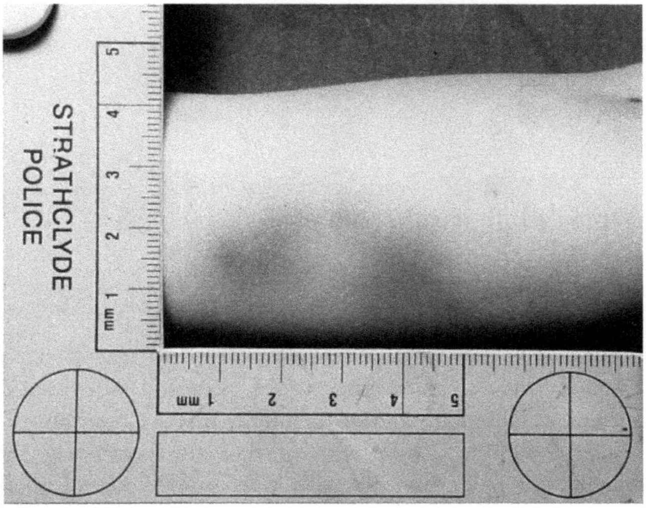

Figure 8.9 Scaled photograph of the arc of marks on the anterior surface of the left forearm taken under the supervision of an odontologist

8.7.2 Physical comparison

The first recorded technique of bite mark analysis was called 'odontoscopy' and was developed by Sörup in 1924 (Ström, 1963). Subsequently, numerous other techniques have been developed; these include using confocal, reflex and scanning electron microscopes, complex computer systems, special light sources, fingerprint dusting powder, 3-dimensional laser scanning of dental casts and overlays (Pretty and Sweet, 2001; Pretty, 2006).

It is widely accepted that the dominant technique currently used for the comparison of the photographs of a bite mark with the dental casts is transparent overlays. Sweet and Bowers (1998) compared five common techniques of producing transparent overlays of the dental casts. The authors used 30 randomly selected study casts to examine tooth rotation and biting surface area. The authors concluded that computer-generated transparent overlays were the most accurate method with respect to the representation of rotation and area; furthermore, they advised this technique over any other method. Sweet and Bowers commented that the accuracy of the computer-generated overlays introduced an objective technique into bite mark analysis; however, they also recognised that the subsequent comparison of the overlay to the photograph of the bite mark was largely a subjective process. Pretty (2006) noted that there are numerous techniques for the production of computer-generated overlays; European odontologists often employ the Naru technique, while American odontologists prefer either the Sweet method or the Bowers modification of it.

Bite mark analysis is the interpretation and comparison of the photographs of a bite mark with the dental casts of a suspect biter. The comparison process consists of two physical comparison techniques, namely, feature-based analysis and superimposition-based analysis (see later).

8.7.3 Principles of physical comparison

Class and individual characteristics

The human dentition demonstrates anatomical features that may be classified as class characteristics and individual characteristics. The class and individual characteristics of the maxillary and mandibular anterior dentitions may be represented in a mark in skin. The representation of class characteristics forms the basis of the identification of the mark as a human bite mark. The representation of individual characteristics forms the basis of the identification of the causal dentition.

The class characteristics of the maxillary and mandibular anterior dentitions are related to the shapes and sizes of the teeth and arches. The incisors usually produce four linear/rectangular marks in the centre of each arc of marks. The maxillary incisors normally produce larger marks than the mandibular incisors. The average dimensions of the incisal edges of upper central and lateral incisors are 8–9 mm and 6–7 mm respectively. The average dimensions of lower central and lateral incisors are less disparate, being 5.5 mm and 6 mm respectively. The canines produce either circular, triangular or diamond-shaped marks towards the end of each arc of marks. The shape of the anterior dental arch is normally described as a catenary curve. The maxillary inter-canine distance is normally larger than the mandibular measurement. The actions of sucking and suckling produce marks in skin that also constitute class characteristics of human bite marks.

The individual characteristics of the maxillary and mandibular anterior dentitions are related to the distinctive features of the incisors and canines. The teeth may be displaced and/or rotated. The incisal/cuspal edges may be distinctive due to fracture, function, developmental abnormality, caries and restorative treatment. The adjacent teeth may be spaced, for example an upper median mid-line diastema.

Metric and non-metric analysis

The terms metric and non-metric analysis are appropriate for use in bite mark analysis nomenclature (Krauss, 1984).

- Metric analysis is the absolute comparison using physical measurements of the class and individual characteristics contained in a bite mark and the dental casts of a suspect.
- Non-metric analysis is the associative comparison of the class and individual characteristics contained in a bite mark and the dental casts of a suspect.

Thus, the terms metric and non-metric analysis are synonymous with objective and subjective analysis respectively. The analysis initially involves a series of fundamental questions that are answered by the odontologist making objective and subjective assessments; these are complementary in nature with a varying proportion of objective and subjective assessments in any given conclusion. The level of objective and subjective assessment will depend on the question posed and the competence of the odontologist.

The questions posed of the presence or absence and the position of individual tooth elements in the bite mark are relatively simple; however, the questions posed of the detail of individual tooth elements are more complex. The questions posed to determine the evidential value of the bite mark are a mixture of relatively simple and complex. The questions posed of the examination of the dental casts are relatively simple. In general terms, the more complex the question, the higher the level of subjective assessment exercised in the conclusion. The level of subjective assessment inherent in the comparison process may be moderated by conducting bite mark analysis on an iterative basis. The comparison process is repeated with a significant time interval or washout period between consecutive comparisons until the subjective assessments are consistent; the number of repeat comparisons required to achieve consistency in the subjective assessments is variable. Clearly, subjective assessment is an unquantifiable and variable factor in bite mark analysis. Duguid and McKay (1981) noted that it was not possible to eliminate the subjective element from bite mark analysis. Indeed, Avon *et al.* (2010) commented that bite mark analysis may be entirely subjective.

The level of objective and subjective assessment in any conclusion also depends on the competence of the odontologist. In general terms, the higher the level of competence, the lower the level of subjective assessment exercised in the conclusion. The competence of the odontologist depends on a natural aptitude that has undergone appropriate training, qualification and subsequent experience. The 'seeing' ability (Rawson *et al.*, 1986b) and the powers of observation of the odontologist are variable and difficult to assess. Nordby (1992) distinguished between seeing and observing: seeing is a physical state, a photochemical excitation that produces a neurological experience; observing is an experience enriched by knowledge, beliefs, values, theoretical commitments, and the goals or purposes for looking in the first place. The odontologist is confronted with the problem of the objective and subjective interpretation of the evidence in a bite mark case. Nordby also distinguished between observation and interpretation: observation involves implicit reasoning, is instant and is a mental experience; interpretation involves explicit reasoning and deliberate thinking. The initial series of fundamental questions and subsequent conclusions provide the basis for the comparison of the photographs of a bite mark with the dental casts of a suspect biter; the comparison involves observing and interpreting points of comparability and incomparability. Comparability is more difficult to observe and interpret than incomparability.

Context effects and observer bias

According to Page *et al.* (2012), context effects are psychological influences on decision making induced by knowledge of extraneous circumstantial information; cognitive bias refers to the psychological sway toward one opinion versus another due to having extraneous information. Context effects give rise to motivational bias and may also give rise to cognitive bias, particularly when there is ambiguity in the choice between two alternative hypotheses. Consequently, odontologists are susceptible to motivational and cognitive bias because of having circumstantial case information and the nature of bite mark evidence respectively. Clearly, context effects can be minimised by limiting the circumstantial case information available to the odontologist prior to bite mark analysis. Page suggested different odontologists collect and analyse the bite mark evidence to further reduce context effects and observer bias in the analysing odontologist.

8.7.4 Feature-based analysis

The analysis involves a number of stages that are conducted in a prescribed sequence: examination of the bite mark photographs, preparation of a predictor of the causal dentition, examination of the dental casts of the suspect biter, and finally comparative study. The entire process is termed 'feature-based analysis'.

Examination of bite mark photographs

Comparison of the photographs with the dental casts of the suspect biter is valid only if the photographs are life-size. The dimensional accuracy of the photographs is confirmed by placing a metric scale against each axis of the rigid, right-angled scale in the photograph. The coincidence of the scales in each axis also verifies that the scale in the photograph is parallel to the film plane.

The examination commences with the recognition and interpretation of the features in the photographs. The odontologist is seeking an explanation for the overall mark and the individual elements in the mark. The initial determinations are that the mark is a human bite mark and it is of a size and shape that is usually seen. The general features that are relevant to comparative analysis are the orientation of the bite mark, the arch centre point, arch size and arch shape; these are recognised by posing the following respective questions:

- Can the maxillary and mandibular arches be oriented in the bite mark?
- Can the arch centre point be determined?
- Can the arch size and inter-canine distance be determined?
- Can the arch shape be determined?

The orientation of the arches is possible because the maxillary arch is usually represented by the larger arc composed of larger individual tooth elements. The arch centre point and arch size may be difficult to assess if the arch representation consists of an incomplete arc. The maxillary and mandibular arch representation is usually oval or almost circular.

The individual tooth elements that may be recorded in the bite mark are the upper and lower central incisors, lateral incisors, canines and first premolars. The

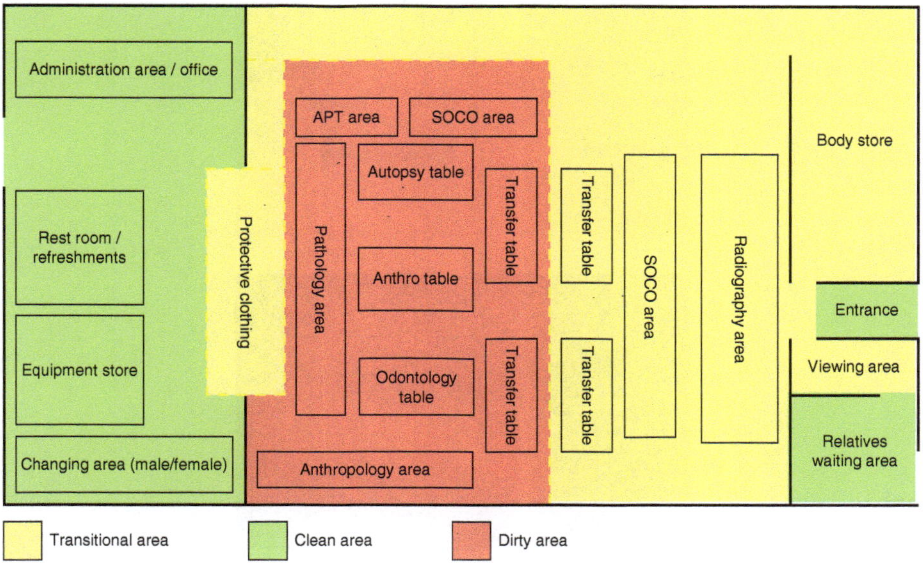

Plate 4.1 Delineation of clean, dirty and transitional areas in a temporary mortuary. APT, Anatomical Pathology Technologist; SOCO, Scenes of Crime Officer

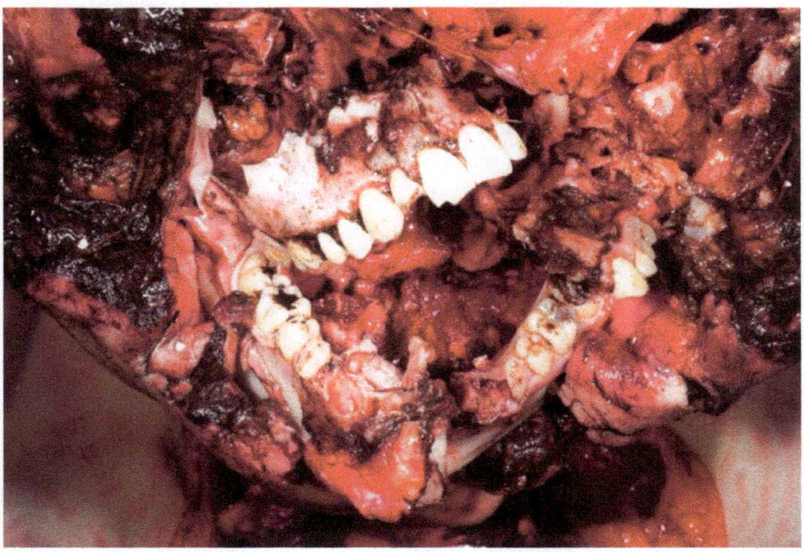

Plate 5.1 Severe facial trauma. Courtesy of Dental Illustration Unit, Cardiff University

Forensic Odontology: An Essential Guide, First Edition.
Edited by Catherine Adams, Romina Carabott and Sam Evans.

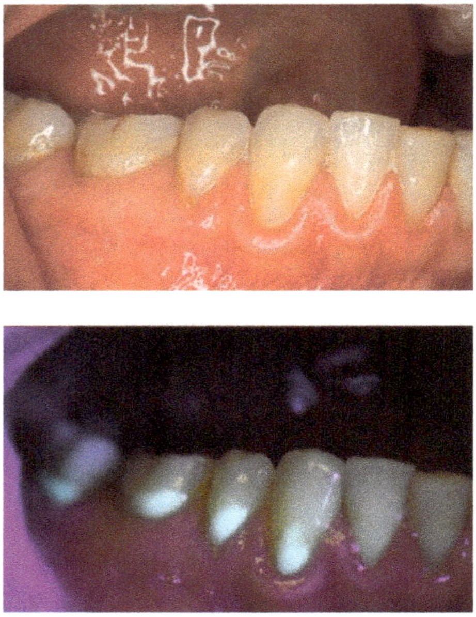

Plate 5.6 Composite fillings seen in normal light and with ultraviolet (395 nm) illumination

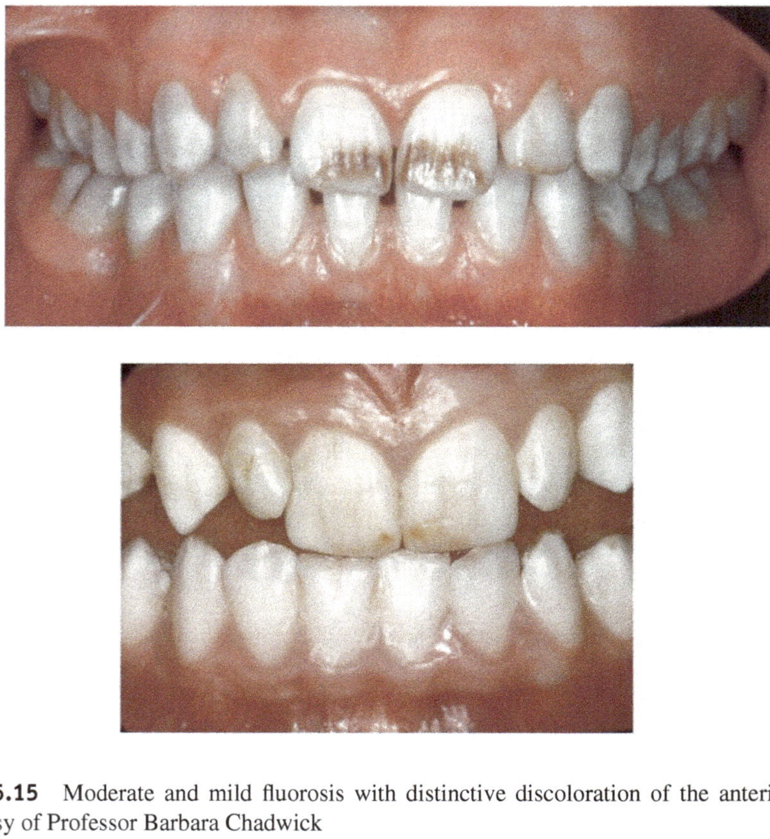

Plate 5.15 Moderate and mild fluorosis with distinctive discoloration of the anterior teeth
Courtesy of Professor Barbara Chadwick

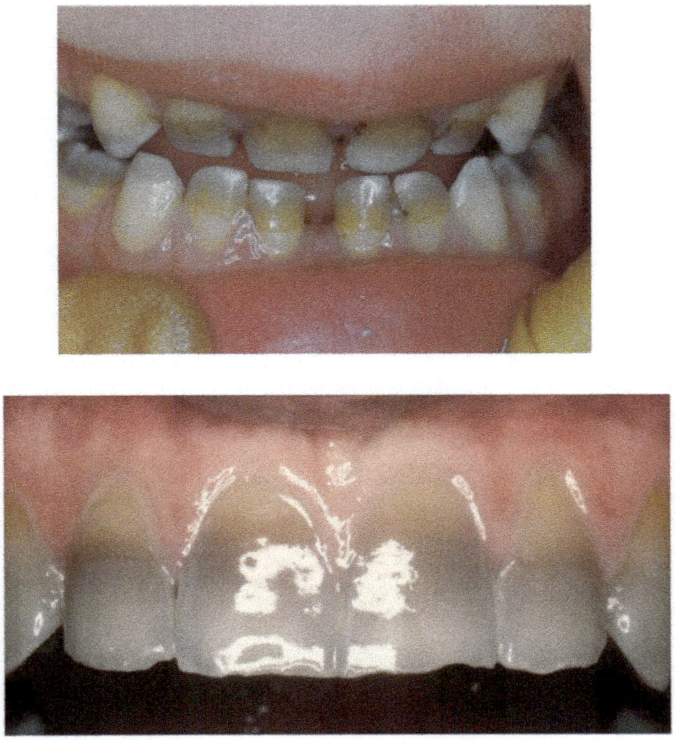

Plate 5.16 Tetracycline staining in deciduous and adult dentition (unrelated cases). Courtesy of Professor Barbara Chadwick

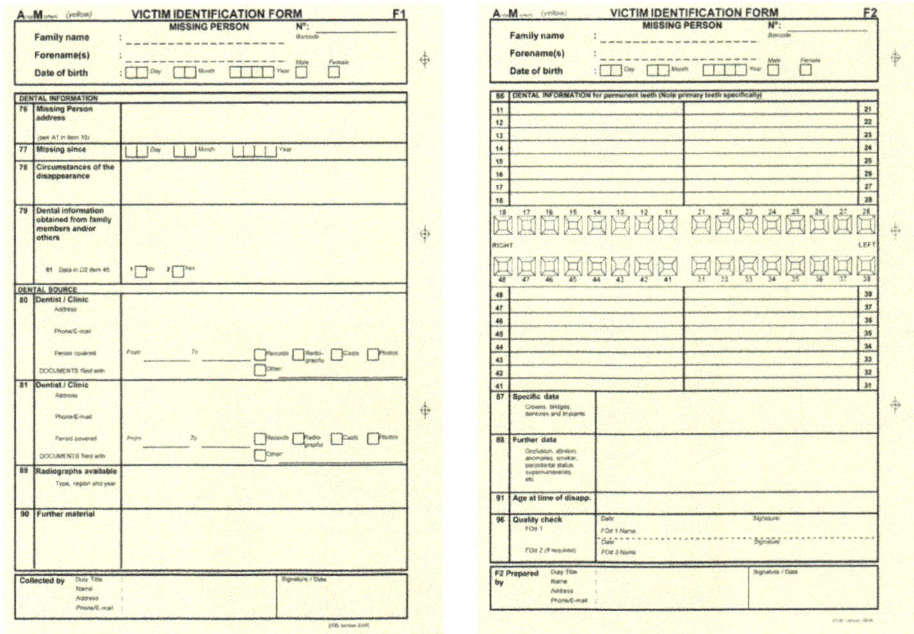

A AM (yellow) VICTIM IDENTIFICATION FORM F1
MISSING PERSON N°:
Family name :
Forename(s) :
Date of birth : Day Month Year Male Female
DENTAL INFORMATION
76 Missing Person address
77 Missing since Day Month Year
78 Circumstances of the disappearance
79 Dental information obtained from family members and/or others
DENTAL SOURCE
80 Dentist / Clinic
81 Dentist / Clinic
89 Radiographs available
90 Further material
Collected by

AM (yellow) VICTIM IDENTIFICATION FORM F2
MISSING PERSON N°:
Family name :
Forename(s) :
Date of birth : Day Month Year Male Female
86 DENTAL INFORMATION for permanent teeth (Note primary teeth specifically)
RIGHT LEFT
87 Specific data
88 Further data
91 Age at time of disapp.
96 Quality check
F2 Prepared by

Plate 6.2 F1 and F2 ante-mortem Interpol forms

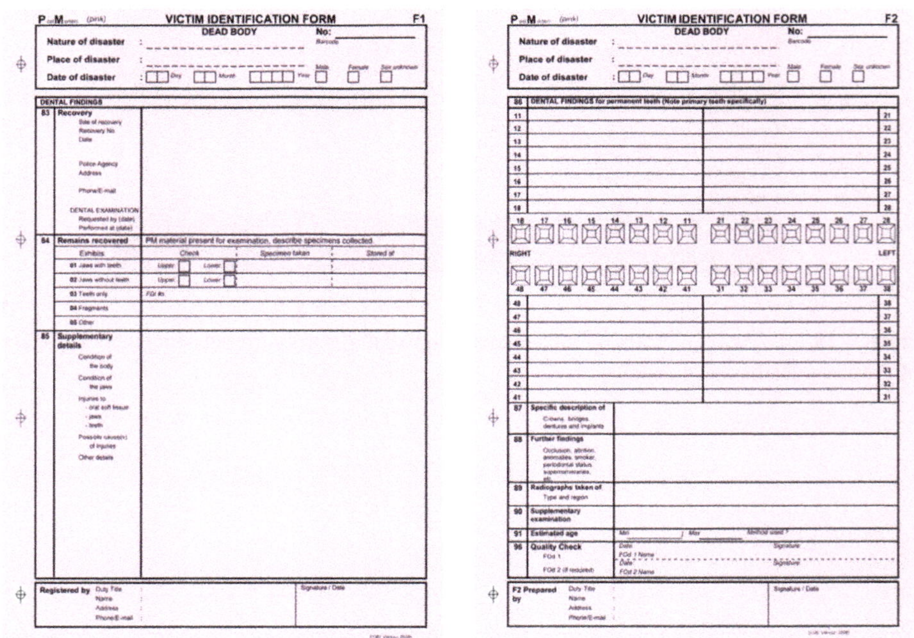

PM (pink) VICTIM IDENTIFICATION FORM F1
DEAD BODY No:
Nature of disaster :
Place of disaster :
Date of disaster : Day Month Year Male Female Sex unknown
DENTAL FINDINGS
83 Recovery
84 Remains recovered
85 Supplementary details
Registered by

PM (pink) VICTIM IDENTIFICATION FORM F2
DEAD BODY No:
Nature of disaster :
Place of disaster :
Date of disaster : Day Month Year Male Female Sex unknown
86 DENTAL FINDINGS for permanent teeth (Note primary teeth specifically)
RIGHT LEFT
87 Specific description of
88 Further findings
89 Radiographs taken of
90 Supplementary examination
91 Estimated age
96 Quality Check
F2 Prepared by

Plate 6.3 F1 and F2 post-mortem Interpol forms

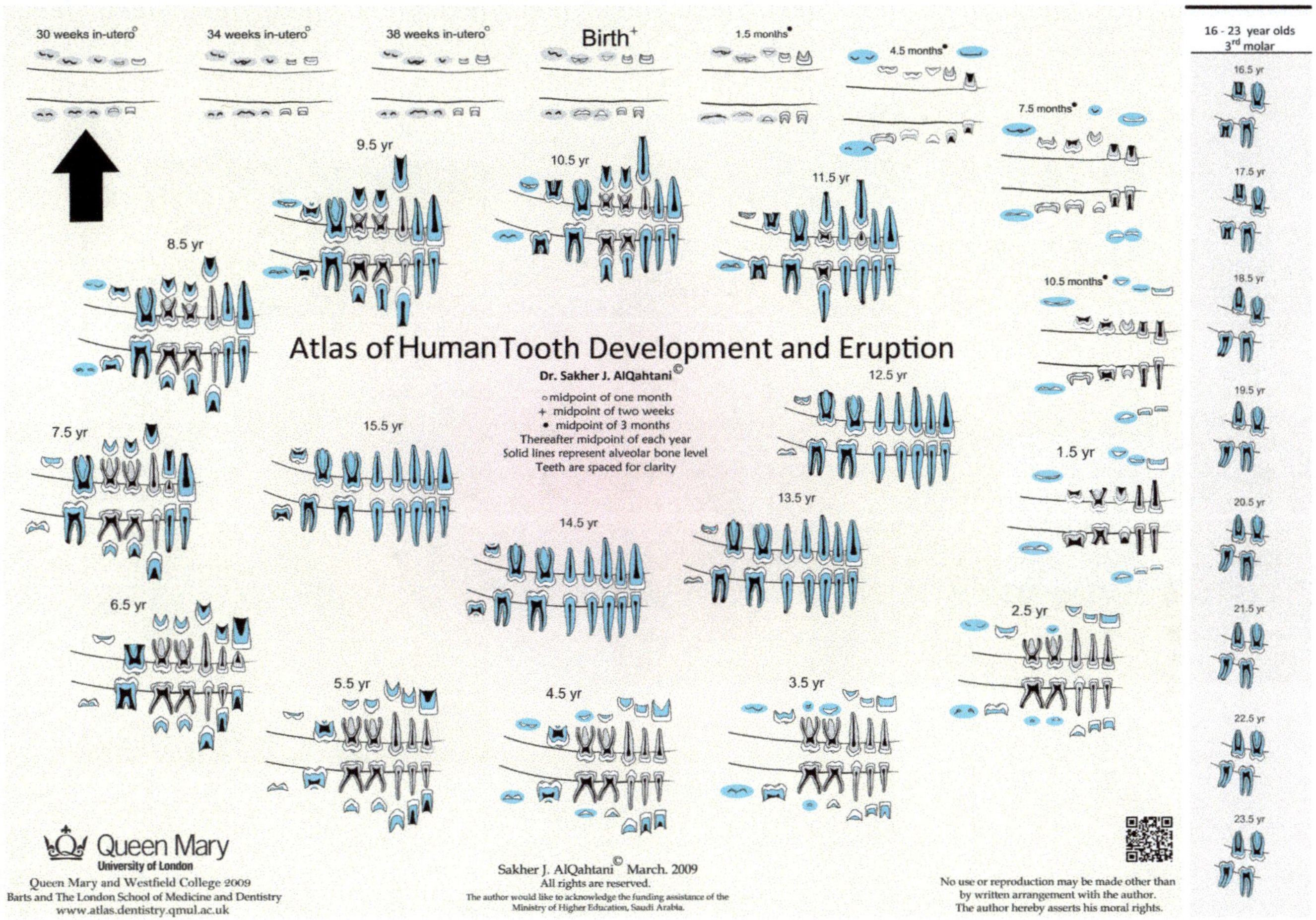

Plate 7.1 Human tooth development and eruption. © 2009: all rights reserved

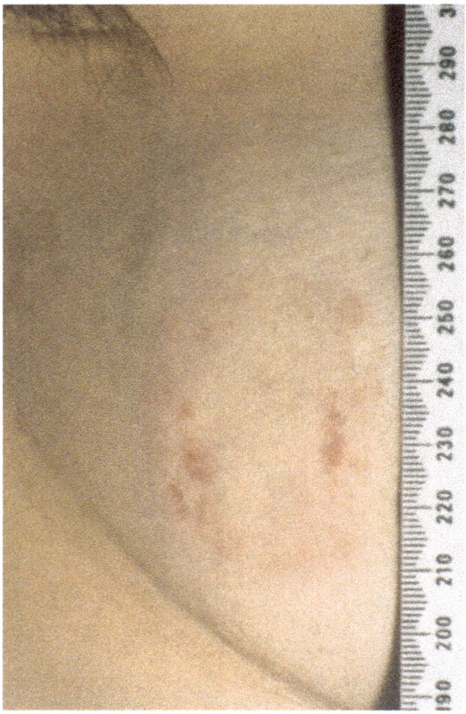

Plate 8.1

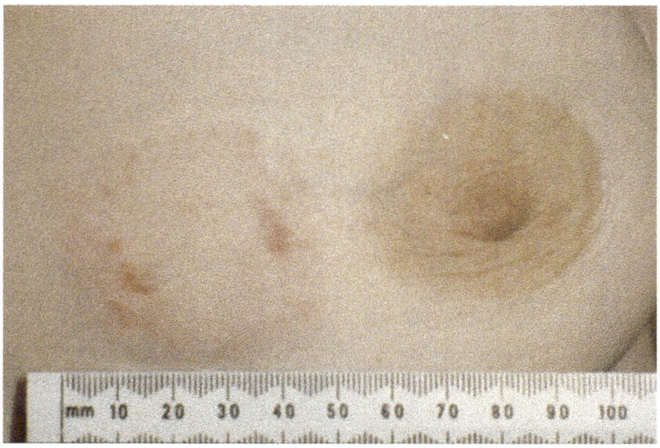

Plate 8.2

Posture distortion in a bite mark on the right breast photographed on successive days with the right arm raised to an unknown position on day 1 (Fig. 8.1) and the arm down by the victim's right side on day 2 (Fig. 8.2). The police photographer was not supervised by an odontologist. The photographs demonstrate posture distortion that produced a significant variation in the size and shape of the bite mark. The variation measures approximately 25% in the vertical axis and 12.5% in the horizontal axis

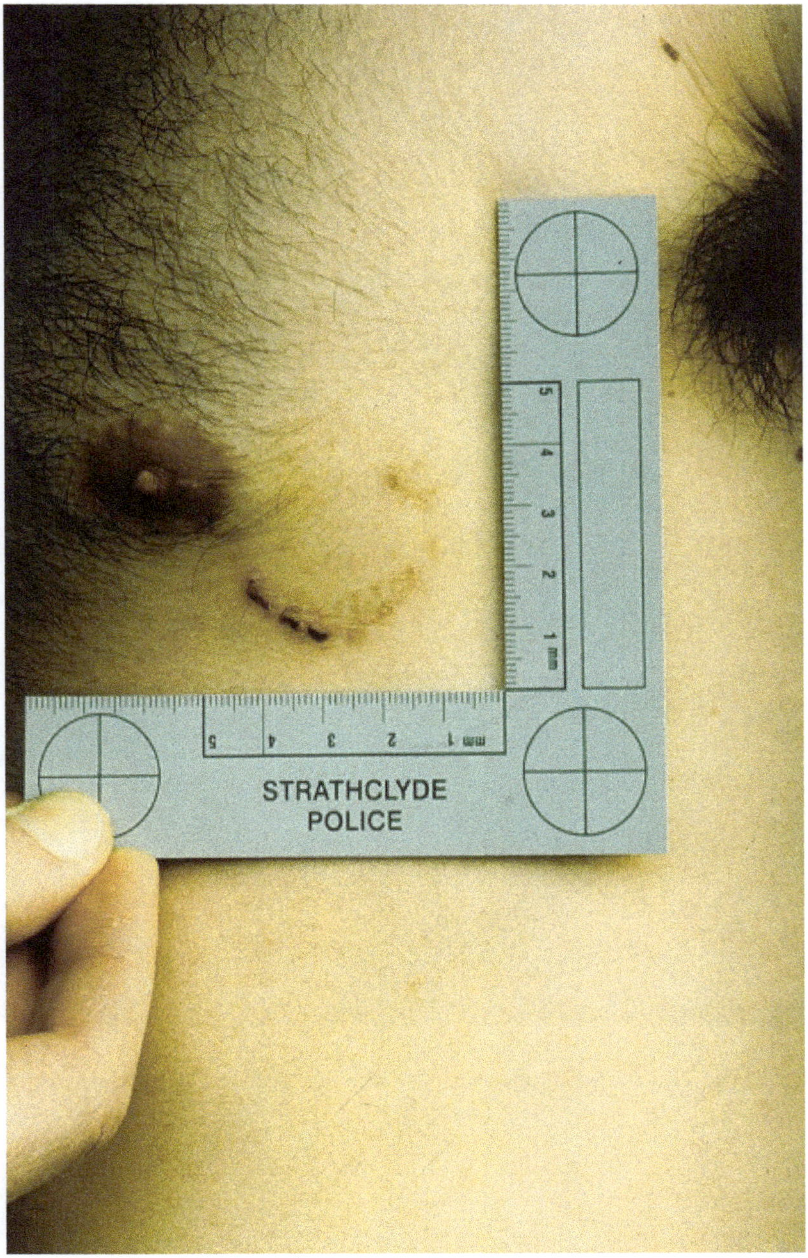

Plate 8.3 The odontologist holds the ABFO no. 2 type scale adjacent to the bite mark. The planes of the scale and bite mark must be parallel and coincident

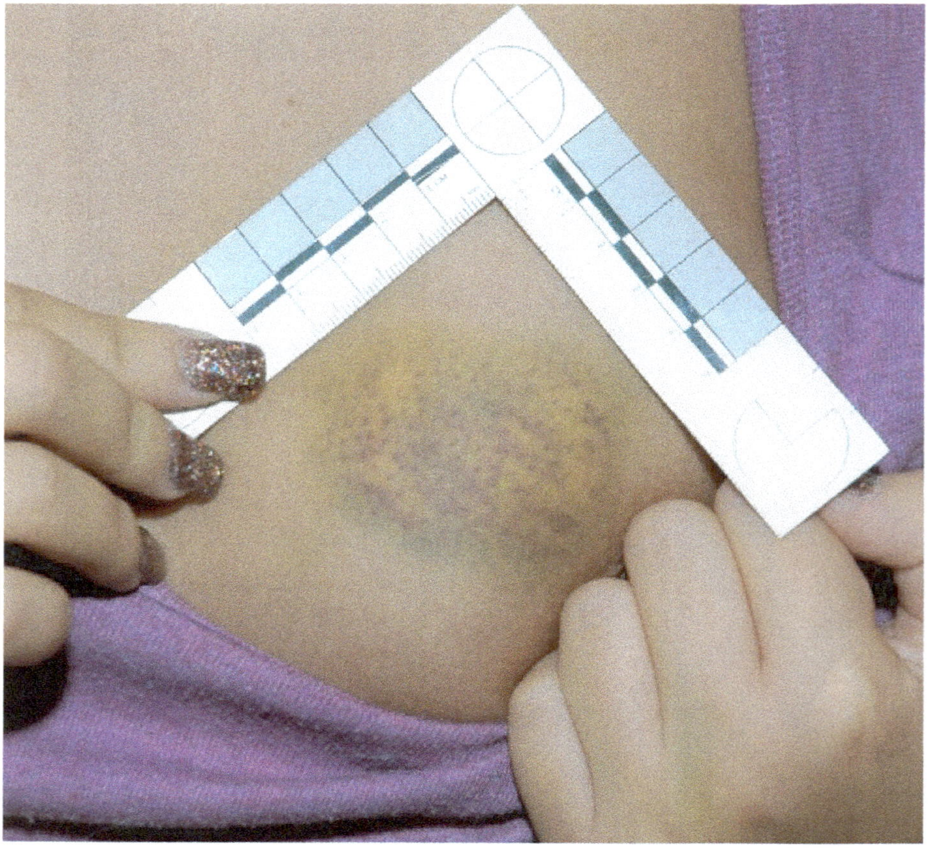

Plate 8.10 Low evidential value bite mark demonstrates a few class characteristics

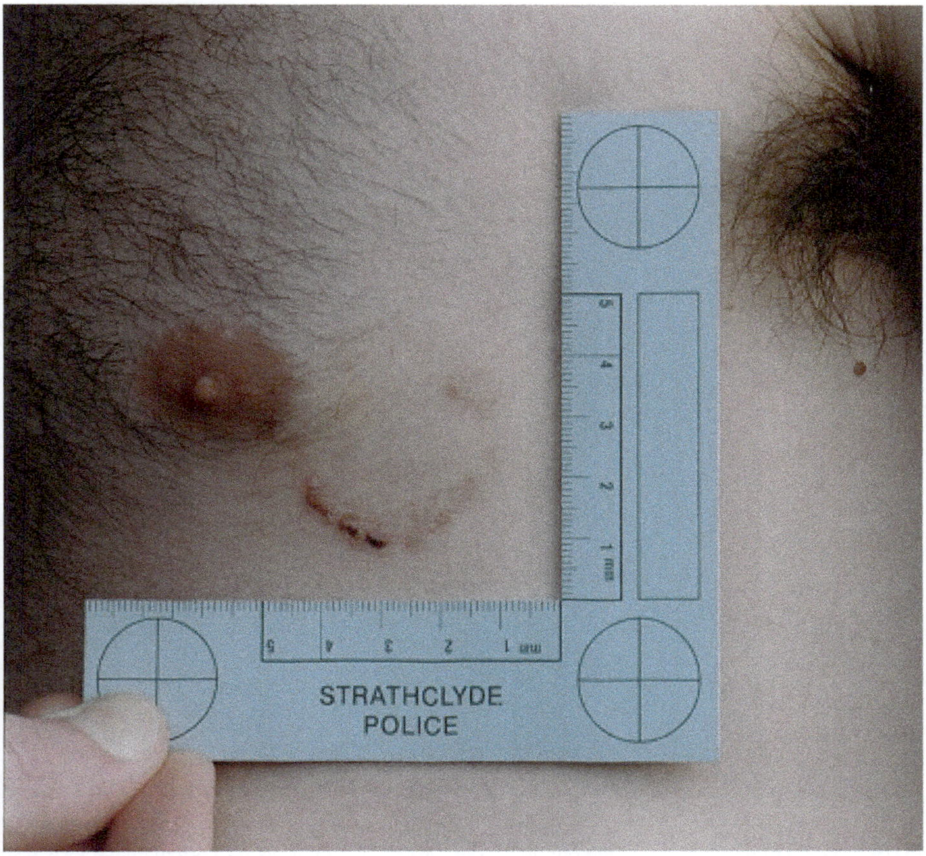

Plate 8.11 Average evidential value bite mark demonstrates a few individual characteristics

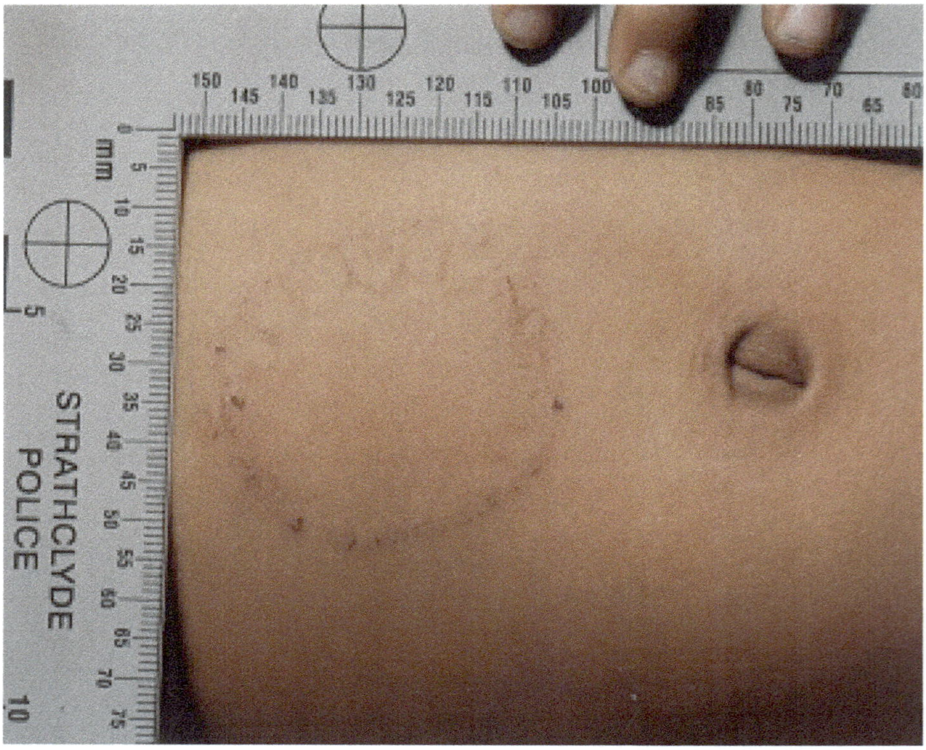

Plate 8.12 High evidential value bite mark demonstrates numerous individual characteristics

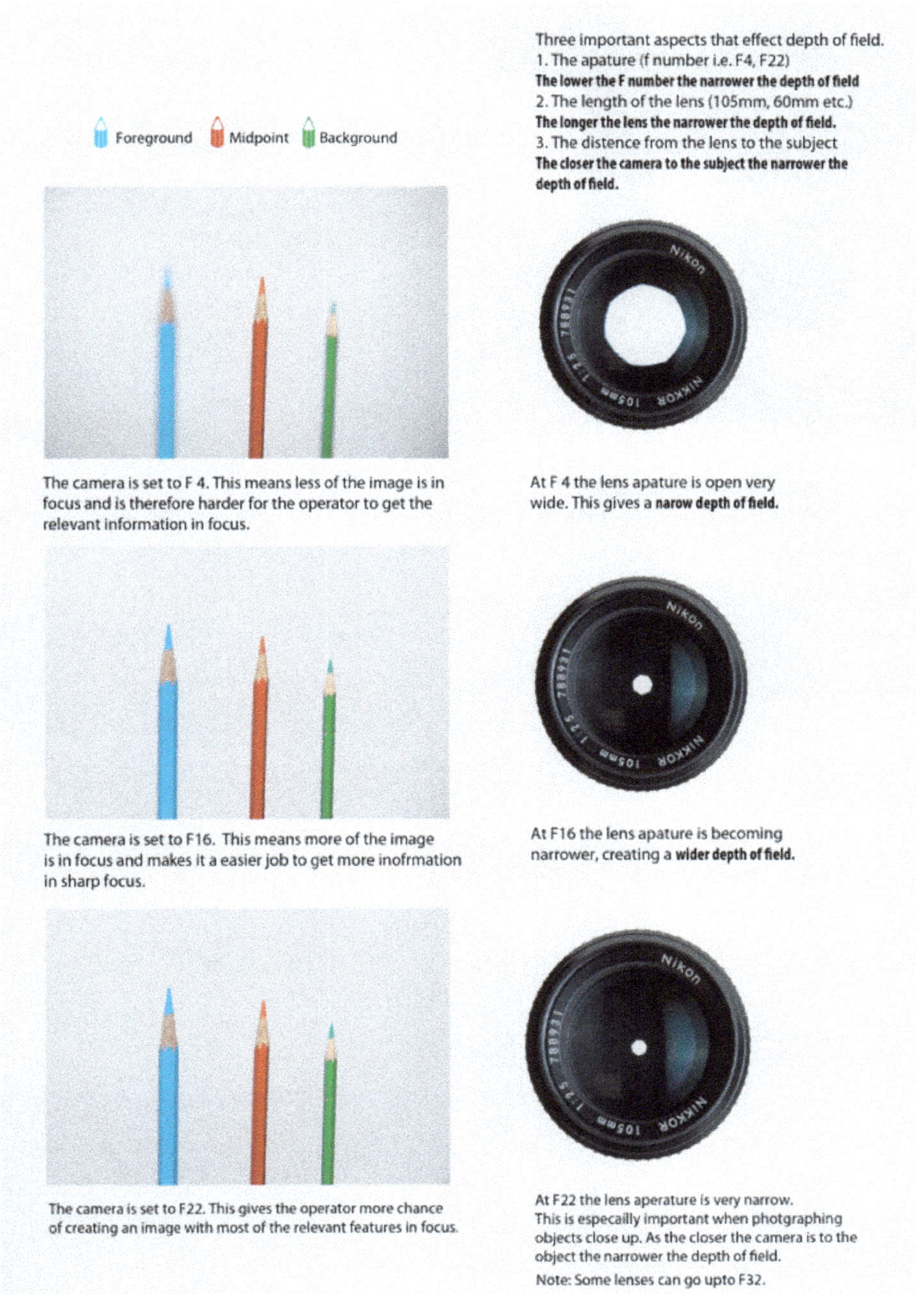

Plate 10.2 Illustration of the effect of depth of field

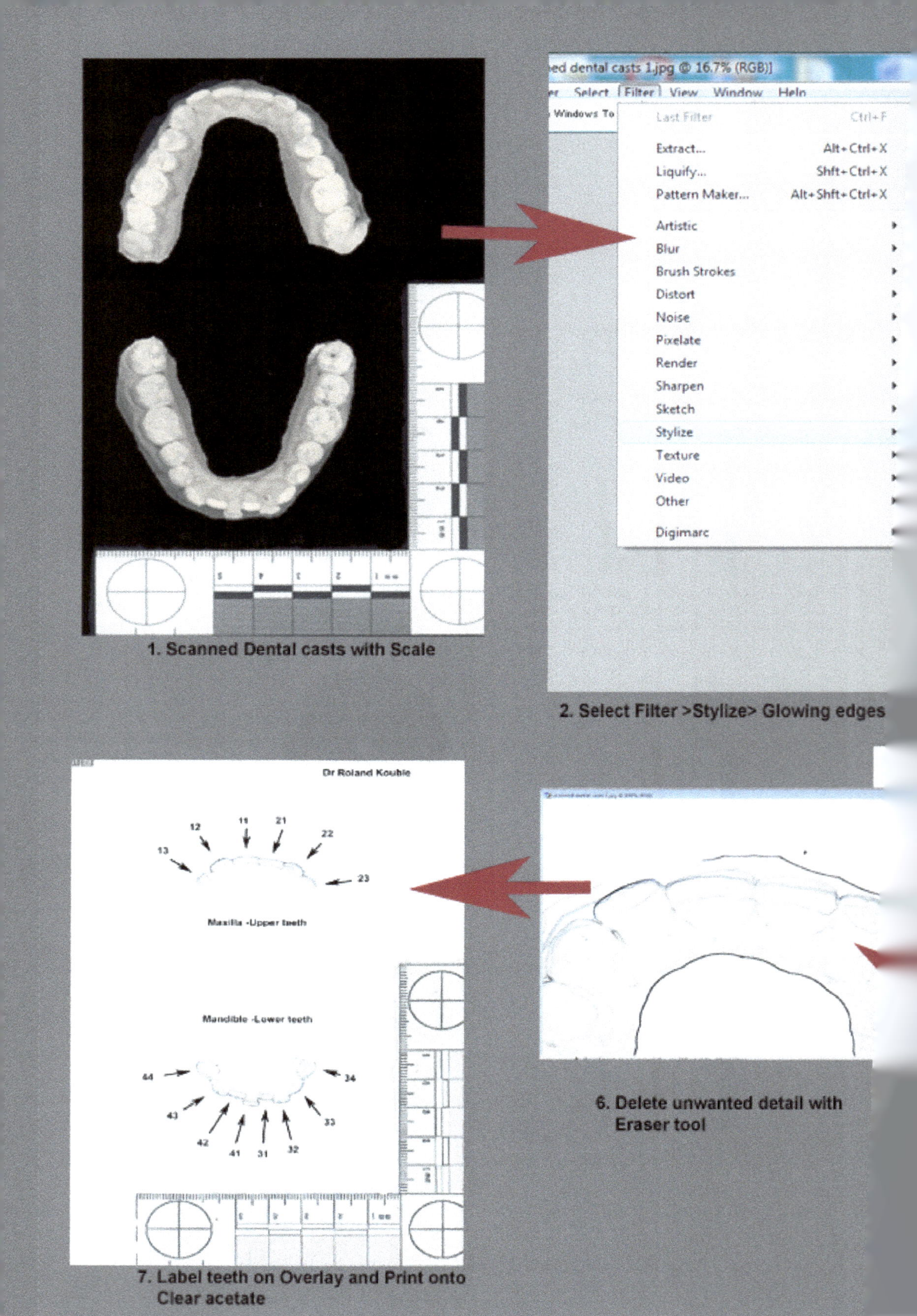

Plate 9.5 Summary of the Glowing Edges technique, showing the step-by-step procedure in overlay production

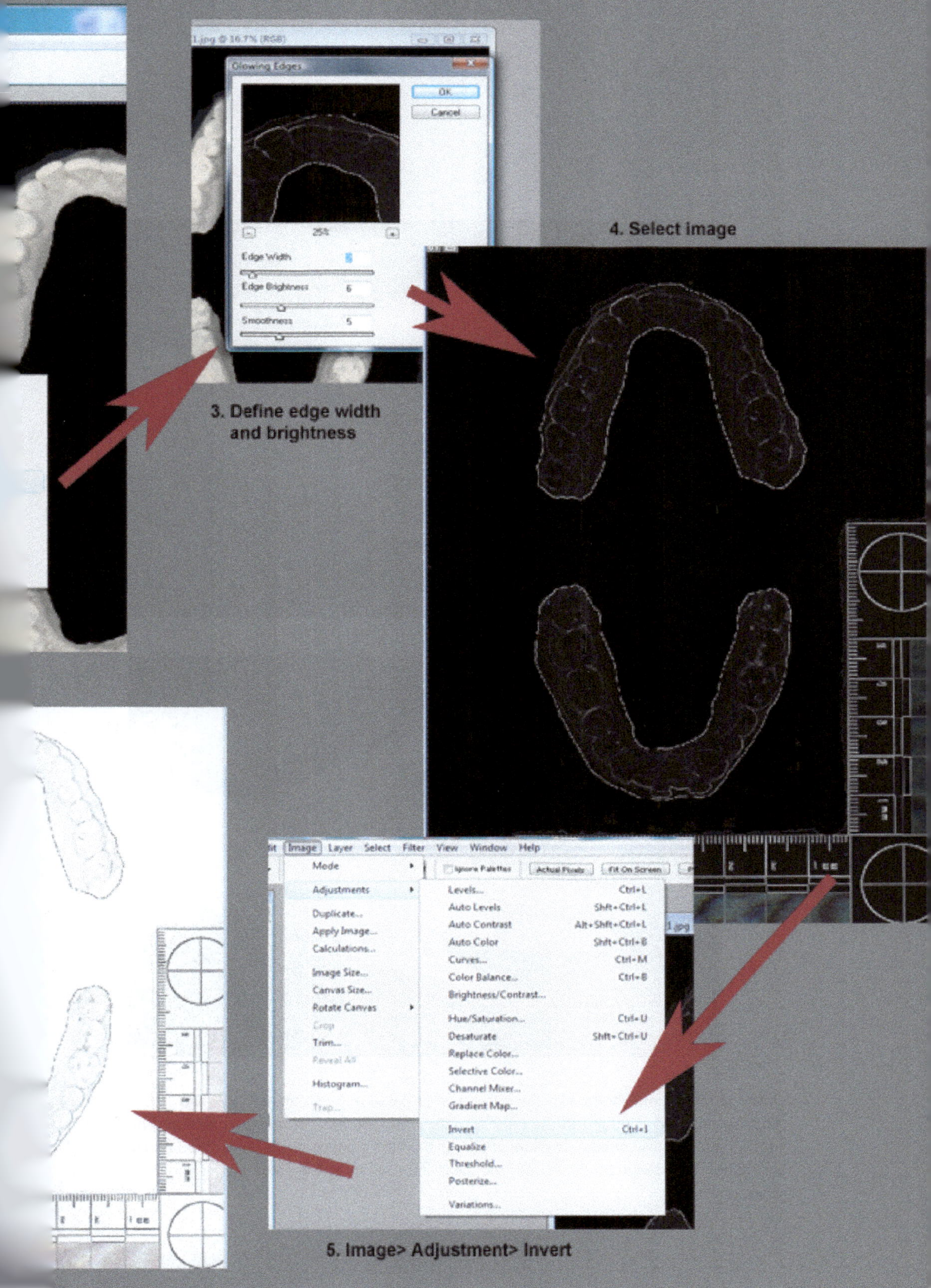
Glowing Edges
OK
Cancel
Edge Width
Edge Brightness
Smoothness
3. Define edge width and brightness
4. Select image
Image
Layer
Select
Filter
View
Window
Help
Mode
Adjustments
Duplicate...
Apply Image...
Calculations...
Image Size...
Canvas Size...
Rotate Canvas
Crop
Trim...
Reveal All
Histogram...
Trap...
Levels... Ctrl+L
Auto Levels Shft+Ctrl+L
Auto Contrast Alt+Shft+Ctrl+L
Auto Color Shft+Ctrl+B
Curves... Ctrl+M
Color Balance... Ctrl+B
Brightness/Contrast...
Hue/Saturation... Ctrl+U
Desaturate Shft+Ctrl+U
Replace Color...
Selective Color...
Channel Mixer...
Gradient Map...
Invert Ctrl+I
Equalize
Threshold...
Posterize...
Variations...
5. Image> Adjustment> Invert

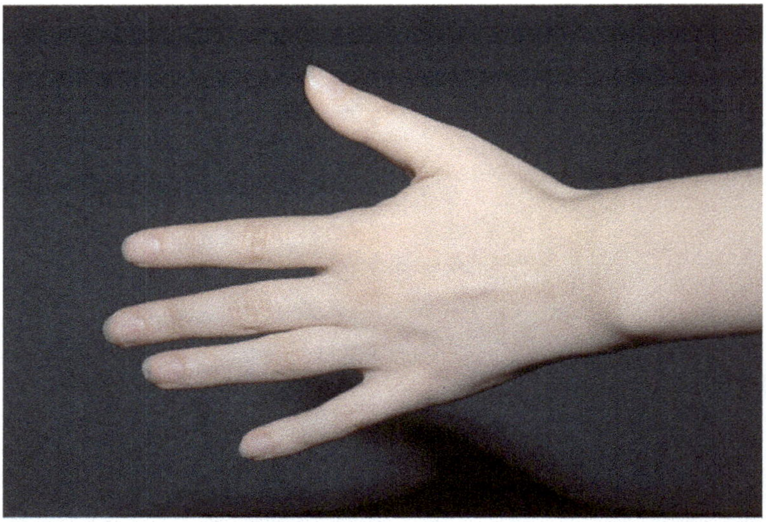

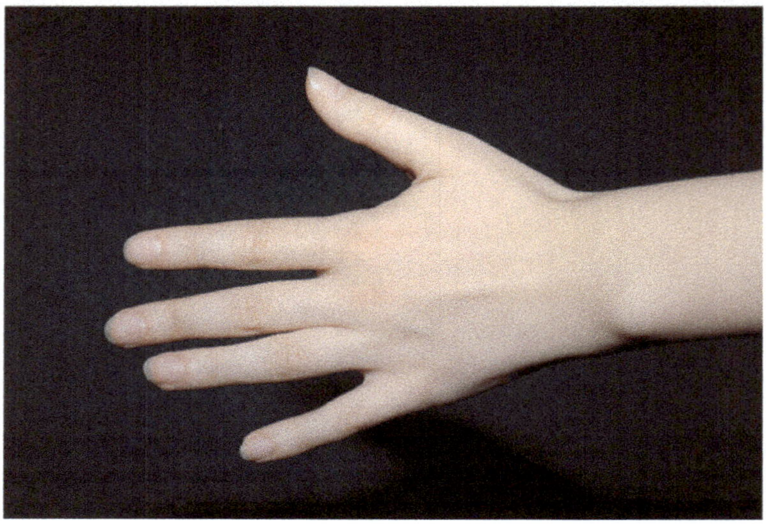

Plate 10.8 Demonstration of the difference in detail and colour in RAW and JPEG capture. The top image is captured in the NEF format, while the bottom image is captured in Nikon's highest quality (lowest compression) JPEG. In the NEF image, notice more detail in background and better tonal range on the skin of the hand. The colour of the green carpet is a more faithful representation

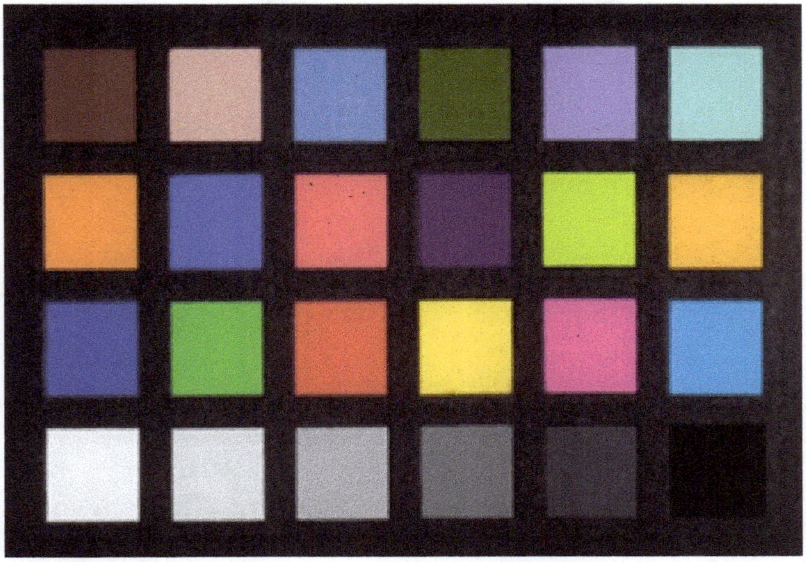

Plate 10.6 Colour checker chart

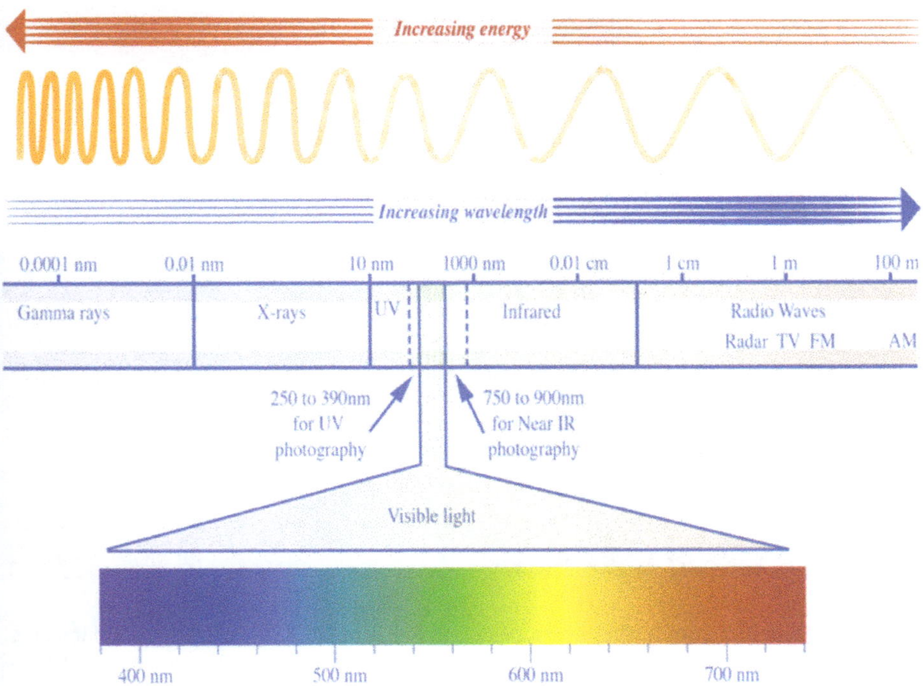

Plate 10.27 The electromagnetic spectrum

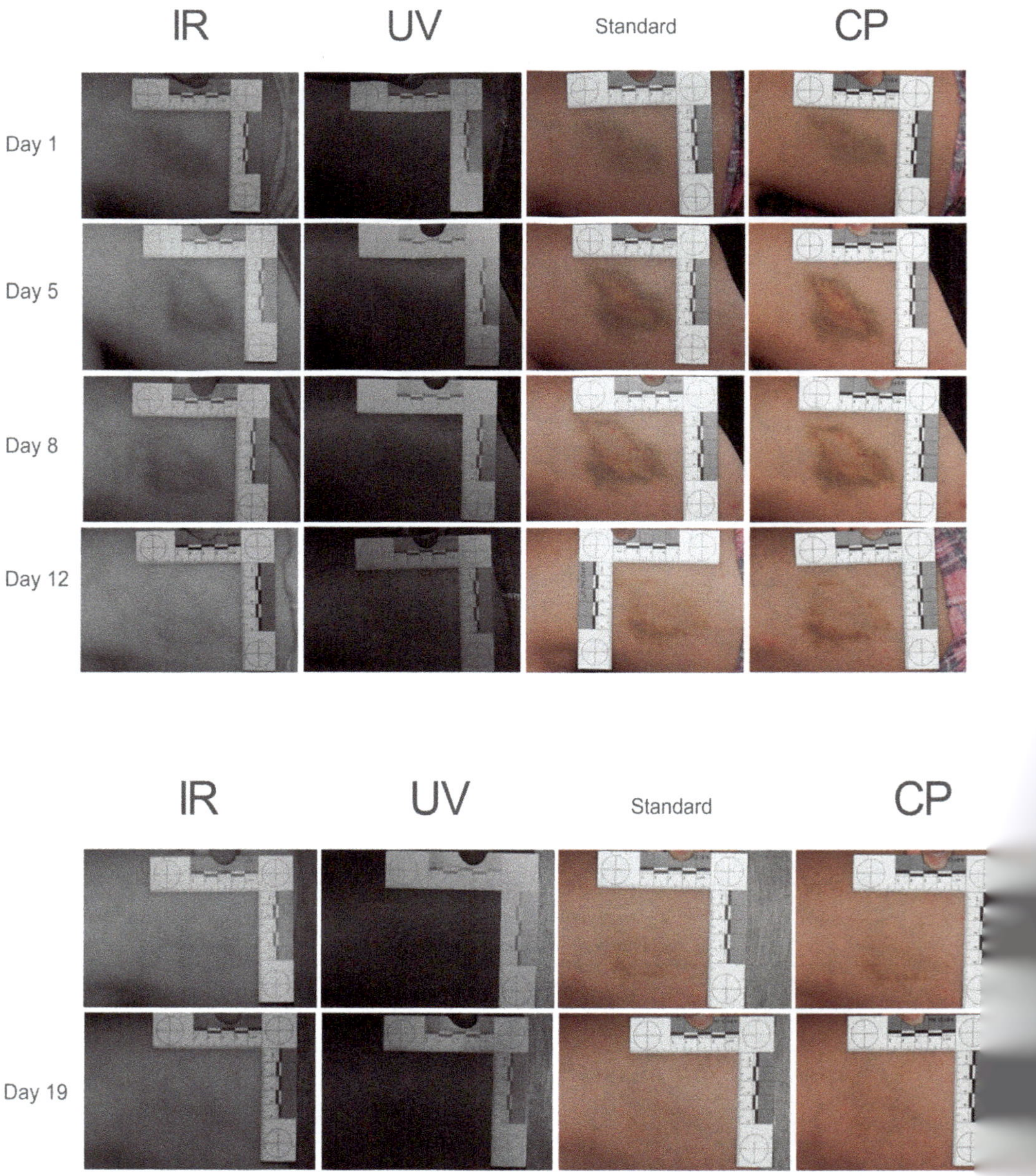

Plate 10.28 Sequence of images over a 19-day period, using IR, UV, CP and standard imaging. Courtesy of child health bruising study, Cardiff University and Medical Research Council

odontologist is attempting to identify the characteristics of the individual elements in the mark. Analysis of the individual tooth elements consists of the recognition and interpretation of the presence or absence, position, rotation and incisal/cuspal detail of each element. The location of the mesial and distal incisal angles of incisors determines their width and centre point. The location of the cusps of canines enables the inter-canine distance to be measured. The cusps of first premolars are rarely recorded. The absence of an individual element may be false; a non-injured space may indicate either an absent tooth or a deficiency in the incisal/cuspal level or the presence of clothing at the time of biting. The recorded detail of an individual element may range from an indistinct mark to a detailed representation of the incisal/cuspal anatomy of a tooth. The number of the individual elements recorded may vary from a few to the complete anterior dentition.

The presence of parallel linear marks that are perpendicular to individual tooth elements is indicative of the movement of the biting edges as they scraped across the surface of the skin; the linear marks are termed 'tooth scrape marks'. The appearance of tongue pressure marks and marks due to other mouth parts may be an indication of the nature of biting. The action of sucking may produce mild diffuse bruising in the centre of a bite mark due to reduced intra-oral pressure that can traumatise the capillaries in the embouched tissue. The presence of the palatal and lingual surface details of a biter is indicative of tongue pressure on the embouched tissue during suckling. The appearance of a butterfly-shaped mark is suggestive of a quantity of tissue having been folded between upper and lower anterior teeth. Multiple bite marks may be superimposed on one another as a result of successive episodes of biting contact at the same anatomical location. The odontologist is attempting to determine the biting mechanism by recognising and interpreting the evidence of the episode of contact between the teeth and skin.

Primary distortion is intrinsic in a bite mark; consequently, the photograph of the bite mark will record an unknown and variable degree of primary distortion. The effects of dynamic and tissue distortion are complex, unpredictable and difficult to recognise and interpret. Secondary distortion may occur subsequent to a bite mark being made and/or during evidence recording; consequently, this affords the odontologist an opportunity to limit the effects of secondary distortion. Time-related distortion in living victims is usually easily recognised since the time elapsed between biting and photography is usually known; however, the interpretation of time-related distortion may be complex. The anatomical location of the bite mark, the number of bite marks, the body position of the victim at the time of biting and photography, whether the victim was alive or dead at the time of biting and photography, the time of biting and photography, the presence and thickness of clothing are significant facts that have to be considered by the odontologist when examining the photographs of the bite mark. An important distinction exists between cases depending on whether or not an odontologist supervises the photographic recording of the bite mark. Photographs taken under supervision may limit the effects of posture and photographic distortion whereas photographs taken without supervision may record an unknown degree of these types of distortion.

The evidential value of a bite mark is related to the gross, class and individual characteristics of the causal dentition that are represented in it. In general terms, marks that demonstrate either gross characteristics or a few class characteristics are of low evidential value; marks that show numerous individual characteristics are of high evidential value. The recognition and interpretation of the features and of distortion in the photographs of the bite mark enables the odontologist to assess the evidential value of the mark. The evidential values may be described simply as low, average and high. Examples of low, average and high evidential value bite marks are illustrated in Figures 8.10, 8.11 and 8.12 respectively.

Preparation of predictor of causal dentition

The recognition and interpretation of the features in the photographs of the bite mark enables the odontologist to prepare a predictor of the dentition that caused the bite mark. The degree of prediction will depend on the evidential value of the bite mark. Marks with a high evidential value will enable detailed and accurate predictors to be prepared; as the evidential value of the mark diminishes, so does the ability to predict the causal dentition. The ability to prepare a predictor adds weight to the evidence and strengthens the opinion of the odontologist. The preparation of a predictor is conducted prior to the odontologist having any knowledge of the dentition of the suspect biter. This sequence of examination provides an element of potential corroboration in the

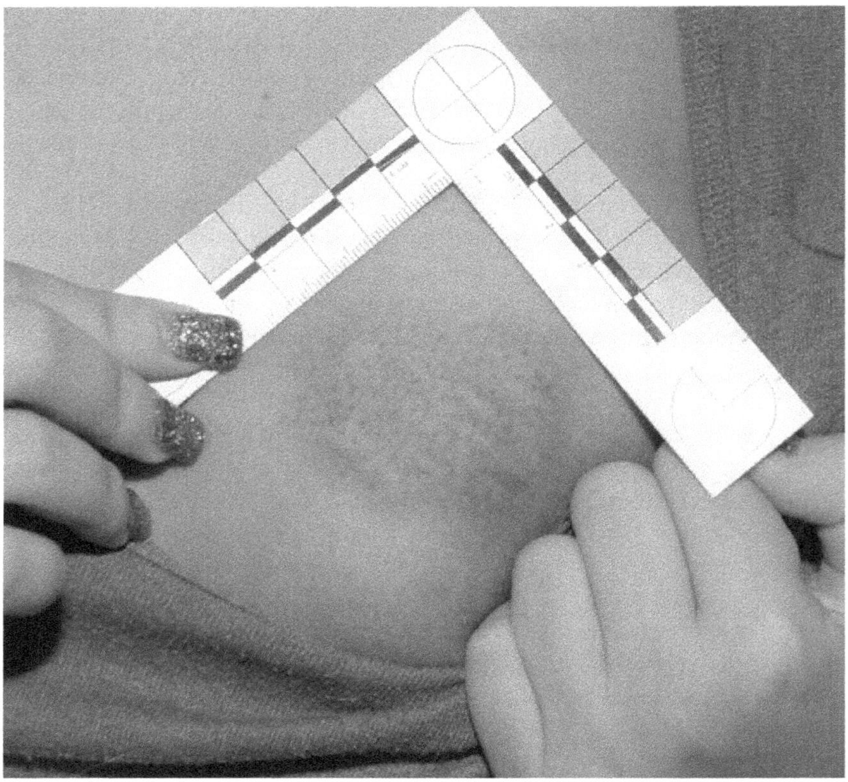

Figure 8.10 Low evidential value bite mark demonstrates a few class characteristics (For colour details, please see colour plate section.)

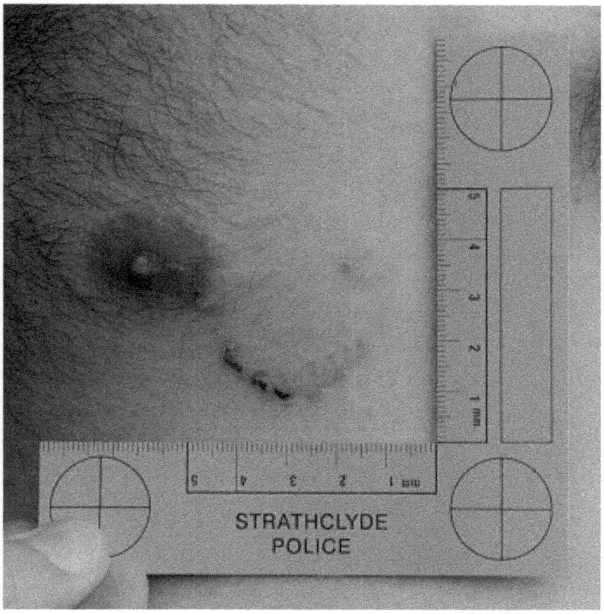

Figure 8.11 Average evidential value bite mark demonstrates a few individual characteristics (For colour details, please see colour plate section.)

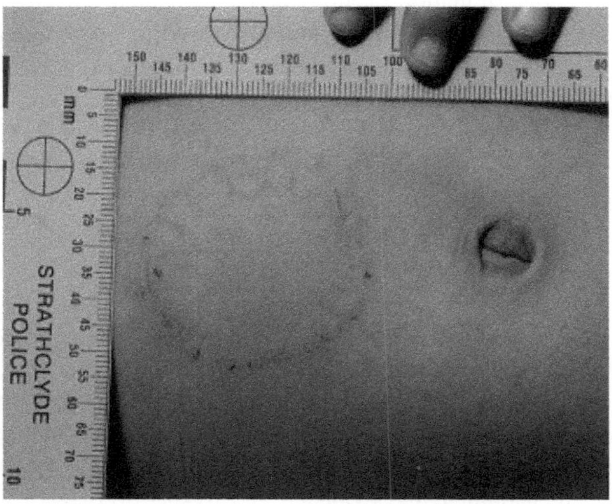

Figure 8.12 High evidential value bite mark demonstrates numerous individual characteristics (For colour details, please see colour plate section.)

comparison of the predictor with the dental casts and in the subsequent comparison of the photographs of the bite mark with the dental casts; this sequence also prevents the preconditioning of the odontologist's knowledge of the biter's dentition. The phenomenon of preconditioning, to prepare beforehand, is avoided by the preparation of a predictor before the examination of the dental casts of the suspect biter. The preconditioning influence due to the preparation of a predictor will be reduced by a significant time interval or washout period prior to the examination of the dental casts.

The prediction of whether the biter is a child or an adult is particularly relevant in cases involving child victims. The prediction is only possible in bite marks demonstrating a high evidential value in respect of inter-canine distance and individual tooth elements. The adult inter-canine distance normally develops by 12 years of age. Consequently, based on this measurement, the age differentiation between child and adult biters is approximately 12 years old. However, the inter-canine distance is variable at 12 years, so only the deciduous inter-canine distance may be relied on to predict a child biter's age. During the development of the mixed dentition, the prediction of age depends on the evidential value of the individual tooth elements in a bite mark. Clearly, the lack of evidential value in a bite mark prevents a valid prediction of the age of the biter.

Examination of dental casts

The examination commences with the recognition and interpretation of the features in the upper and lower dental casts of the suspect biter. The general features that are relevant to comparative analysis are the determination of arch size by measuring the inter-canine distance and determination of arch shape. The detailed features that form the basis of comparison are the presence or absence, position, rotation and incisal/cuspal anatomy of the individual teeth. The incisal edges of the incisors and the cusps of the canines and first premolars are examined in detail. The incisal and cuspal anatomy may demonstrate a variety of distinctive features; incisal edge tubercles, attrition, fracture, defective incisal restorations, caries, peg-shaped, fixed or removable prosthesis. The level of the incisal edges and cusps is examined and any variations are noted.

Comparative study

The comparative study commences with the comparison of the predictor of the causal dentition with the findings of the examination of the dental casts of the suspect biter. The evidential value of the bite mark will determine the degree of prediction; high values enable detailed and accurate predictors to be compared with the dental casts. When this comparison is positive it provides an element of corroboration of opinion that adds significant weight to the evidence and to the strength of opinion. As the evidential value of the mark diminishes, so does the ability to predict the causal dentition; consequently the comparison with the dental casts becomes more limited.

The comparative study continues with the comparison of the findings of the examinations of the bite mark photographs with those of the dental casts. The points of comparison are the orientation of arches, arch centre point, arch size, arch shape and individual tooth features; these features are the presence or absence, position, rotation and incisal/cuspal anatomy of each tooth. The comparative study provokes a number of questions at this stage:

- Are the oriented arches comparable?
- Are the individual tooth elements in the bite mark comparable with the teeth of the biter?
- Are the distinctive tooth elements in the bite mark comparable with the distinctive teeth of the biter?
- Are there individual elements in the bite mark that are incomparable with the teeth of the biter?
- Is the representation of the biting mechanism comparable with the dentition and/or mouth parts of the biter?

The answers to these questions will result in degrees of comparability and of incomparability. When all the answers are comparable and none is incomparable, the comparison is considered positive. A positive comparison provides an additional element of corroboration of opinion that adds further significant weight to the evidence and to the strength of opinion. When the answers are a combination of comparable and incomparable, the comparison is contradictory; this is appropriately reflected in the weight of evidence and strength of opinion in the case.

The level of subjective assessment inherent in the comparison process may be moderated by conducting feature-based analysis on an iterative basis. The analysis is repeated with a significant time interval or washout period between consecutive analyses until the opinion is consistent and cannot be developed any further. The number of repeat analyses required to achieve consistency of opinion is variable. The concluding opinions in feature-based analysis are expressed in a range of conclusions that are designed to reflect the evidential value of the bite mark, the weight of evidence and the strength of opinion in the case.

In general terms, the degree of soft tissue injury in a bite mark is consistent with the force applied by the biting edges of upper and lower front teeth. The force may be described as mild, moderate or severe:

- mild force is consistent with bruising and abrasion
- moderate force is consistent with abrasion and laceration
- severe force is consistent with laceration and avulsion.

Bite marks often demonstrate more than one type of tissue injury. The odontologist describes the degree of tissue injury and indicates the degree of causal force.

The stages of examination of the bite mark photographs, preparation of a predictor of the causal dentition, examination of the dental casts of the suspect biter and comparative study are repeated for each bite mark. The feature-based analysis will result in an opinion for each bite mark. Multiple bite marks may be caused by either a single suspect biter or an unknown biter or biters or a combination of both possibilities. Multiple bite marks may occur in single or multiple victims.

The stages of examination of the dental casts of the suspect biter and comparative study are repeated for each suspect biter. The feature-based analysis will result in an opinion for each suspect biter. Multiple suspect biters may have caused single or multiple bite marks in single or multiple victims.

Feature-based analysis is extremely complex in cases involving multiple bite marks and/or multiple suspect biters. In these cases, the exclusion of a suspect as having caused the bite mark is usually the simpler conclusion to reach. The exclusion of a suspect or suspects assists the investigators in redirecting the search for the biter. A bite mark case that presents with a single suspect biter may be referred to as having a *closed population*; this contrasts with a case that presents with multiple suspect biters as having an *open population*.

More than one odontologist may conduct feature-based analysis independently in a case. The opinions may be corroborative which mutually strengthens the opinions in the case; conversely, the opinions may be contradictory which mutually weakens the opinions. It is generally accepted that two competent odontologists reporting independently in a bite mark case serve the interests of forensic odontology and justice.

8.7.5 Superimposition-based analysis

The role of superimposition-based analysis is to provide appropriate visual corroboration of the findings of feature-based analysis. The techniques are described in Chapter 9.

8.8 Feature-based analysis conclusions

The initial examination of the alleged/suspected bite mark determines whether it can be identified as a human bite mark. The initial conclusions are simple and significant: either *inclusion* which continues the involvement of the odontologist, or *exclusion* which redirects the investigation.

The initial conclusion of the identification of a human bite mark justifies further examination that specifically considers the evidential value of the bite mark. The evidential value may be reflected in three initial conclusions: possible bite mark, probable bite mark or positive bite mark.

- A low evidential value supports the conclusion of a possible bite mark – teeth or another factor possibly caused the mark.
- An average evidential value supports the conclusion of a probable bite mark – teeth more probably than another factor caused the mark.
- A high evidential value supports the conclusion of a positive bite mark – teeth caused the mark.

Clearly, evidential values demonstrate a range that is more varied than these three conclusions; the objective of these initial conclusions is to indicate the applicability of feature-based analysis to investigators at an early stage in a case.

In applicable bite mark cases, feature-based analysis is conducted by the odontologist who assesses the evidential value of the bite mark and weight of evidence and subsequently forms an opinion in the case. The opinion is initially expressed in one of three categories of general conclusion: exclusion of the suspect, limited conclusion, or inclusion of the suspect.

8.8.1 Exclusion of the suspect

When the comparison of the predictor of the causal dentition with the findings of the examination of the dental casts of the suspect biter is incomparable, this supports exclusion of the suspect. Similarly, when the comparison of the findings of the examination of the bite mark photographs with those of the dental casts is incomparable, this further supports the exclusion of the suspect. In essence, when all of the features in the photographs of the bite mark are incomparable with the dental casts of the suspect biter, the appropriate general conclusion is the exclusion of the suspect as the biter in the case. In effect, the detailed comparisons of the features of the bite mark with the dental casts of the suspect biter show that these teeth do not provide an explanation for the features observed in the bite mark.

The obvious consequence of the exclusion of a single suspect in a case is that the biter remains unidentified. The evidential value of the bite mark may justify feature-based analysis; the mark may demonstrate a degree and type of tissue injury that may indicate the degree of causal force. These observations and opinions may be important in the further investigation of the case. In cases with multiple suspect biters, the exclusion of suspects assists the identification of the biter. Clearly, the exclusion of a single suspect or multiple suspects assists the investigators in redirecting the search for the biter.

Previously it was thought that bite mark analysis was of greater assistance as an exclusionary process rather than an inclusionary process (Ström, 1963; Gustafson, 1966; Dinkel, 1974; Vale *et al.*, 1976). However, the development of bite mark analysis has enabled odontologists to make significant progress in the contribution of the inclusionary process. Certainly the exclusion of a suspect as having caused the bite mark is usually the simpler conclusion to reach.

8.8.2 Limited conclusion

When the features in the photographs of the bite mark consist of only class characteristics, the general conclusion is limited to identifying it as a bite mark. The conclusion is limited to stating that the mark is of a size and shape that is suggestive of a human bite mark. In effect, the absence of individual characteristics in the mark prevents a valid comparison with the teeth of a suspect biter. However, the bite mark may demonstrate a degree and type of tissue injury that may indicate the degree of causal force; these observations and opinions may provide corroboration of other evidence in the case.

8.8.3 Inclusion of the suspect

When the features in the photographs of the bite mark and in the dental casts are comparable, the appropriate general conclusion is the inclusion of the suspect as the biter in the case. In effect, the detailed comparisons of the features of the bite mark with the dental casts of the suspect biter may demonstrate varying degrees of comparability which are described in three specific conclusions: possible, probable, or positive. The specific conclusions reflect the odontologist's strength of opinion in the case.

- *Possible biter*. A weak opinion is expressed as a possible biter, which reflects a non-specific comparison with no detail between the bite mark and teeth. In essence, feature-based analysis has demonstrated general comparability between the bite mark and the dental casts; the comparability is of a general nature and lacks any detailed features.
- *Probable biter*. A moderate opinion is expressed as a probable biter, which reflects a specific comparison with limited detail between the bite mark and teeth. In essence, feature-based analysis has demonstrated specific comparability between the bite mark and the dental casts; the comparability is of a specific nature with limited detailed features.
- *Positive biter*. A strong opinion is expressed as a positive biter, which reflects a specific and detailed comparison between the bite mark and teeth. In essence, feature-based analysis has demonstrated specific comparability between the bite mark and the dental casts; the comparability is of a specific nature with detailed features.

The specific conclusions are designed to reflect the odontologist's strength of opinion in the case. Aitken and MacDonald (1979) noted that classified bite mark characteristics on large sections of the population were unavailable, and this statement remains true today. Consequently, it is important to recognise that the specific conclusions are not based on scientific data.

Finally, the odontologist describes the degree and type of tissue injury and indicates the degree of causal force. These observations and opinions may corroborate the specific conclusions.

8.9 Feature-based analysis report

The various stages in the investigation of a forensic bite mark are collated in a feature-based analysis report that depends on the contemporaneous notes for case information. The report is structured to reflect the sequence of the different stages in the investigation of a bite mark. Consequently, the report is formatted in five sections: introduction, examination of alleged/suspected bite mark, dental examination of suspect biter, comparison of alleged/suspected bite mark with suspect biter, and conclusions.

- *Introduction*. This section commences with a brief curriculum vitae of the odontologist with particular reference to relevant qualifications and experience. The introduction notes the name and designation of the person who made the initial request for assistance with the investigation of the alleged/suspected bite mark and the date of the request. The general location of the injury and the victim's name are noted along with details of the photographic prints and other case material that was supplied to the odontologist.

- *Examination of alleged/suspected bite mark.* The anatomical location and dimensions of the mark are recorded. An initial opinion is expressed whether the mark is of a size and shape that is suggestive of a human bite mark. The detailed examination commences with the recognition and interpretation of the features in the photographs of the bite mark; this enables the preparation of a predictor of the dentition that caused the bite mark. There is an attempt to determine the biting mechanism by recognising and interpreting the evidence of the episode of contact between the teeth and skin. The degree and type of tissue injury is recorded and the degree of causal force is indicated. An initial conclusion of whether the mark can be identified as a human bite mark is expressed; this will determine the validity of a comparative study.
- *Dental examination of suspect biter.* The location and date of the dental examination of the suspect are noted; this also includes details of the dental impressions and of the continuity of evidence in the production of the dental casts. The findings of the detailed examination of the features in the upper and lower dental casts of the suspect biter are recorded.
- *Comparison of alleged/suspected bite mark with suspect biter.* The comparison of the photographs of the alleged/suspected bite mark with the dental casts of the suspect biter is conducted in two stages of comparative study. First, the comparison of the predictor of the causal dentition with the findings of the examination of the dental casts of the suspect biter is detailed. Second, the comparison of the findings of the examinations of the bite mark photographs with those of the dental casts is also detailed. A specific conclusion regarding the identification of the biter is expressed.
- *Conclusions.* This section commences with an initial conclusion of whether the mark can be identified as a human bite mark. The findings of comparative study and a specific conclusion regarding the identification of the biter are recorded. Finally, the degree and type of tissue injury is recorded and the degree of causal force is indicated.

The report contains a combination of factual and opinion evidence. Expert witnesses are granted the privilege of expressing opinions on matters in which they are qualified. Consequently, the feature-based analysis report constitutes expert witness evidence. The primary responsibility of the expert witness is to assist the court, irrespective of the instructing party in a case. In order to assist the court, the report must be able to be understood by lay people; this is achieved by using basic vocabulary and reducing technical terms. In addition, the format and content of the report should be logical and concise respectively; the format reflects the sequence of the different stages in the investigation of the bite mark. Finally, to complete its assistance to the court, the report must withstand cross-examination.

Photographs of the bite mark and dental casts of the suspect biter are submitted as court productions in the case. The productions are signed and dated by the odontologist to demonstrate the continuity of the evidence.

8.10 Limitations of bite mark analysis

The comparison of bite marks in human skin with a dentition has had a long and controversial history. The first bite mark investigation to appear in the literature was in 1874 (Skrzeezkas, 1874). Much of the initial research in bite mark analysis was conducted in Scandinavia. The first significant case in the UK was *HM Advocate v Hay* (Harvey *et al.*, 1968); subsequently, Butler (1973) stressed the value of the bite mark evidence.

In the United States the first bite mark case was reported in 1954 (*Doyle v State*, 159 Tex. C.R. 310, 263 S.W.2d 779 (1954)). In perhaps the most compelling article on the legal implications of bite mark evidence, Hale (1978) questioned both the reliability of bite mark comparisons and the general acceptance of bite marks in the scientific community. Hale suggested that bite mark evidence should be excluded from court because of the lack of scientific reliability and the highly prejudicial nature of the evidence with the possibility of the failure of bite mark evidence to satisfy the Frye rule (*Frye v United States*, 293 F. 1013, 1014 (D.C. Cir. 1923)). The Frye case established guidelines for the admissibility of scientific evidence related to new techniques. Therefore, in order to satisfy the Frye rule, the scientific principle must be recognisable, the principle must be sufficiently established and the principle must have gained acceptance in the field to which it belongs (Whatmough and Nuckles, 1992). Neufeld and Colman (1990) stated that, in order to be admitted as evidence, a forensic test should satisfy three criteria: the underlying scientific theory must be considered valid by the scientific community; the technique itself must be known to be reliable; and the technique must be shown to have been properly applied in the particular case.

Various techniques for the comparison of a bite mark in skin with a dentition had been described in court and legal decisions suggested acceptance of the procedures used (Levine, 1982). However, some techniques had gained more acceptance than others which was partly due to certain legal decisions (*Frye v United States*, as above; and *California v Kelly*, 17 Cal. 3d 24 (1976)). Using the rationale of the Frye and Kelly precedents, the admission of bite mark evidence had been based on assessing the weight of the evidence rather than the admissibility of the bite mark evidence itself (Beckstead *et al.*, 1979). The development of bite mark analysis had led to its acceptance by the scientific and legal communities (Levine, 1982; Whatmough and Nuckles, 1992). Farrell *et al.* (1987) suggested that the validation of new comparison techniques was facilitated by the scientific evidence that had previously validated the science of the comparison of fingerprints. In the United States by 1986, 192 cases had been cited in the legal literature and there were no references in the scientific or legal literature to a case in which bite mark testimony had not been allowed. However, a review of trial transcripts revealed that distortion and the interpretation of distortion were the main factors in contentious cases (Rawson *et al.*, 1986a). Consequently, the American Board of Forensic Odontology established formal guidelines to aid in the handling of bite mark evidence in 1984 (American Board of Forensic Odontology Inc., 1986). Subsequently, the American Academy of Forensic Sciences and the American Board of Forensic Odontology (ABFO) studied and rationalised the major concerns in bite mark analysis and testimony. Those items considered most important for the development of scientifically founded standards were uniqueness, consistency and accuracy in matching, methods for evidence collection and analysis, classification of tissue, analysis of distorted marks and expertise of the odontologist as demonstrated by certification and experience. In 1997 the American Society of Forensic Odontology published the ABFO *Guidelines and Standards* for forensic odontology; the sections related to bite marks established methods for collection of bite mark evidence, analysis and relevant terminology (American Society of Forensic Odontology, 1997).

In 1988, Zarkowski stated in a legal review that bite mark analysis had never progressed through the rigorous scientific examination that was common to other sciences, to determine its accuracy or reliability.

The admissibility of scientific evidence was ruled on in the landmark case of *Daubert v Merrell Dow Pharmaceuticals*, 509 U.S. 579 (1993). The court stated that, for expert opinion to be admissible, the testimony must be both relevant and reliable: *relevant opinion* had a bearing on the facts of the case, while *reliable opinion* was based on a scientific method. Reliability of scientific evidence was to be based on scientific validity. To guide in this matter, the Daubert court outlined four non-definitive factors regarding scientific evidence: whether the theory can be and has been tested; the theory's error rate; whether the theory has been subjected to peer review and publication; and whether the theory has met with general acceptance in the scientific community. At present, the scientific literature and published research evidence relating to bite mark analysis lacks peer-reviewed publications supporting its current use, including data on error rates and reliability; consequently, bite mark analysis is not able to completely satisfy the Daubert ruling. Despite this fact, bite mark evidence has continued to be admitted in cases under Daubert.

Differences in opinion regarding the context of bite mark analysis continued to be expressed, and there were those who suggested re-evaluating the technique of bite mark analysis (Aksu and Gobetti, 1996). However, according to Saferstein (1995), bite mark analysis is an inexact science whose evidential value is not underpinned by large, statistically relevant numbers but rather depends on the identification and comparison of class and individual characteristics. Kieser *et al.* (2007) commented that bite mark analysis, in common with other forensic comparative techniques, relies on a number of variable characters that must often be evaluated in an inductive (experience based) rather than a deductive (mathematical) manner.

The rules on the admissibility of expert witness testimony in the United States include the Frye rule, the Daubert ruling and the Federal Rules of Evidence. Unfortunately, the courts have not applied the rules on the admissibility of bite mark evidence, so there have been a number of cases in the United States that relied on flawed bite mark analysis resulting in false convictions that were ultimately overturned following DNA analysis (Bowers, 2006). Clement and Blackwell (2010) noted that lawyers now argued that bite mark methodology had never undergone sound scientific validation and had never been critically scrutinised in order to legitimately satisfy the appropriate rules for admissibility, such as the Frye or Daubert rules as applied in certain states of the US. The authors suggested that the absence of scientific principles in bite mark analysis had been partly responsible for creating a divergence of expert opinions in bite mark cases; the most notable example of disagreement between experienced odontologists was the Norwegian case, *Public Prosecutor v Torgersen* (1958).

Pretty and Sweet (2010) commented on the National Academy of Sciences report entitled *Strengthening Forensic Science in the United States: A Path Forward* (2009). The report referred to the judicial use of forensic science and the state of science itself. In terms of judicial responsibility the report stated:

> Much forensic evidence, including bite mark, firearm and tool mark identification, is introduced in criminal trials without any meaningful scientific validation, determination of error rates or reliability testing to explain the limits of the discipline.

This statement related to the failure of judges to ensure that only forensic evidence that satisfied the rules on the admissibility of expert witness testimony was admitted in court. Indeed, Barsley (2010) commented that, to date, no case on appeal had ever held as inadmissible the opinion of an odontologist based on a lack of scientific or technical standing in the field of odontology. Referring to bite mark identification, the report cited the lack of empirical evidence for the uniqueness of the human dentition, the movement of skin and its ability to record any asserted uniqueness and the nature of photographic analysis as problematic areas. The report stated:

> Reliability is one of the pillars of scientific inquiry, that a scientist's results can be reproduced by other scientists. There are several studies in which bite mark experts plying their craft in controlled laboratory tests have shown widely differing results and a high percentage of false positive matches.

With respect to bite mark evidence, the report concluded:

> Although the majority of forensic odontologists are satisfied that bite marks can demonstrate sufficient detail for positive identification, no scientific studies support this assessment and no large population studies have been conducted. In numerous instances, experts diverge widely in their evaluations of the same bite mark evidence.

The National Academy of Sciences report highlighted two major concerns regarding bite mark analysis in the United States: the lack of reliability of the scientific evidence; and the failure to ensure that the evidence satisfied the rules on the admissibility of expert witness testimony. The current concern regarding the lack of reliability of the evidence is not a new development; this concern has been a constant feature in the history of bite mark analysis in various different countries. Indeed, Hale in 1978 questioned both the reliability of bite mark comparisons and the general acceptance of bite marks in the scientific community. Clearly the concerns in bite mark analysis that were reported in 1978 have continued to the present day. Aitken and MacDonald (1979) noted that classified bite mark characteristics on large sections of the population were unavailable, and this statement remains true today. The recognition of the absence of scientific evidence to validate the identification of an individual to the exclusion of all others on the basis of the comparison of a bite mark in human skin with teeth has finally produced a paradigm shift in the analysis of bite marks. The current efficacy of bite mark analysis should rely on the available scientific evidence and limit expert opinions accordingly. The future efficacy of bite mark analysis will depend on determining the reliability of the scientific evidence and the competence of odontologists. Hypothesis-driven research is required to determine the reliability of the scientific evidence that will validate the expert opinions expressed in bite mark case reports and in court testimony.

8.11 References

Aitken C. and MacDonald D. G. (1979) An application of discrete kernel methods to forensic odontology, *Journal of the Royal Statistical Society* **28**: 55–61.

Aksu M. N. and Gobetti J. P. (1996) The past and present legal weight of bite marks as evidence, *American Journal of Forensic Medicine and Pathology* **17**: 136–140.

Altmeyer B. K., Williams D. E. and Sams V. (1985) Treatment of severe self-injurious and aggressive biting, *Journal of Behavioural Therapy and Experimental Psychiatry* **16**: 159–167.

American Board of Forensic Odontology Inc. (1986) Guidelines for bite mark analysis, *Journal of the American Dental Association* **112**: 383–386.

American Society of Forensic Odontology (1997) ABFO guidelines and standards. In: *Manual of Forensic Odontology*, 3rd rev. edn. Grimsby, Ontario: Manticore Publishers, pp. 299–357.

Avon S. L., Victor C., Mayhall J. T. and Wood R. E. (2010) Error rates in bite mark analysis in an in-vivo animal model, *Forensic Science International* **201**: 45–55.

Barbanel J. C. and Evans J. H. (1974) Bite marks in skin–mechanical factors, *Journal of the Forensic Science Society* **14**: 235–238.

Barsley R. E. (2010) Odontology as a forensic science, the North American experience, *Forensic Science International* **201**: 5–7.

Beckstead J. W., Rawson R. D. and Giles W. S. (1979) Review of bite mark evidence, *Journal of the American Dental Association* **99**: 69–74.

Bernstein M. L. (1985) Two bite mark cases with inadequate scale references, *Journal of Forensic Sciences* **30**: 958–964.

Borgula L. M., Robinson F. G., Rahimi M., Chew K. E. K., Birchmeier K. R., Owens S. G., Kieser J. A. and Tompkins G. R. (2003) Isolation and genotypic comparison of oral streptococci from experimental bitemarks, *Journal of Forensic Odontostomatology* **21**: 23–30.

Bowers C. M. (2006) Problem-based analysis of bitemark misidentifications: the role of DNA, *Forensic Science International* **159**: 104–109.

Bowers C. M. and Pretty I. A. (2009) Expert disagreement in bitemark casework, *Journal of Forensic Sciences* **54**: 915–918.

Burton D. J., Chiafail J. G. and Davis R. G. (1981) Human bites to the face: management, review of the literature, and report of a case, *Journal of the American Dental Association* **102**: 192–194.

Bush M. A., Miller R. G., Bush P. J. and Dorion R. B. J. (2009) Biomechanical factors in human dermal bitemarks in a cadaver model, *Journal of Forensic Sciences* **54**: 167–176.

Butler O. H. (1973) The value of bite mark evidence, *International Journal of Forensic Dentistry* **1**: 23–24.

Chambers English Dictionary (1989) 7th edn. London: Chambers, and Cambridge University Press.

Clement J. G. and Blackwell S. A. (2010) Is current bite mark analysis a misnomer? *Forensic Science International* **201**: 33–37.

Dahlberg A. A. (1960) Clinical ageing patterns in teeth of different population groups. In: *Ageing. Some Social and Biological Aspects*, Proceedings of the Chicago symposium 1959. Publication no. 65 of the American Association for the Advancement of Science, p. 357.

Dinkel E. H. (1974) The use of bite mark evidence as an investigative aid, *Journal of Forensic Sciences* **19**: 535–547.

Duguid R. and McKay G. S. (1981) Bite length measurements and tooth-to-arch relationships obtained from dental casts using an X,Y-digitiser and computer, *Journal of the Forensic Science Society* **21**: 211–223.

Farrell W. L., Rawson R. D., Steffens R. S. and Stephens D. (1987) Computerised axial tomography as an aid in bite mark analysis: a case report, *Journal of Forensic Sciences* **32**: 266–272.

Garven H. S. D. (1965) The skin. In: *A Student's Histology*, 2nd edn. Edinburgh: Livingstone, pp. 305–353.

Gresham G. A. (1986) Wounds. In: *Colour Atlas of Wounds and Wounding*. Lancaster: MTP Press, pp. 9–27.

Gustafson G. (1966) Bite marks. In: *Forensic Odontology*. London: Staples Press, pp. 140–165.

Hale A. (1978) Admissibility of bite mark evidence, *Southern California Law Review* **51**: 309–334.

Harvey W. (1976) Bites and bite-marks. In: *Dental Identification and Forensic Odontology*. London: Henry Kimpton, pp. 88–123.

Harvey W., Millington P., Barbanel J. C. and Evans J. H. (1976) Experimental human bite-marks. In: *Dental Identification and Forensic Odontology*. London: Henry Kimpton, pp. 124–135.

Harvey W., Butler O., Furness J. and Laird R. (1968) The Biggar murder, *Journal of the Forensic Science Society* **8**: 155–219.

Hyzer W. G. and Krauss T. C. (1988) The bite mark standard reference scale–ABFO no. 2, *Journal of Forensic Sciences* **33**: 498–506.

Keiser-Nielsen S. (1967) Forensic odontology–a survey. Paper presented at the FDI/ERO meeting, Vienna.

Kieser J. A., Bernal V., Waddell J. N. and Raju S. (2007) The uniqueness of the human anterior dentition: a geometric morphometric analysis, *Journal of Forensic Sciences* **52**: 671–677.

Krauss T. C. (1984) Photographic techniques of concern in metric bite mark analysis, *Journal of Forensic Sciences* **29**: 633–638.

Levine L. J. (1977) Bite mark evidence, *Dental Clinics of North America* **21**: 145–158.

Levine L. J. (1982) Bite mark evidence. In: *Outline of Forensic Dentistry*. Chicago: Year Book Medical, pp. 112–127.

Ligthelm A. J. and de Wet F. A. (1983) Recognition of bite marks: a preliminary report, *Journal of Forensic Odontostomatology* **1**: 19–26.

MacDonald D. G. (1974) Bite mark recognition and interpretation, *Journal of the Forensic Science Society* **14**: 229–233.

MacFarlane T. W., MacDonald D. G. and Sutherland D. A. (1974) Statistical problems in dental identification, *Journal of the Forensic Science Society* **14**: 247–252.

Mann R. J. (1977) Human bite marks of the hand: twenty years of experience, *Journal of Hand Surgery* **2**: 97–107.

Miller R. G., Bush P. J., Dorion R. B. J. and Bush M. A. (2009) Uniqueness of the dentition as impressed in human skin: a cadaver model, *Journal of Forensic Sciences* **54**: 909–914.

Neufeld P. J. and Colman N. (1990) When science takes the witness stand, *Scientific American* **262**: 18–25.

Nordby J. J. (1992) Can we believe what we see, if we see what we believe?–Expert disagreement, *Journal of Forensic Sciences* **37**: 1115–1124.

Page M., Taylor J. and Blenkin M. (2012) Context effects and observer bias–implications for forensic odontology, *Journal of Forensic Sciences* **57**: 108–112.

Pretty I. A. (2003) A web-based survey of odontologist's opinions concerning bitemark analyses, *Journal of Forensic Sciences* **48**: 1117–1120.

Pretty I. A. (2006) The barriers to achieving an evidence base for bitemark analysis, *Forensic Science International* **159**: 110–120.

Pretty I. A. (2007) Development and validation of a human bitemark severity and significance scale, *Journal of Forensic Sciences* **52**: 687–691.

Pretty I. A. and Sweet D. (2001) The scientific basis for human bitemark analyses–a critical review, *Science and Justice* **41**: 85–92.

Pretty I. A. and Sweet D. (2010) A paradigm shift in the analysis of bitemarks, *Forensic Science International* **201**: 38–44.

Rahimi M., Heng N. C., Kieser J. A. and Tompkins G. R. (2005) Genotypic comparison of bacteria recovered from human bite marks and teeth using arbitrarily primed PCR, *Journal of Applied Microbiology* **99**: 1265–1270.

Rawson R. D. (1982) A method of classification and analysis of distorted patterns in human bite marks. In: *American Academy of Forensic Sciences*, Colorado Springs, Colorado, p. 65.

Rawson R. D. and Brooks S. (1984) Classification of human breast morphology important to bite mark investigation, *American Journal of Forensic Medicine and Pathology* **5**: 19–24.

Rawson R. D., Koot A., Martin C., Jackson J., Novosel S., Richardson A. and Bender T. (1984a) Incidence of bite marks in a selected juvenile population: a preliminary report, *Journal of Forensic Sciences* **29**: 254–259.

Rawson R. D., Ommen R. K, Kinard G., Johnson J. and Yfanits A. (1984b) Statistical evidence for the individuality of the human dentition, *Journal of Forensic Sciences* **29**: 245–253.

Rawson R. D., Vale G. L., Herschaft E. E., Sperber N. D. and Dowell S. (1986a) Analysis of photographic distortion in bite marks: a report of the Bite Mark Guidelines Committee, *Journal of Forensic Sciences* **31**: 1261–1268.

Rawson R. D., Vale G. L., Sperber N. D., Herschaft E. E. and Yfantis A. (1986b) Reliability of the scoring system of the American Board of Forensic Odontology for human bite marks, *Journal of Forensic Sciences* **31**: 1235–1260.

Saferstein R. (1995) In: *Criminalistics–an introduction to forensic science*, 5th edn. Englewood Cliffs, NJ: Prentice-Hall.

Scott J. H. and Symons N. B. B. (1972) The form and relations of human teeth. In: *Introduction to Dental Anatomy*, 6th edn. Edinburgh: Churchill Livingstone, pp. 3–42.

Sheasby D. R. and MacDonald D. G. (2001) A forensic classification of distortion in human bite marks, *Forensic Science International* **122**: 75–78.

Simpson K. and Knight B. (1985) Types of injuries and wounds. In: *Forensic Medicine*, 9th edn. London: Edward Arnold, pp. 48–70.

Skrzeezkas R. (1874) Betreffend die verletzung, zeige fingel usw, *Vierteljahrliche gerichtlich Medizinischer*, **21**.

Sobel M. N. and Perper J. A. (1985) Self-inflicted bitemark on the breast of a suicide victim, *American Journal of Forensic Medicine and Pathology* **6**: 336–339.

Sognnaes R. F., Rawson R. D., Gratt B. M. and Nguyen N. B. T. (1982) Computer comparison of bitemark patterns in identical twins, *Journal of the American Dental Association* **105**: 449–451.

Sopher I. M. (1976) Bite mark analysis. In: *Forensic Dentistry*. Springfield, IL: Charles C. Thomas, pp. 125–152.

Sopher I. M. (1977) The dentist and the battered child syndrome, *Dental Clinics of North America* **21**: 113–122.

Stimson P. (1982) Photographic distortion in bite marks. In: *American Academy of Forensic Sciences*, Colorado Springs, Colorado, p 64.

Stols G. and Bernitz H. (2010) Reconstruction of deformed bite marks using affine transformations, *Journal of Forensic Sciences* **55**: 784–787.

Ström F. (1963) Investigation of bite-marks, *Journal of Dental Research* **42**: 312–316.

Sweet D. and Bowers C. M. (1998) Accuracy of bite mark overlays: a comparison of five common methods to produce exemplars from a suspect's dentition, *Journal of Forensic Sciences* **43**: 362–367.

Sweet D., Lorente J. A., Lorente M., Valenzuela A. and Villanueva E. (1997) An improved method to recover saliva from human skin: the double swab technique, *Journal of Forensic Sciences* **42**: 320–322.

Vale G. L. and Noguchi T. T. (1983) Anatomical distribution of human bite marks in a series of 67 cases, *Journal of Forensic Sciences* **28**: 61–69.

Vale G. L., Sognnaes R. F., Felando G. N. and Noguchi T. T. (1976) Unusual three-dimensional bite mark evidence in a homicide case, *Journal of Forensic Sciences* **21**: 642–652.

DeVore D. T. (1971) Bite marks for identification?–A preliminary report, *Medicine, Science and the Law* **11**: 144–145.

Warnick A. J., Biedrzycki L. and Russanow G. (1987) Not all bite marks are associated with abuse, sexual activities, or homicides: a case study of a self-inflicted bite mark, *Journal of Forensic Sciences* **32**: 788–792.

Whatmough L. N. and Nuckles D. B. (1992) Bite mark evidence: increasing acceptance with a qualified expert witness, *Legal Medicine* 49–78.

Whittaker D. K. (1975) Some laboratory studies on the accuracy of bite mark comparison, *International Dental Journal* **25**: 166–171.

Whittaker D. K. and MacDonald D. G. (1989) Bite marks in flesh. In: *A Colour Atlas of Forensic Dentistry*. London: Wolfe Medical, pp. 108–119.

Zarkowski P. (1988) Bite mark evidence: its worth in the eyes of the expert, *Journal of Law and Ethics in Dentistry* **1**: 47–57.

9

Bite marks – II

Roland Kouble
Dental Surgeon and Forensic Odontologist, Sheffield, UK

9.1 Guidelines for bite mark analysis

The analysis of bite mark evidence needs to be undertaken with a systematic impartial approach by the odontologist. Clear guidelines have been published by various organisations, including the British Association for Forensic Odontology (BAFO) and the American Board for Forensic Odontology (ABFO). The BAFO guidelines present a synopsis of good practice procedures (BAFO, 2010).

Bite mark analysis basically comprises three fundamental elements:

- assessment of the bite mark injury
- assessment of the dentition of the suspected biter/biters
- comparison of the features seen in the injury with the characteristics seen in the suspected biter's dentition.

9.2 Collection of evidence

The collection of evidence in a suspected bite mark case involves photographs with a scale, swabbing for the biter's saliva and /or DNA analysis, and occasionally impressions of the bitten surface if indentations are present, as well as a visual examination of the injury. Any estimation of the age of the injury should be approached with extreme caution or, better still, avoided completely, as ageing bruises is an inaccurate procedure, and the appearance of colours within bruises is very variable (Dailey and Bowers, 1995). An examination also needs to be made of the contour and elasticity of the skin at the site of injury. The position of the victim during the attack will also yield important information as to the extent of the distortion in the bite mark. Other important information such as history of a bleeding diathesis in the victim also will need to be recorded.

Forensic Odontology: An Essential Guide, First Edition.
Edited by Catherine Adams, Romina Carabott and Sam Evans.

In England and Wales, evidence collected from the suspect must be obtained according to sections 62–64 of the *Police and Criminal Evidence Act 1984*. Impressions of the suspect's dentition are classed as intimate samples and therefore need to be authorised by a senior ranked police officer and to have the informed and signed consent of the suspect before being taken. Swabs for saliva or DNA analysis are not classed as intimate samples and therefore do not need consent according to the Act (English and Card, 2001).

9.3 Assessment of the suspected bite mark injury

Assessment of the suspected bite mark usually involves the examination of life-size photographic prints which usually come in the form of JPEG images. The photographs should be taken with a right-angled scale parallel to the film plane. There is further discussion of bite mark photography in Chapter 10.

During collection of the evidence, examination of the injuries on the victim should also be performed if possible, and this may yield further information regarding the orientation of the bite and any likely postural or anatomic distortion that may affect the injury and the photographic images. Examination of the injury should involve metric analysis of the bite mark, which can be undertaken using a ruler *in vivo* or digitally by computer from scanned photographs (Johansen and Bowers, 2000).

Bite marks can exhibit so-called 'class' characteristics, which are clearly recognisable features such as the shape produced by certain teeth. Incisor teeth generally produce rectangular marks and the two central incisor marks tend to be the longest rectangular shapes produced; these features would be considered class characteristics of incisor teeth. Upper incisor teeth produce larger marks than lower incisor teeth and this is another example of a class characteristic (Stimson and Merzt, 1997). The shape and size of the upper and lower arches is another class characteristic that can allow the orientation of a bite mark injury to be determined. Contusion or suck-mark injuries are a class characteristic of human bite marks as they are produced by negative pressure from suction and tongue thrusting during the act of biting. Animals do not produce the suction injuries and this type of mark is usually associated with sexual crimes and abuse of the vulnerable person (Knight, 1996).

Individual characteristics in a bite mark are features that are distinct from what we expect to be the norm, such as rotated teeth, displaced teeth, fractured biting edges on teeth, peg-shaped lateral incisor teeth and tooth spacing (Figure 9.1).

It is important to examine the area of the suspected bite mark not just for lesions caused by the teeth but also for skin blemishes or other alterations in the skin colour and surface that could be mistaken to be part of the injury.

An estimate of the *inter-canine distance* should be attempted from life-size images of the bite mark injury. This can be done directly *in vivo* on the victim's skin and digitally using software such as Adobe Photoshop®.

Inter-canine distances are a useful class characteristic feature in human bite mark analysis. The average male inter-canine distance in the maxilla is 33.93 mm ±2.3 mm and the mandibular measurement is 26.58 mm ±1.97 mm. In females this is somewhat smaller as expected, measuring 32.67 mm ±2.18 mm for the maxilla and

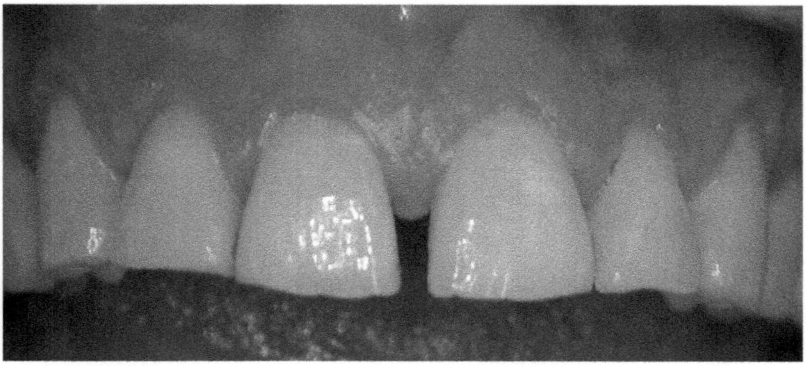

Figure 9.1 Upper midline diastema: an individual characteristic

25.73 mm $\pm$1.69 mm for the mandible. These data are from a longitudinal study of 486 boys and girls who were observed at half-yearly intervals, and the measurements quoted here are for 12-year-olds (Van der Linden, 1983).

Various studies report differing values for inter-canine distance because of the differences in the reference criteria used to obtain the measurement, and size of the samples used in the studies (Bernstein, 2005, Barsley and Lancaster, 1987; Burris and Harris, 1998). Inter-canine distances are a useful class characteristic in bite mark analysis as they may allow orientation of the injury by showing which part of the injury was caused by upper teeth and by lower teeth. Inter-canine distances can also be used to exclude a suspect. Trying to determine whether the mark is more likely to have been made by an adult ($>$12 years in terms of the developmental stage of the dentition) or child can be attempted, but this must be carried out with caution because of the overlap of the size of values of inter-canine distances in children and adults.

Once analysis of the bite mark has been carried out then the investigator must decide on the extent and quality of the evidence. Clearly defined conclusions have been advised in the BAFO and ABFO guidance. The five conclusions that one can reach are as follows:

- *Exclusion.* The injury is not a bite mark.
- *Insufficient.* There are insufficient details within the injury to permit either identification or exclusion of a bite mark.
- *Possible.* An injury showing a pattern that may or may not have been caused by teeth. The injury may have been caused by other factors but biting cannot be ruled out.
- *Probable.* The pattern of the injury strongly suggests or supports an origin from teeth but could conceivably be caused by something else.
- *Definite.* There is no reasonable doubt that teeth created the injury.

It cannot be overstated how important it is to recognise an injury that has low forensic significance and should not be over-analysed or over-interpreted. Sadly, cases where marks have been over-interpreted where there is poor forensic evidence has clearly led to some of the wrongful convictions recently highlighted by the Innocence Project in North America.

9.4 Examination of the dentition of the suspected biter/biters

After examining the bite mark the odontologist should then analyse the dentition of the suspect. A tooth-by-tooth analysis of the suspect's dentition in the form of plaster casts needs to then be studied and the findings should be recorded before any comparison is made between the casts and the victim's injury. The presence of absence of teeth should be recorded as well as tooth rotations, tooth displacements, fractured tooth biting edges, unusual anatomy and restorations.

Metric analysis is also carried out in the form of inter-canine distance measurements on the casts or digital scans of the casts. The suspect's dental casts should be scanned using a flatbed scanner to subsequently produce a hollow volume overlay that can be used for comparison with the injury.

9.5 Bite mark comparisons

9.5.1 Feature-based analysis

Bite mark comparison can be undertaken using numerous techniques; but having made an effective list of all the features in the bite mark injury and another list with the characteristics seen in the suspect's dentition, the two can be compared for points of correspondence or agreement. Likewise, points of discrepancy must also be explained. By carrying out a comparison of the recorded features one can approach the analysis in an open-minded fashion rather than attempting to make an overlay fit the bite mark. During the comparison of the two sets of findings the odontologist takes consideration of the effects of dynamic distortion, tissue distortion, time-related distortion, postural distortion and the effects of photography on the image.

Consideration should also be made of the effects of biting through clothing and the biting mechanism itself.

Once a comparison of the recorded features in the bite mark injury and the suspect's dentition have been made, then demonstration of the various points of correspondence or disagreement can be confirmed using an overlay.

9.5.2 Comparison with overlays and dental casts

Bite mark comparison techniques can be divided into *direct and indirect methods* (Ciapparelli and Hughes, 1992). Direct techniques involve the use of a plaster cast or photographs of the suspect's dentition compared with photographs of the bite mark (Furness, 1968). Indirect comparisons involve the use of transparent overlays to represent the suspect's teeth.

Much research has been done on creating new and varied methods of producing bite mark overlays. Overlays can be produced simply by placing an acetate sheet over a plaster cast of the suspect's teeth and tracing the biting edges, but this has been criticised as the process of hand tracing can introduce error and bias (Pain, 1997). Tracings have also been made from artificial bite marks made using a cast of the suspect's teeth on the skin of the victim and the skin of an anatomically similar volunteer in an attempt to reproduce the same amount of distortion as shown in the original bite mark photograph. Dailey devised a method of producing photocopier-generated overlays which still involved an element of hand tracing. Techniques where hand tracing is involved introduce an element of bias and subjectivity, and even the thickness of the pen nib can affect the accuracy of the tracing.

Sörup used a method based on printing techniques (Humble, 1933). The teeth on a cast were inked and, using several stages of a printing method, an overlay of the inked biting edges was produced on transparent paper. The method was very complicated involving many stages and many likely errors.

A modified method of Dailey's technique (Kouble and Craig, 2004) was developed, which also involved inking the biting edges of a plaster cast of the suspect's dentition and then producing 1:1 xerographic copies directly on to acetate (Figure 9.2).

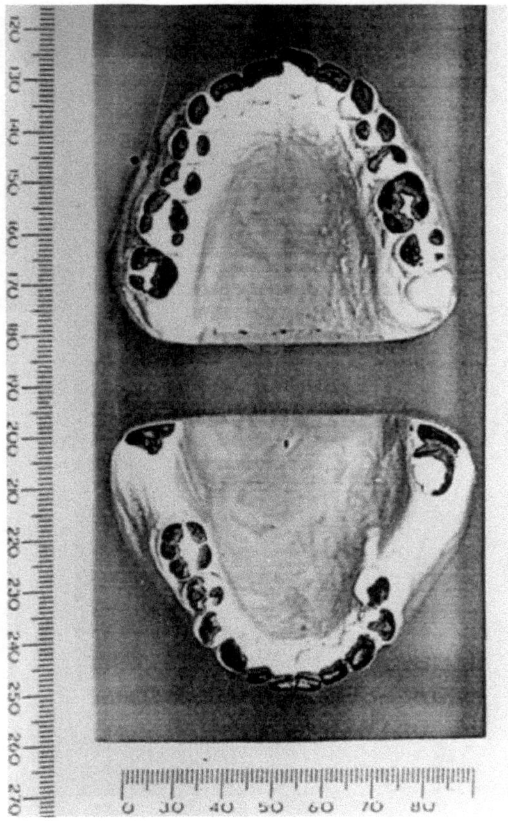

Figure 9.2 Example of a photocopier-generated overlay

Other techniques have also been tried to remove some of the subjectivity involved in producing overlays. Bite marks have been produced in wax and the resulting indentations filled with radiopaque particles to produce radiographs that can in turn be used to produce overlays or transparencies. However, the area of the indentations produced will be dependent on the pressure used to produce the imprint in the wax, a significant and uncontrolled variable.

Very accurate overlays have been produced using computerised axial tomography to scan casts of a suspect's teeth (Farrel *et al.*, 1983). The overlays produced via this method can show the biting edge profiles of the teeth at varying levels or depths, a feature that may more accurately reflect the bite marks that result when different pressures are used.

Scanning electron microscopy has also been used to analyse bite marks to study distinctive details that may not be identified visually by an examiner in the bite mark injury or the plaster casts (David, 1986).

At present the standard method of overlay production involves computer-based techniques (Sweet and Bowers, 1998) that make use of scanned images of the dental casts (Figure 9.3). These scanned casts are then used to produce a hollow volume

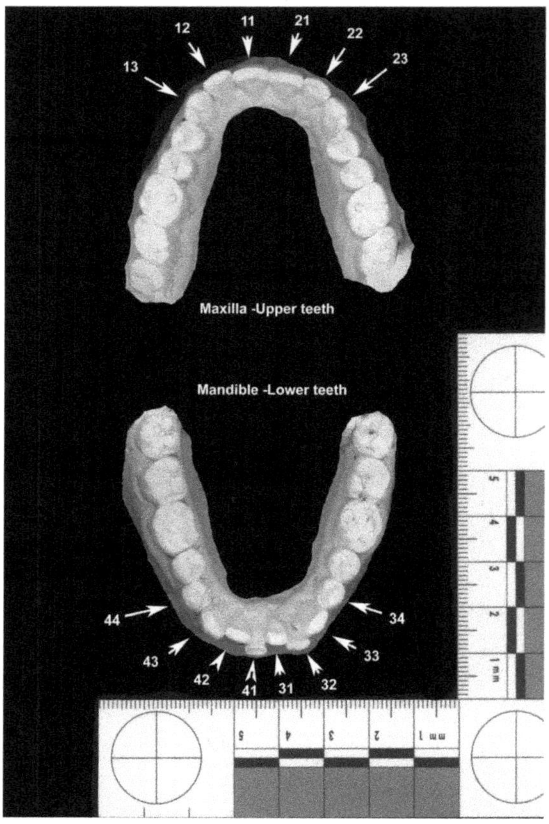

Figure 9.3 Scanned dental casts

overlay of the biting edges of the teeth which can then be superimposed on to the image of the injury.

There are two basic techniques that use Adobe Photoshop® software to fabricate overlays (McNamee *et al.*, 2005). The first method makes use of the Magic Wand tool. The Magic Wand cursor is placed on the biting edges of each tooth and the area is then selected. This selected area will contain pixel tones that are adjacent with the same or similar values depending on the tolerance setting of the Magic Wand tool. This outlined perimeter for each tooth biting edge is then defined using a two-pixel black line, creating the overlay. These computer-based techniques have been shown to be more accurate than other techniques for overlay production in a study by Sweet and Bowers (1998). They found that, when looking at biting edge profile areas and tooth rotation representations on overlays produced by five different techniques, the most reproducible method was computer-based.

However, the process of defining biting edge profiles digitally requires the actions of the investigator which introduces an element of subjectivity.

Another method of overlay production using Adobe Photoshop® software used predominantly in Europe uses differences in contrast levels in the cast image and the Glowing Edges filter (McNamee *et al.*, 2005). The investigator selects Filters, Stylize and Glowing Edges filter in Adobe Photoshop®. The Glowing Edges filter selects and highlights the edges of the casts and teeth, after which the image is inverted and any unwanted areas are deleted to leave the outline of the biting edges of the teeth required for analysis (Figure 9.4). One could argue that this method also involves some level of subjectivity during the process of deleting the 'unwanted' detail. However, the biting edges are not selected by the investigator but independently selected by the Glowing Edges filter – although this does not appear to make much difference as both methods have been shown to be equally reliable.

The Glowing Edges technique is summarised in Figure 9.5, showing the step-by-step procedure in overlay production.

With improvements in computer scanning technology, the production of overlays should become even less subjective. Hollow volume overlays can be set at different levels of the biting edge plane, allowing the biting edge profile to be analysed in more detail (Figure 9.6). This is particularly useful in cases where there are teeth with differential wear patterns and malocclusions that allow certain biting edges to create a deeper impact into a bitten substrate.

9.5.3 Conclusion

Once the investigator has carried out his/her analysis of the injury and the suspect's teeth, and made the comparison, then a conclusion should be reached. Once again there are clear guidelines published by BAFO (2010) as to how these should be stated in the odontology report:

- *Excluded.* There are discrepancies between the bite mark and the suspect's dentition that exclude the individual from having make the mark.
- *Inconclusive.* There is insufficient forensic detail or evidence to draw any conclusion on the link between the suspect's dentition and the bite mark.

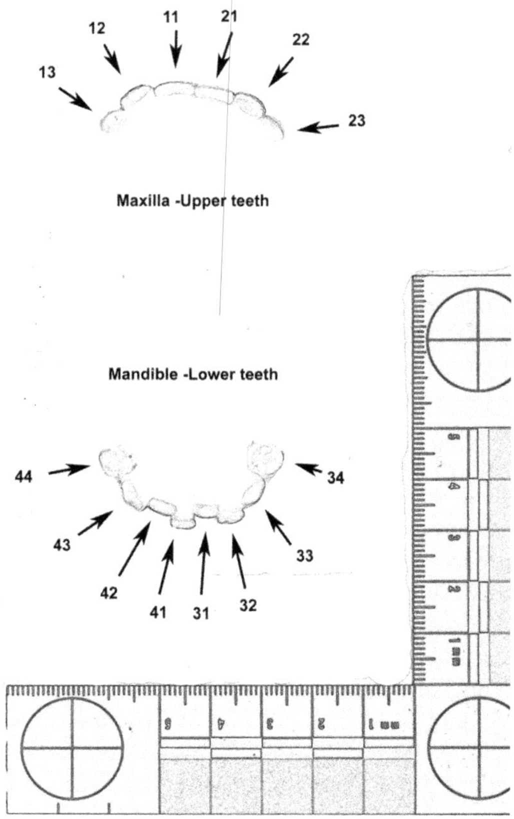

Figure 9.4 Bite mark overlay produced using the Glowing Edges technique

- *Possible biter.* Teeth like the suspect's could be expected to create a mark like the one examined, but so could other dentitions.
- *Probable biter.* The suspect most likely made the bite. Most people in the population would not leave such a bite.
- *Reasonable medical certainty.* The suspect is identified for all practical purposes by the bite mark. Any expert with similar training and experience, evaluating the same evidence, should come to the same conclusion of certainty.

9.5.4 Open and closed populations

In certain circumstances when comparing multiple suspects with a bite mark injury it may be useful to qualify one's conclusions with regard to the number of potential suspects who could be implicated. For example, if a bite mark is of moderate forensic value and there are no distinctive characteristics present within the injury, and two suspects' dentitions are being compared, then you may conclude that one of the suspects is a possible biter if the potential pool of suspects could include many other

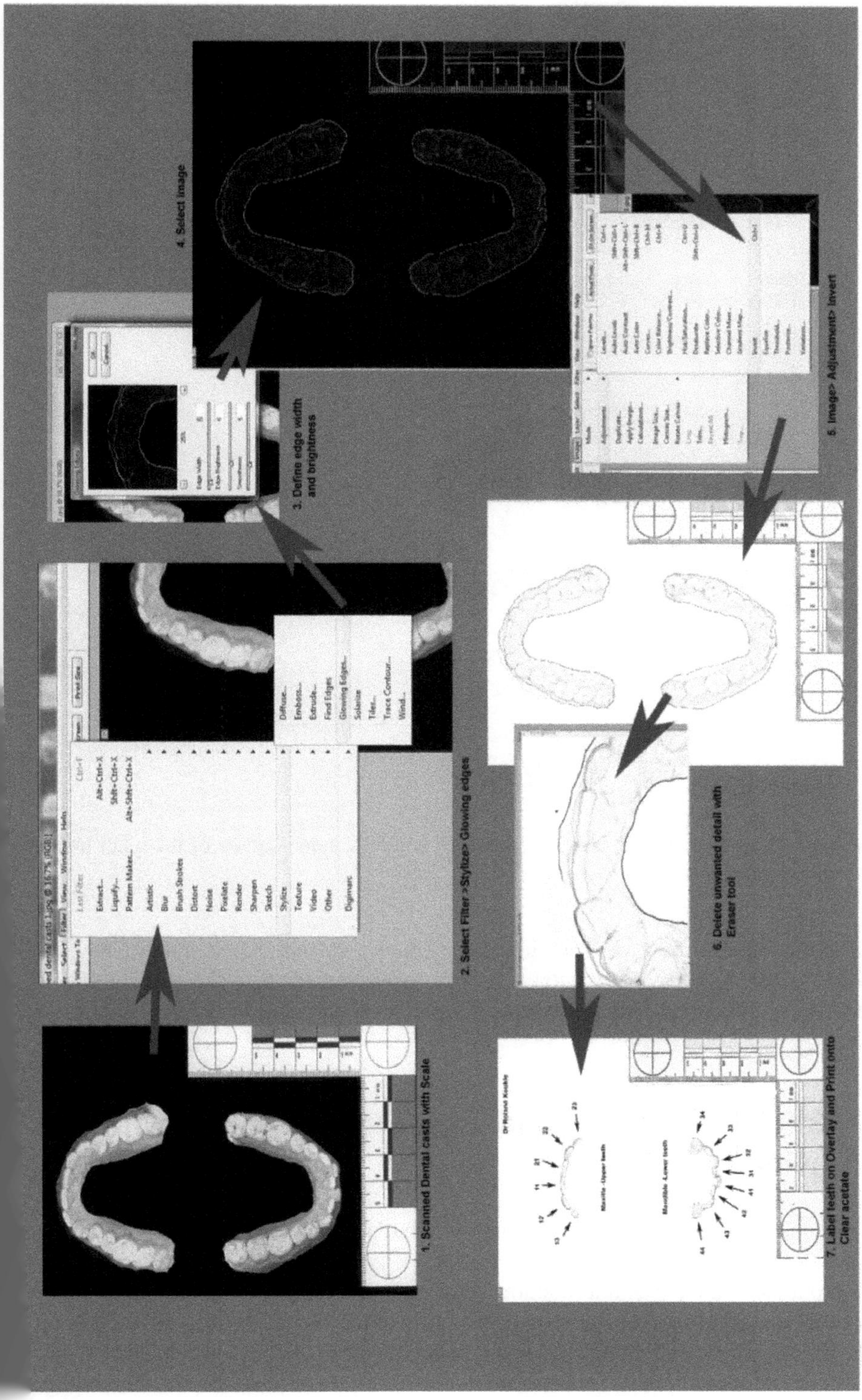

Figure 9.5 Summary of the Glowing Edges technique, showing the step-by-step procedure in overlay production (For colour details, please see colour plate section.)

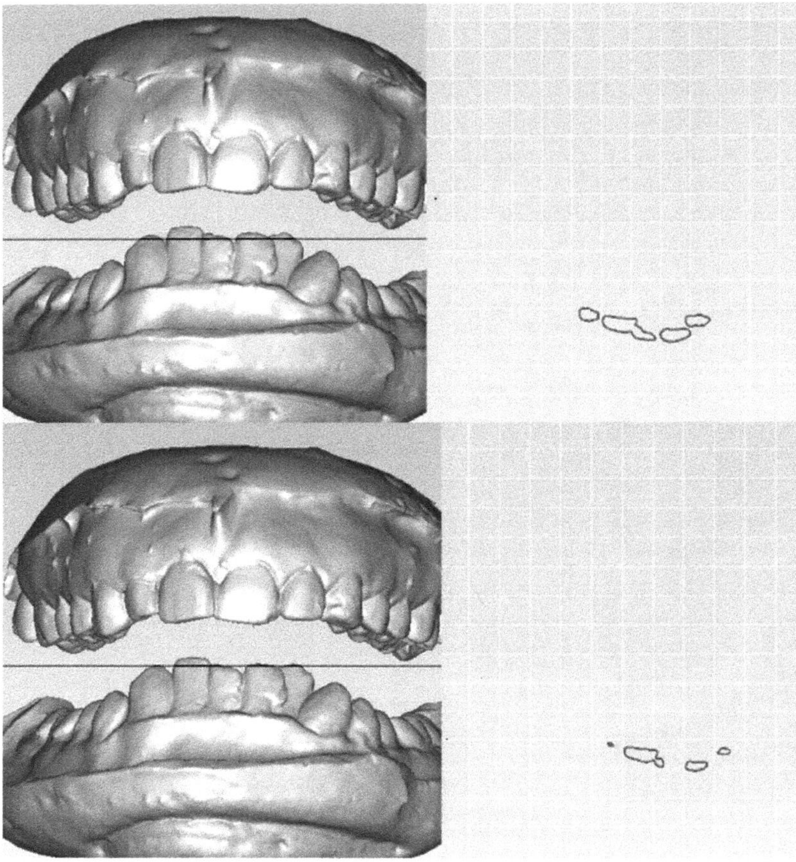

Figure 9.6 Three-dimensional scanned casts with hollow volume outline of the tooth biting edges at different planes

people (an *open pool of suspects*). However, if only two individuals could have left the mark (a *closed pool of suspects*) then you may conclude that the suspect was a probable biter given that only two suspects could have inflicted the bite.

9.6 Bite mark reports and presentation of evidence to a court

Report writing is covered in detail in Chapter 3, but a bite mark report should contain certain important elements.

The report should have an introduction to the case with a timeline of the events starting with the date and time of the initial contact by either the police or solicitor. There should also be a list of all the evidence and materials received, such as copies of statements from witnesses, expert reports and copies of photographs/exhibits. The report should give a description of the injury and the expert's interpretation of the injury. Copies of the images of the injuries with labels should be included in the report to further highlight the investigator's interpretation of the injury. Using the BAFO guidelines, the injury should be classified as an excluded, possible, probable or definite bite mark. As discussed, a feature-based analysis is recommended as the method of choice for bite mark analysis. This can then lead onto a comparison of the features seen in the bite mark and those seen in the suspect's dentition. The results of features comparison and the results of the comparisons using the overlays should be discussed and presented in the report.

It is just as important to highlight discrepancies between the teeth and the bite mark as it is to identify corresponding features. Any discrepancy will need to be explained in the report and cannot be overlooked. If one is unsure about the causation of a mark then this should be stated rather than ignored.

The conclusions can then finally be presented at the end of the report clearly and concisely. It is important to note that the report should present the expert's opinion and explanation of how that opinion was reached. Using the BAFO guidelines, one can then express that opinion with the levels of certainty discussed previously in such a way that a lay person reading the report should be able to understand the facts and conclusions.

Bite mark case work will in some cases require the expert to attend court to give evidence. This can be disruptive to practitioners who run their own practice and difficult for practitioners who are either employed or self-employed associates. It is important to communicate with the witness care team so that time can be booked in advance where possible to facilitate both parties. Odontologists are regarded as expert witnesses in court rather than professional witnesses. Giving evidence for the first time can be stressful, but keeping a cool head and sticking to your own field of expertise is important to avoid getting into difficulties.

Both your report and spoken evidence should be given in an objective and unbiased manner, without the use of too much specialist language, to be as clear as possible.

9.7 References

Barsley R. E. and Lancaster D. M. (1987) Measurement of arch widths in a human population: relation of anticipated bite marks, *Journal of Forensic Science* **32**(4): 975–982.

Bernstein M. L. (2005) Nature of bitemarks. In: Dorion R. B. J. (ed.), *Bitemark Evidence*. New York: Marcel Decker, pp. 59–80.

British Association for Forensic Odontology (BAFO) (2010) *Guidelines for Good Practice in Bite Mark Investigation and Analysis*.

Burris B. G. and Harris E. F. (1998) Identification of race and sex from palate dimensions, *Journal of Forensic Science* **43**(5): 959–963.

Ciapparelli L. and Hughes P. (1992) Bite marks in tissue and in inanimate objects: analysis and comparison. In: Clark D. H. (ed.), *Practical Forensic Odontology*. Oxford: Wright, pp. 149–177.

Dailey J. C. and Bowers C. M. (1995) Ageing of bitemarks: a literature review. In: Bowers C. M. and Bell G. L. (eds), *Manual of Forensic Odontology*, 3rd edn. American Society of Forensic Odontology, pp. 184–190.

David T. J. (1986) Adjunctive use of scanning electron microscopy in bite mark analysis: a three-dimensional study, *Journal of Forensic Science* **31**(3): 1126–1134.

English J. and Card R. (2001) Identification methods. In: *Butterworth's Police Law*, 7th edn. London: Butterworth, pp. 147–150.

Farrell W. L., Rawson R. D., Steffens R. S. and Stephens D. (1987) Computerised axial tomography as an aid in bite mark analysis: a case report, *Journal of Forensic Science* **32**(1): 266–272.

Furness J. (1968) A new method for the identification of teeth marks in cases of assault and homicide, *British Dental Journal* **124**(6): 261–267.

Humble B. H. (1933) Identification by means of teeth, *British Dental Journal* **54**: 528–536.

Johansen R. J. and Bowers C. M. (2000) *Digital Analysis of Bite Mark Evidence using Adobe Photoshop*. Forensic Imaging Services.

Knight B. (1996) Forensic dentistry for the pathologist. In: *Forensic Pathology*. London: Arnold, pp. 517–530.

Kouble R. F. and Craig G. T. (2004) A comparison between direct and indirect methods available for human bite mark analysis, *Journal of Forensic Science* **49**(1): 111–118.

McNamee A. H., Sweet D. and Pretty I. (2005) A comparative reliability analysis of computer-generated bitemark overlays, *Journal of Forensic Science* **50**(2): 1–6.

Pain S. (1997) Murderous molars, *New Scientist* (special suppl.): 14–16.

Stimson P. C. and Merzt C. A. (1997) Bite mark techniques and terminology. In: Stimson P. C. and Merzt C. A. (eds), *Forensic Dentistry*. New York: CRC Press, pp. 137–159.

Sweet D. and Bowers M. (1998) Accuracy of bite mark overlays: a comparison of five common methods to produce exemplars from a suspect's dentition, *Journal of Forensic Science* **43**(2): 362–367.

Van der Linden F. (1983) Numerical and graphical information concerning development of the dentition. In: *Development of the Dentition*. Chicago: Quintessence, pp. 161–199.

10

Forensic photography and imaging

Sam Evans
School of Dentistry, Cardiff University, UK

10.1 Introduction

This chapter aims to provide information for both the novice and the professional photographer to successfully to acquire images that may be needed for subsequent analysis. Some sections are more in-depth and are there to supplement the knowledge of those with more experience.

Imaging of the patterned bruise of a bite mark is one of the few variables in the process of bite mark analysis that the investigator can control. The technique and equipment employed by the operator will greatly influence the quality of the photographic evidence. Timing is an important factor too. Over time, bruises are likely to fade, although it is conceivable that a bruise can be photographed too soon as it may not be fully developed. These factors make it difficult to ascertain a clear pattern from which the forensic odontologist can analyse the relevant features.

The author suggests that, where possible, a qualified forensic odontologist and professional photographer with a comprehensive understanding of this field work together to achieve the best quality images for analysis. If that arrangement is not possible, then this section will provide information on the basic requirements on how to obtain the necessary images. Each step will be explained, from camera equipment advice to the correct positioning of the camera in relation to the bite mark.

10.2 The photography of bite marks

As stated in the British Association of Forensic Odontology's *Guide for Good Practice in Bite Mark Investigation and Analysis* (BAFO; www.bafo.org.uk), it is good practice, where possible, to photograph bite marks in the presence of a forensic odontologist. In the UK there are five professional groups that may record bite mark injuries for further analysis by forensic odontologists: the first two groups are well trained and

Forensic Odontology: An Essential Guide, First Edition.
Edited by Catherine Adams, Romina Carabott and Sam Evans.

experienced in image capture, while the other three will have generally received less training and have accumulated less experience. The groups are:

- police forensic photographers
- clinical (hospital) photographers
- scene of crime (SOC) officers (crime scene investigators)
- forensic experts (forensic odontologists and pathologists)
- clinicians (paediatricians etc.).

Within each group there are varying degrees of success in the recording of the evidence. However, regardless of ability, even well-trained and experienced professionals will still produce a certain amount of photographic distortion (introducing measurement error) in the image capturing process owing to the limitations of 2-dimensional (2D) technology. This is most apparent in the reduction of the 3-dimensional (3D) structure of the human body into the 2D space of the digital camera.

Forensic photography demands consistently accurate results when depicting an object in its 2D representation. Consistency is required in the framing of the object in the centre of the image, the sharpness of the focus and, within the limitations of the camera, absence of photographic distortion. The consistency of the colour and the tonal range are equally important. Care must also be taken to eliminate any unwanted or distracting shadows. To achieve these results the quality of the equipment is very important. High-end digital single-lens-reflex (DSLR) cameras are routinely used, equipped with a range of lenses and separate flash systems.

One area not often discussed is the end-product of digital imaging, the digital print or the on-screen image. Issues surrounding colour representation and reproducibility are the most variable. The same image on different monitors can look very different if the monitors are not professionally calibrated. Further variability can be introduced when the digital image is printed: often the printed image does not represent what appears on screen. This can be quite a complex problem to rectify, but it is not necessarily a problem that will commonly affect the forensic analysis of patterned injuries. It is, nonetheless, an important issue to be aware of.

Canon and Nikon are two DSLR manufacturers whose products are used by most forensic photographers. Both companies provide a range of suitable cameras, lenses and flash systems. The latest digital SLR cameras have very high pixel counts. Currently, Nikon's D3x at 24.5 megapixels, the Nikon D800E at 36.3 megapixels and Canon's EOS-1Ds Mark III at 22.3 megapixels represent the pinnacle. (Some medium-format cameras – used in photographic studios, mostly for portraits and fashion – have pixel counts of up to 60 megapixels. The Hasselblad digital range is an example.)

As the power of the computer processor will inevitably increase and change over time, so will the sensitivity and capabilities of the sensor in the digital camera. Although the quantity of pixels is very important to the amount of information recorded by the camera, it is only part of the story (dynamic range and pixel noise are also important). The quality and build of the lens is also an important factor in capturing the right levels of detail. Control over detail and thus consistency is needed for forensic analysis. The right lens will limit the photographic distortion (not taking into account operator error). There are many different types of lenses available to the operator; however, most are unsuitable for use in photographing bite marks or other patterned bruises. Lenses used with DSLRs mostly fall into two categories: prime or zoom, which have varying focal lengths. The focal length relates to the distance between the film plane (in digital cameras, the sensor) and the focal point of the lens (the optical centre of the end of the lens). The focal length is usually measured in millimetres.

- *Prime lenses* have a fixed focal length. For example, a 105 mm lens can provide the fine detail that may be needed to demonstrate individual teeth marks accurately. Lenses like the 60 mm allow the photographer to get relatively close to the subject (bite mark injury) and still retain the required 90-degree angle needed for limitation of angular distortion. A lens with a lower focal length, such as a 20 mm, will introduce noticeable barrel distortion and should be avoided.
- *Zoom lenses* do not have a fixed focal length but instead have a range. An 18–55 mm or 18–105 mm lens is commonly supplied with a camera when sold as a kit. The focal length will be changed if using non-full-frame sensors (more detail is given later in the chapter).

Zoom lenses should be avoided when photographing bite marks. When using a zoom lens, the operator can often change the focal length without realising. Using such equipment will likely result in poor consistency, as the objects in a sequence of images would be of varying sizes. Furthermore, changing the position of the zoom lens to a short focal length may introduce visual aberrations, such as barrel and pin-cushion (curvilinear) distortion. Langford (1975) describes it as a variation in magnification across the image plane. A lens with a focal length less than 50 mm will start to introduce some distortion. Furthermore, a poor-quality lens can create such distortion. Barrel distortion creates a sphere-like distortion of the image (Figure 10.1). However, visually obvious distortion would only occur when using lenses with very short focal lengths.

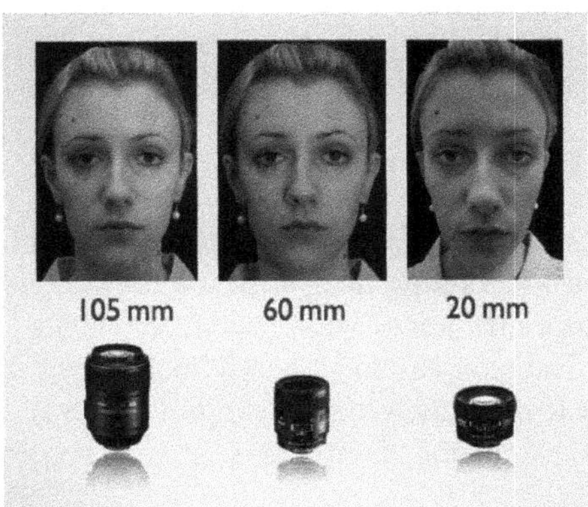

Figure 10.1 Demonstration of barrel distortion. With thanks to J. Oliver

An important aspect of photography that applies to all cameras and all operators of varying abilities is *depth of field*. The depth of field describes the area in the image that is in focus, from the foreground to the background. Figure 10.2 demonstrates the important aspects of depth of field and how it can affect the relevant detail in the image.

10.3 Relevant equipment

For best results, professional or semi-professional grade cameras, lenses and flash systems should be used. This ensures the quality and precision needed, especially when concerning detail, sharpness of focus, quality of tonal range and control over distortion introduced by the camera. As mentioned above, when photographing bite marks the single most important aspect is the control over photographic distortion. When choosing equipment the operator must consider not just the type of camera but the quality and type of lens. The level of quality needed in a lens is usually only available in the SLR camera systems (Figure 10.3). Although mobile phones with cameras have become ubiquitous, they should be considered a last resort for use in recording patterned injuries such as a bite mark. Despite the fact these devices have sensors with large pixel counts, the lenses used are likely to have short focal lengths (equivalent to around 30 mm in an SLR camera). The lens distortion and the likelihood of pixel noise and lack of tonal range in a digital image produced by a mobile phone will reduce the quality of the photographic evidence. However, in certain circumstances and with an understanding of the limitations of the technology, a mobile phone may be the only option available to the operator and may provide important information to the investigation.

The digital single-lens-reflex camera

There are many types of digital camera available, from entry level to high-end cameras used by professional photographers (e.g. Nikon D series, Canon EOS series). There are some subtle differences between the entry level and professional cameras, ranging from the quality of the build to the ability to capture images in low light settings.

Lenses

As mentioned already, the type of lens is instrumental in providing consistent images with minimal distortion for forensic analysis. Furthermore, if it is necessary to take images at a close distance then a lens with macro capabilities is required. Such a lens allows the operator to focus on an object barely inches away, giving a great amount of detail. Some non-SLR cameras, such as compact cameras, have a macro function but this often works only when the zoom lens is set to a short focal length, thus giving barrel distortion.

Some high quality micro system cameras may be fitted with adequate lenses that are suitable for photography of bite marks. To maintain consistency it is advantageous

Three important aspects that affect depth of field.
1. The aperture (f number i.e. F4, F22)
The lower the F number the narrower the depth of field
2. The length of the lens (105mm, 60mm etc.)
The longer the lens the narrower the depth of field.
3. The distance from the lens to the subject
The closer the camera to the subject, the narrower the depth of field.

Foreground Midpoint Background

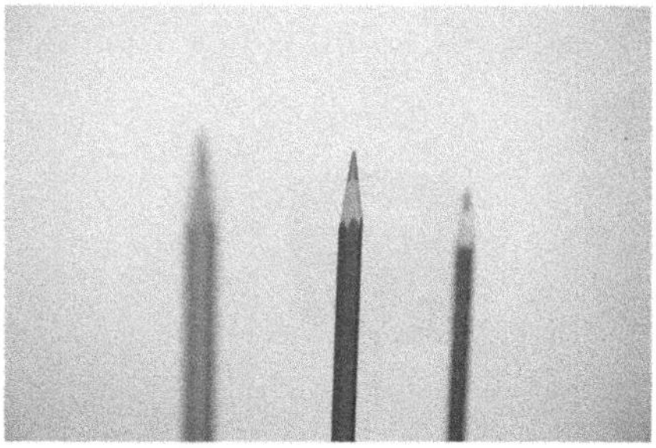

The camera is set to F 4. This means less of the image is in focus and is therefore harder for the operator to get the relevant information in focus.

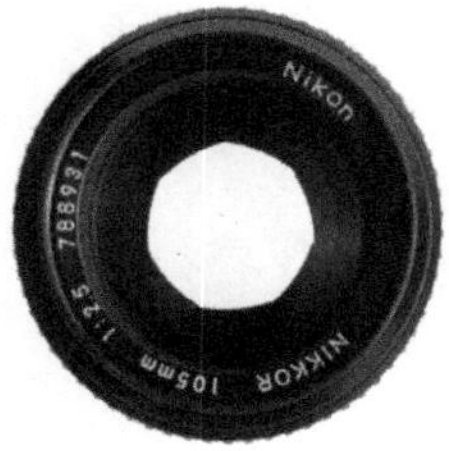

At F 4 the lens aperture is open very wide. This gives a **narow depth of field.**

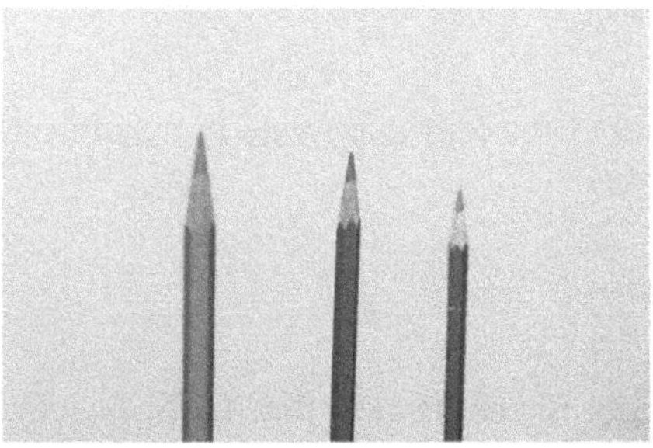

The camera is set to F16. This means more of the image is in focus and makes it an easier job to get more information in sharp focus.

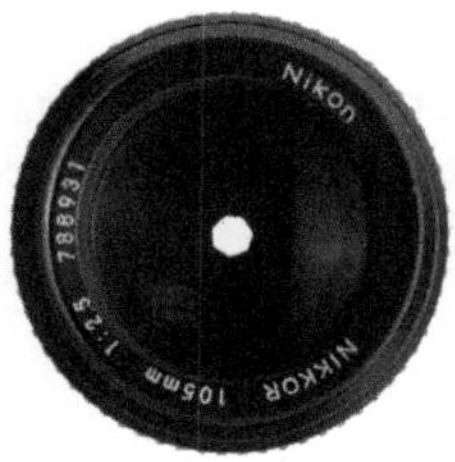

At F16 the lens aperture is becoming narrower, creating a **wider depth of field.**

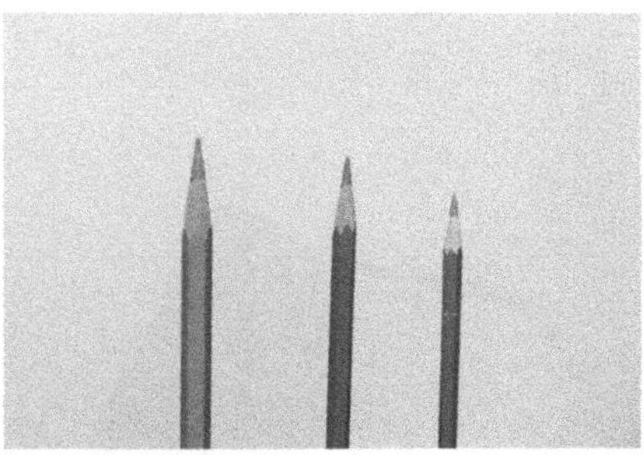

The camera is set to F22. This gives the operator more chance of creating an image with most of the relevant features in focus.

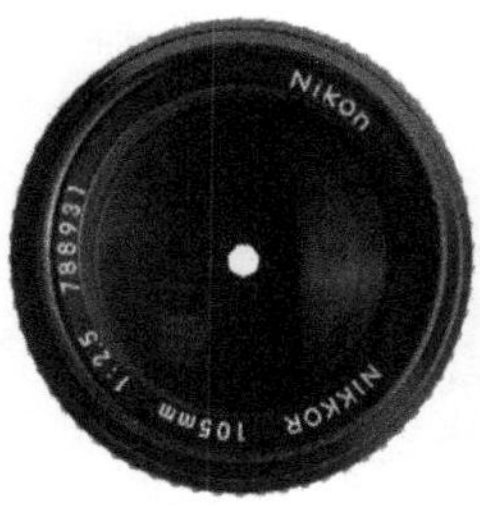

At F22 the lens aperture is very narrow.
This is especially important when photographing objects close up, as the closer the camera is to the object the narrower the depth of field.
Note: Some lenses can go up to F32.

Figure 10.2 Illustration of the effect of depth of field (For colour details, please see colour plate section.)

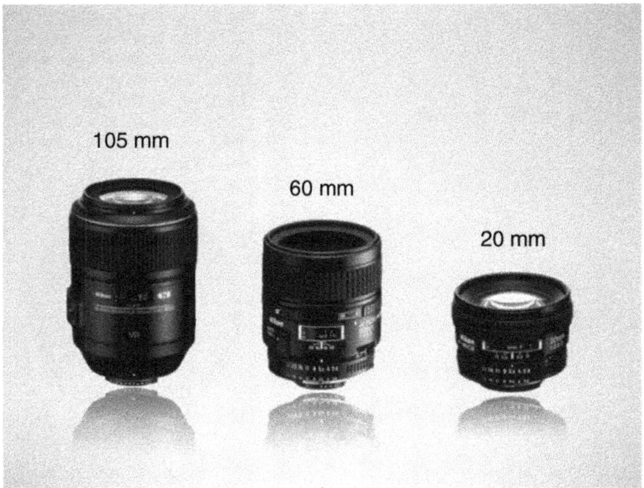

Figure 10.3 A range of lenses

to use lenses that have markings on the barrel of the lens that relate to magnification ratios, or distance in metres or in feet.

Flash devices

When photographing bite marks it is strongly recommended that flash devices be used (Figure 10.4). Many cameras have a built-in flash, but it is inadvisable to use

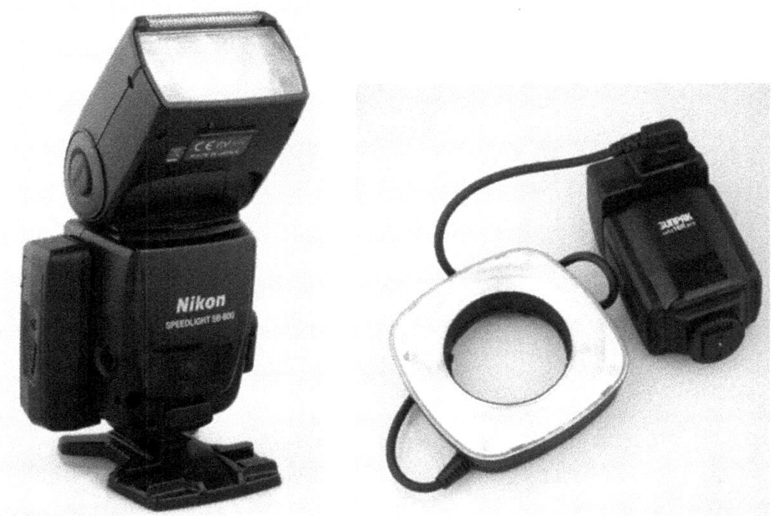

Figure 10.4 Suitable flash devices

this facility. When photographing a bite mark the camera is relatively close to the subject, which results in the light that is emitted from the built-in flash to cause unwanted shadows and over-exposure, which may then obscure important information.

Many textbooks suggest that it is ideal to have a mounted flashgun on each side of the camera to give even illumination. However, when photographing small bruises from a close distance, reasonable results can be obtained with a suitable single flashgun or ringflash if properly positioned. (If large scenes, such as a whole room, need illumination then two flashguns may be required.)

An accurate scale

A rigid scale, such as the ABFO no. 2, L-shaped scale (Figure 10.5), is *essential* for the photography of any patterned injury (Hyzer and Krauss, 1998). The scale, when placed correctly, allows the investigator to make consistent measurements of the bruise. Without this scale being placed correctly and photographed with the injury, the subsequent measurements will be subject to error. The analysis will consequently be affected and may result in inadmissible evidence for court.

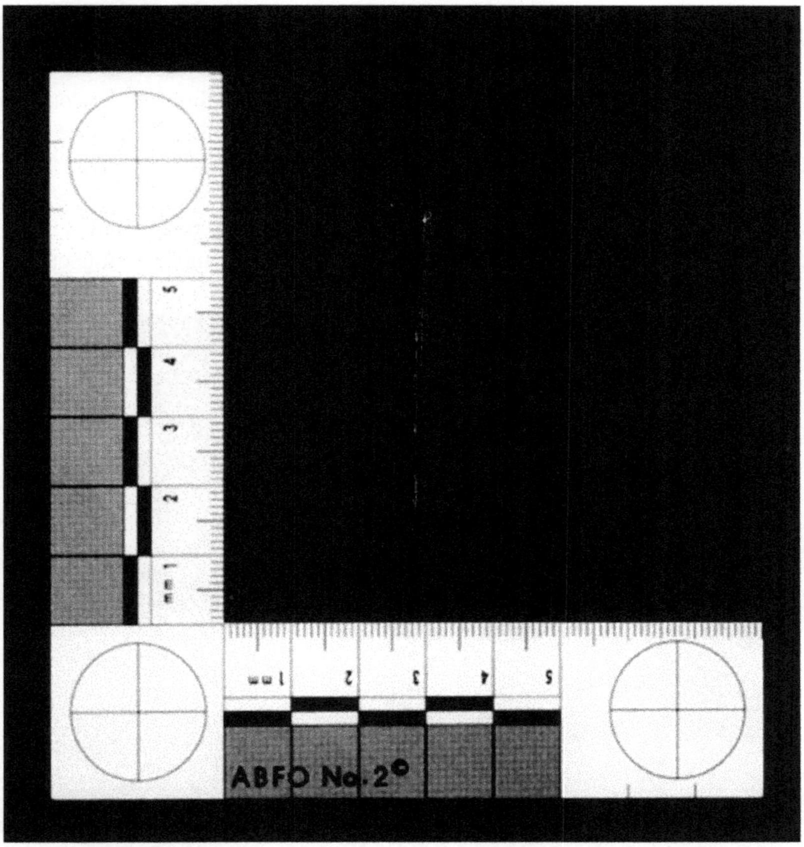

Figure 10.5 The ABFO no.2 scale

Research has shown that some caution should be applied when using scales for forensic analysis (Payne-James, 2012). Not all rulers are created equally. Very small variations will likely be present between different scales and subtle bias in the measurements may be introduced. When taking photographs of the bite mark and making recordings of the suspect's dental cast, it may be pertinent to use the same scale, to minimise any unwanted measurement error. All scales should have a matt finish to reduce reflections.

An accurate colour chart

To ensure correct colour calibration in the image via a computer, an accurate colour chart will be needed when photographing the bite mark. A mini colour checker will be the most practical. Digital photographs are made up of pixels, and each pixel has a colour value related to its red, green and blue content. Good-quality colour charts have the red, green and blue (RGB) value for each colour with the accompanying documentation (Figure 10.6).

The use of a colour chart is well described in a guideline publication from the Scientific Working Group on Imaging Technologies:

> The purpose of colour balancing is to render colours in the scene faithfully. For example, a colour test target having known colours can be placed in the scene prior to recording the image. ... It is commonly assumed that the colour of other objects in the scene will be rendered accurately as well. Improper colour balance can render colours inaccurately, causing objects to appear to have the wrong color.

For consistent results a colour chart should be visible in every image that is taken. This is because slight changes in the distance between the flash and the subject will have

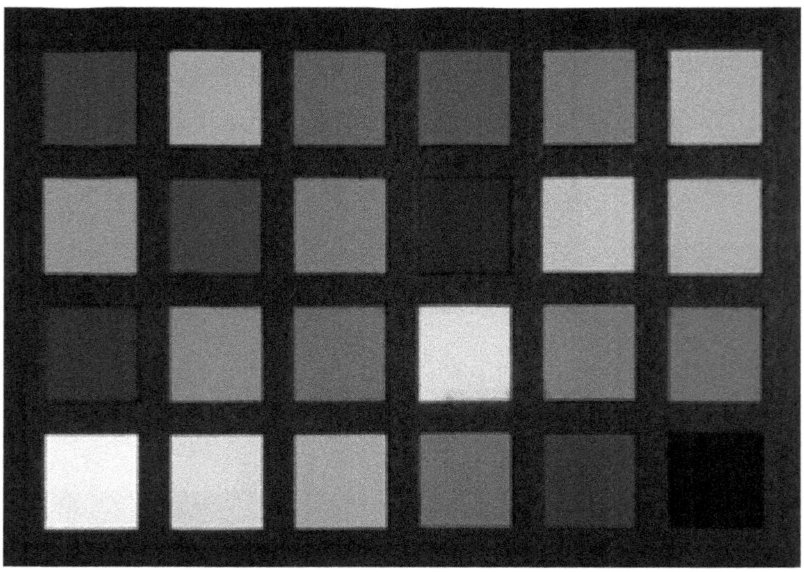

Figure 10.6 Colour checker chart (For colour details, please see colour plate section.)

an influence on the brightness within the image and thus will create slight variance in the colour. Nonetheless, any noticeable impact this variation has on the process of bite mark analysis will be speculative.

Using colour charts can help calibrate images for colour balance. However, because there are many variables to account for, it would be inadvisable to use photography as a tool to interpret colour and to correlate any forensic significance to the colour of the bruise, especially in terms of ageing (Maguire *et al.*, 2005).

Recap of relevant equipment

Figure 10.7 shows a typical camera case and equipment. It contains all the equipment mentioned above.

10.4 Digital image file formats

It is likely that most, if not all, high-end digital cameras have the function to capture and then transfer the digital image in a very minimally compressed (or lossless compression) format, which the operator can determine. The type of compression here

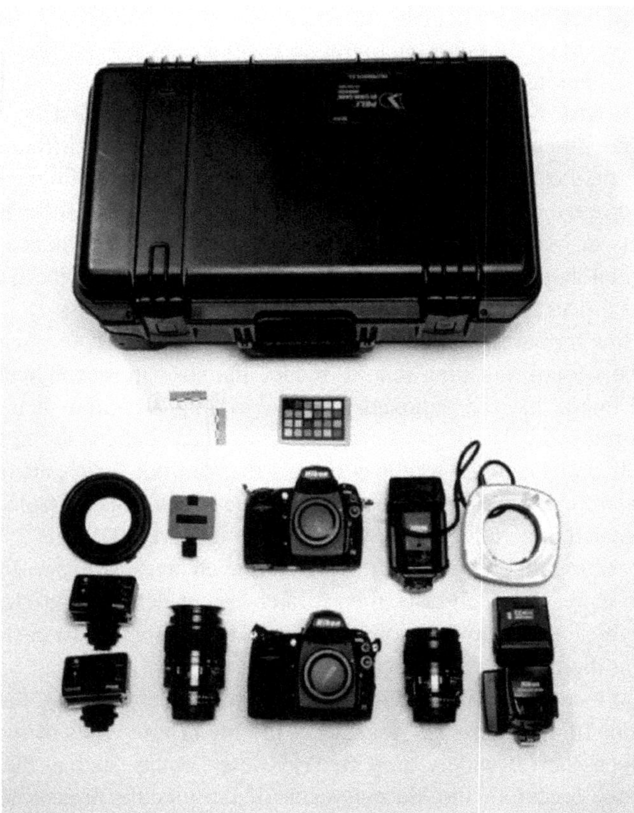

Figure 10.7 Typical camera case and equipment

refers to the act of reducing the file's size in megabytes. This is done by the removal of pixels from the image, so some definition is lost. The Select Committee on Science and Technology's report in 1998 suggested that there should not be a strict command for any particular file format:

> We recommend that evidence should not necessarily be inadmissible because it does not conform with some specific technological requirement.

A particular format cannot be insisted upon as technology will inevitably advance and develop. However, it is important to state that file formats using high levels of compression should be avoided, by 'using an appropriate file format to capture different scenes without compromising the image quality' (ACPO and NPIA, 2007). Furthermore, guidelines published in the United States by the Federal Bureau of Investigation suggest adjusting the digital camera's capture settings to the 'highest quality possible' (FBI Laboratory, 2005).

The lossless (little compression) type of format used by the camera will most likely be either the TIF (Tagged Image File) format or a RAW image format. Each manufacturer has their own proprietary RAW image format. Currently, two commonly used examples are the Canon RAW version (CRW and CR2) and the Nikon electronic format (NEF). The ability to use RAW image files is an important component for the forensic application, as it gives an unfettered image, described by some as the 'digital negative'. Many forensic photographers will use only RAW files when creating photographic evidence.

The Nikon's NEF format, the 16-bit NEF file (the original/first copy), cannot be manipulated. The file can only be saved as a working copy, in a different format (e.g. an 8-bit TIFF or the lossy (heavy compression) JPEG (Joint Photographic Experts Group)). The original cannot be overwritten by image processing software. The use of lossless formats such as the NEF means that the integrity of the evidence is maintained as all the original data are reconstructed faithfully at all stages in the workflow, from the viewing to the archiving of the image.

The JPEG file format uses a heavier compression (although the amount of compression can be varied), meaning that, to reduce the size (in megabytes), parts of the data from the image file are removed. It is the coding algorithm that decides what information is removed. The JPEG format can introduce changes to the appearance of the image itself. For example, artefacts (pixels that did not form part of the original image) appear around the edges of an object in the digital image. Colour changes or colour loss are also affected by lossy compression (Figure 10.8).

The greater the lossy compression, the greater the changes. If image enhancement is needed (e.g an increase of contrast), then further loss of detail is introduced. Changes brought about by image compression may cause issues for the forensic investigator when analysing the images.

An important factor when using RAW image formats is proprietary; they are susceptible to problems in the future use (legacy) of the file. These types of file will need to be copied as open-source (widely supported) lossless formats, such as the TIFF format. A problem in the legacy of the file may occur if the manufacturer ceases to support

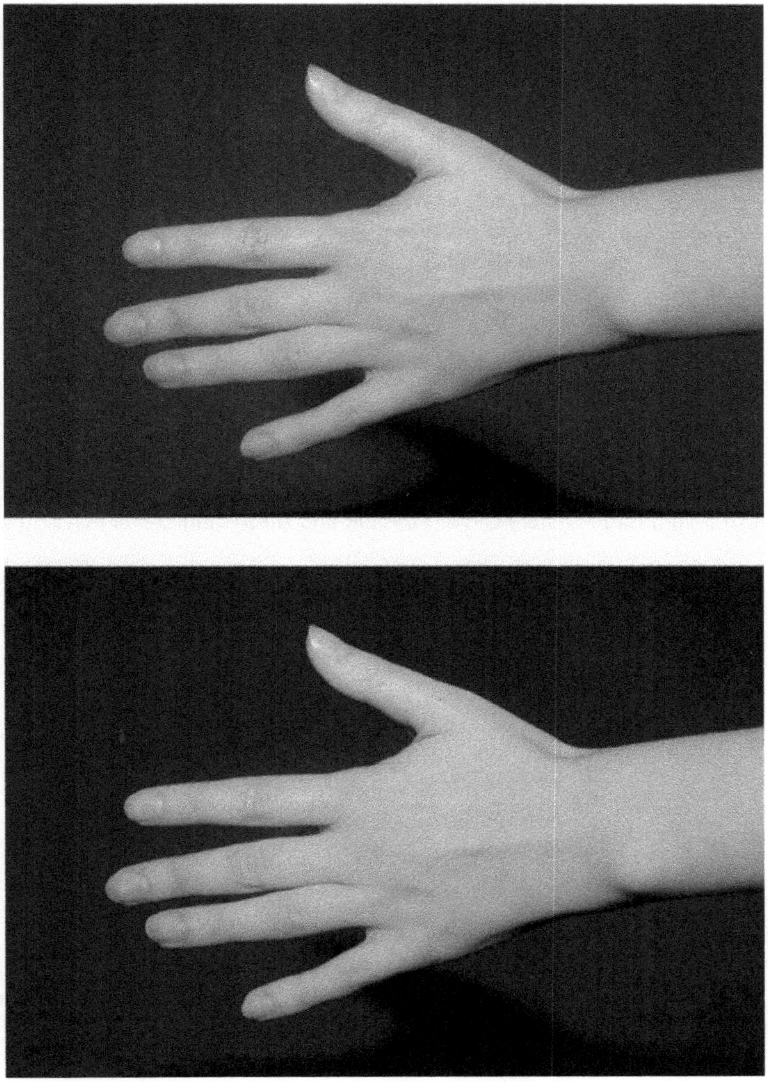

Figure 10.8 Demonstration of the difference in detail and colour in RAW and JPEG capture. The top image is captured in the NEF format, while the bottom image is captured in Nikon's highest quality (lowest compression) JPEG. In the NEF image, notice more detail in background and better tonal range on the skin of the hand. The colour of the green carpet is a more faithful representation (For colour details, please see colour plate section.)

such technology, so the files may become unreadable in the future. This scenario is very unlikely to happen; but as the digital image is used as evidence in court, the case may be re-examined many years after the initial trial and all data will need to be available. It may be a useful analogy, when discussing legacy issues, to refer to changes in digital storage media: how many people now have access to floppy disk drives?

Table 10.1 RAW and JPEG formats compared

Benefits	Drawbacks
RAW format	
All recorded data retained	Large file size (megabytes, MB)
Cannot be overwritten	proprietary file format
Unprocessed ('digital negative')	
Greatest tonal range	
JPEG format	
Smaller file size (megabytes, MB)	High level of compression
Open-source format	Can introduce artefacts
	Can introduce colour shift
	Compresses each time file is saved
	Loss of tonal range

Table 10.1 summarises the relative benefits and disadvantages of RAW and JPEG formats.

10.5 Guidance for preparation of equipment for forensic photography

There are a few basic steps to follow prior to photography, which are required for best practice in gathering photographic evidence.

Camera maintenance

After some use the SLR camera will benefit from maintenance. The interchangeable lens system means that it is inevitable that fragments of dust will get on to the various components, especially when lenses are changed frequently. Those pieces of dust will appear as very small marks/spots on photographs, and may on occasion obscure parts of the bite mark. Removal of the dust can be a difficult procedure and should be performed by those who are experienced in such tasks. The chances of dust getting on to the components can be reduced if care is taken when the lens is changed.

Batteries for camera and flash devices should, of course, be kept fully charged.

Verify camera date and time

This will ensure that the correct date and time is embedded within the digital images (as 'metadata'). It is important in terms of evidence integrity that the date in the image's metadata does not conflict with information given in any statements made. The metadata can be accessed in databases or image editing software.

Image file format setting

To ensure that the least amount of compression is applied, the camera, regardless of model or make, should have the 'quality setting' set to the greatest quality available.

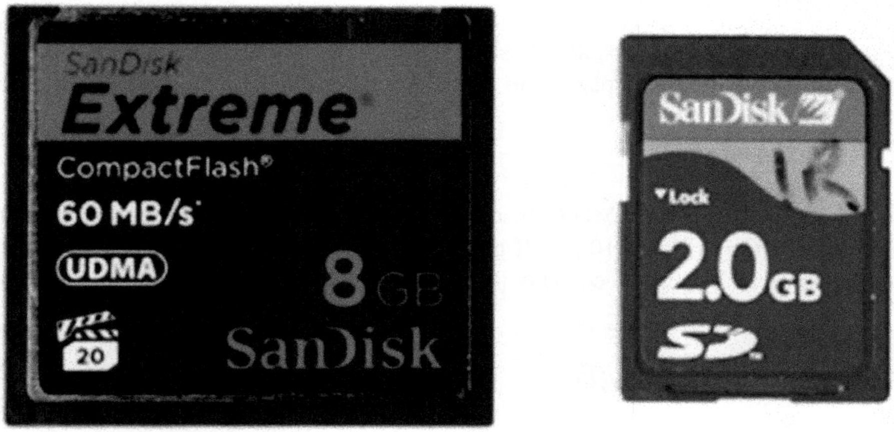

Figure 10.9 Examples of compact flash (CF) and secure digital (SD) cards

Memory card formatting

Depending on the model of camera, the external memory/media that is put into the camera will likely be either a Compact Flash (CF) or Secure Digital (SD) card (Figure 10.9). When starting a forensic case, the memory card should be reformatted; this will remove all earlier data and thus prevent the mixing of forensic cases on the memory card.

10.6 Photographing a bite mark

10.6.1 Minimising image distortion

A fundamental component in the process of photographing a bite mark – or any patterned injury – is the correct positioning of the camera to the injury.

Forensic analysis of patterned injuries is severely affected by *distortion*. This can be categorised into two types: primary and secondary (Sheasby and MacDonald, 2001).

- *Primary distortion* is due to the process in action at the time of impact, which includes two categories: dynamic (the interaction of the implement and skin) and tissue (stretching and swelling of the skin etc.).
- *Secondary distortion* is broken down into three categories: time-related changes, body position, and photographic distortion.

Photographic distortion is one of the few controllable variables in the whole process of the forensic analysis. Any distortion in the image may hamper attempts to produce viable evidence for court. Evans *et al.* (2012) have reported that if a wound or a feature on the body is photographed at more than a 15-degree angle to the perpendicular, then there will be visible distortion and thus change the pattern that is being investigated.

Certain main types of photographic distortion are prevalent in photographing patterned injuries, described in detail by Bowers and Johansen (2000) and demonstrated below. To try to avoid such errors, the following steps in correct 'camera-to-scale-to-injury' placement should be adhered to.

Type 1 distortion

The film plane (CCD or CMOS sensor) of the camera *must be perpendicular to the plane of the injury* (Figure 10.10). If the photographer fails to achieve this, then type 1 distortion will be introduced. This is also called *angular distortion* (Figure 10.11).

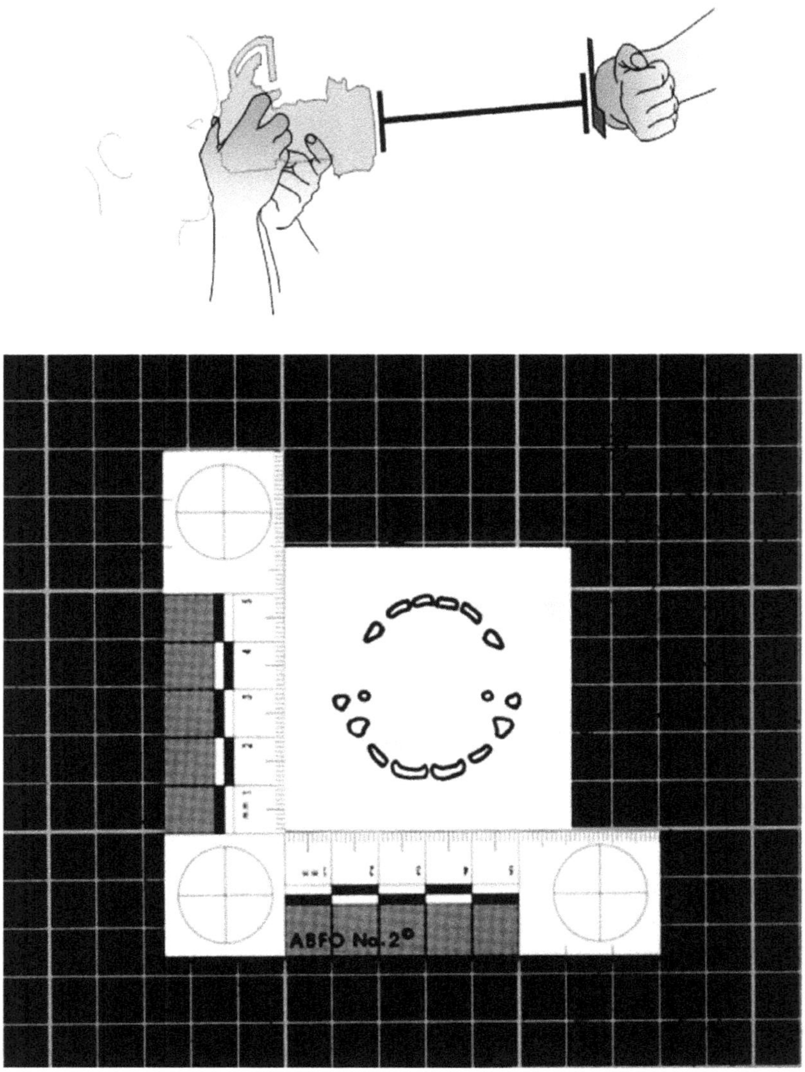

Figure 10.10 Correct positioning of a scale – no distortion produced

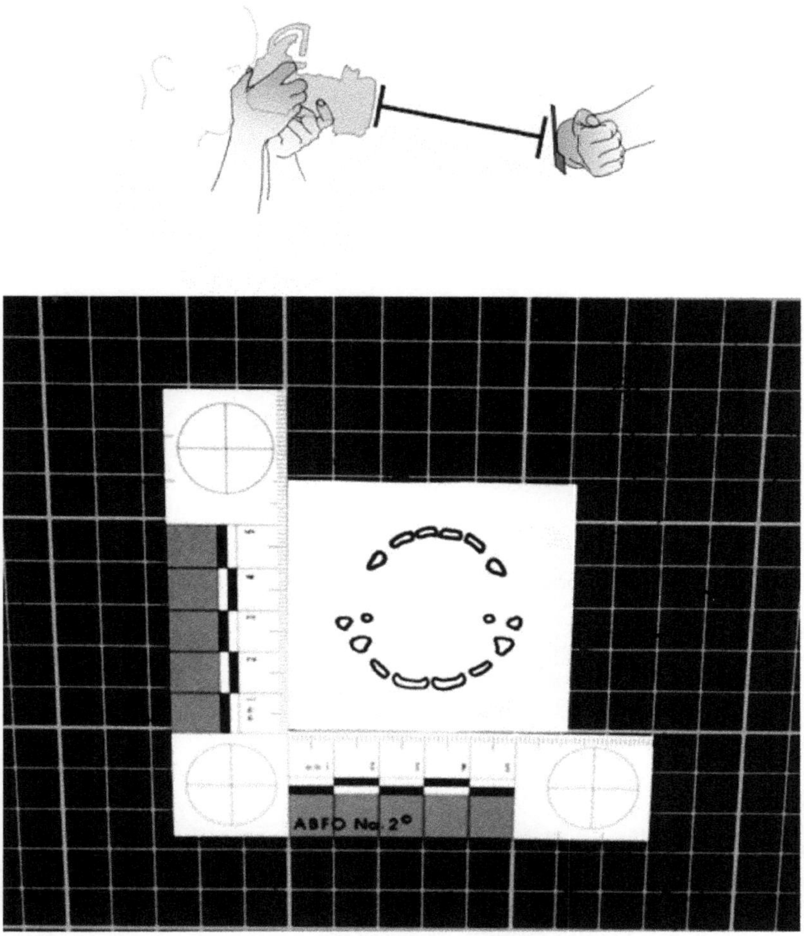

Figure 10.11 Incorrect positioning of a scale, producing type 1 (angular) distortion

The use of a 60 mm lens with the DSLR camera might make it easier to obtain images that are perpendicular to the injury and the scale; less distance will be required to stay at the correct position than when using a 105 mm lens. However, it should be noted that using a 105 mm lens might be preferable if the photographer needs to have a safer working distance.

Type 2 distortion

The scale should be placed on the surface of the skin (Figure 10.12). This will ensure the scale is on the same plane as the injury. If the scale is not on the same plane as the injury then there will be type 2 distortion (Figure 10.13).

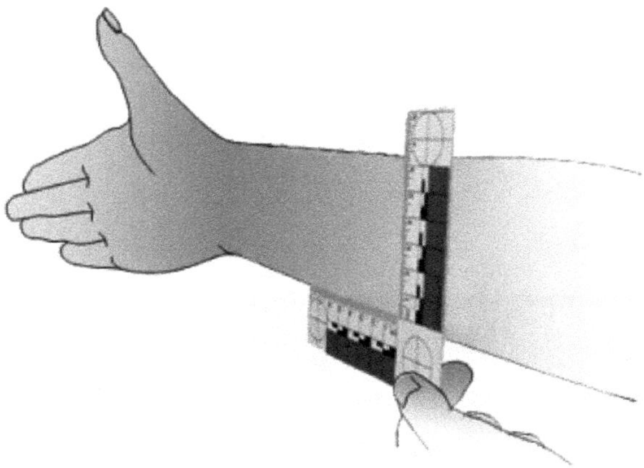

Figure 10.12 Correct positioning of a scale – no distortion produced

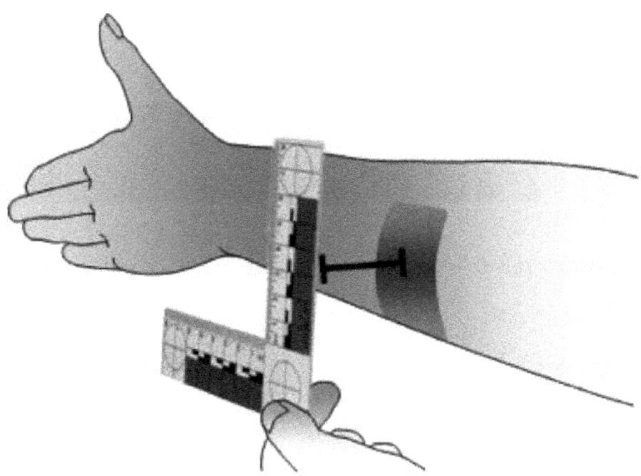

Figure 10.13 Incorrect positioning of a scale, producing type 2 distortion

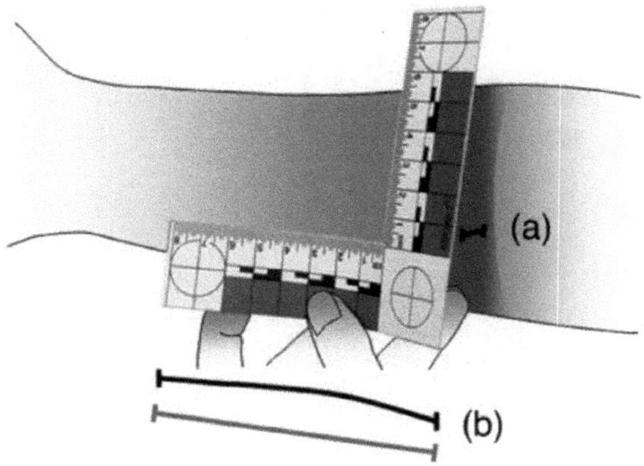

Figure 10.14 Incorrect handling of a scale: (a) orientation, and (b) bending

Types 3 and 4 distortion

Applying too much pressure when the scale is placed next to the injury can warp a portion of the scale. Furthermore, if the scale is tilted it will cause error. Figure 10.14 shows incorrect orientation and bending of the scale.

10.6.2 Can distortion be corrected?

When using the ABFO no. 2 scale it is important to include all of the circles to help the operator identify any angular distortion present in the image. It has been mentioned in some research studies that such distortion can be digitally corrected. However, any digital 'correction' of an image with angular distortion may result in the interpolation of the pixels. If interpolation takes place, then the digital evidence falls under the banner of 'reconstruction'. According to National Policing Improvement Agency guidance (NPIA, 2007), reconstruction can be applied only as a graphical interpretation and cannot be presented as a true image.

As mentioned by Sheets and Bush (2010):

> Non-affine (local) transformation tools are offered and may be used arbitrarily to alter all or portions of an image. However, no mathematical description of what is changing in an image is provided to the operator when using these tools. Results from this study indicate that it is not advisable to perform arbitrary alterations to an image of a bitemark.

If the operator intends to correct for angular distortion with the use of the circles, further issues arise. The scale and the bite mark are 3-dimensional structures in 3D space, whereas the photograph is analysed in 2-dimensional space. It will be difficult to know

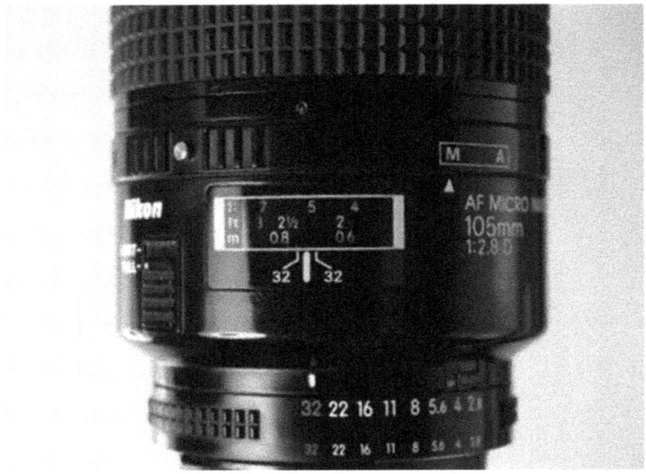

Figure 10.15 Magnification ratios 1:1, 1:2, 1:3 etc

from analysing the circles if there is not only angular distortion along the vertical axis but also angular distortion along the horizontal axis. Any geometric correction using the circles in the photograph would have to take these factors into account. It is advisable to use caution when applying geometric restoration to the image of a bite mark or patterned injury, without a thorough understanding of the digital process involved.

10.6.3 Magnification ratios: a tool for consistency

One benefit of using a professional camera and lens is the ability to have consistency in setting the lens magnification. Using the same magnification ratio for each image in a sequence keeps the object the same size in the frame. The operator can make a note of the magnification ratio when photographing the subject, allowing the operator to repeat images at a later date and the subject will be the same size in the frame. To focus, the operator should move the camera back and forth to the subject until the object in the frame is in sharp focus. The magnification ratios can be found on the barrel of the lens (Figure 10.15). A drawback of using a compact camera is that it is unlikely to have ratio markings on its lens.

Different camera models can have an effect on the magnification ratio. Most modern DSLRs will have what is described as a full-frame sensor, meaning the sensor is approximately the same size as the 35 mm film camera frame. Some DSLRs have smaller sensors which, when using the same lens type, crop the frame – making it appear that the magnification has changed. If the camera has a lens that is designed specifically for a smaller sensor, then there should not be a significant change.

10.6.4 Sequence of images when photographing a bite mark

For best practice, the accepted order of taking images should be followed. To preserve the continuity of the sequence all images must be kept. It is very important that none of the images are deleted, even if mistakes (exposure, poor focus) are made. Questions may be asked of the evidence if images appear to be missing from the sequence. There is *never* an acceptable reason to delete images; even if some images do not depict important information, the continuity of the sequence should be preserved. To ensure that the images are in sequence, the operator will need to check in the camera's menu system that 'file number sequence' (or similar) is activated.

1. Take an image of the person's ID (patient label, consent form, etc.). This image is needed to link images of injuries to the person being photographed.
2. Take a 'location shot' showing the injury and identifying its anatomical area, without a scale (e.g. the whole arm, or full face or leg). This image should illustrate the bruising with the surrounding area, so the viewer will be able to ascertain the anatomical position of the injuries.
3. Take close-up shots of the injury, including the whole of the scale. All three circles of the ABFO no. 2 scale must be shown, helping identify any angular distortion. It is crucial that any angular distortion be reduced by following the positioning suggested earlier, enabling accurate pattern analysis to be performed on these images.
4. If the injury is on a curved surface, then multiple views (at least three) will be needed. When photographing a patterned injury on a curved surface, such as the edge of a forearm or bicep, it is vital that the photographer takes images from at least three different positions (Figure 10.16). The camera must remain perpendicular to the injury and scale for all images. If the injury is on an area like the chest, the position of the body should be taken into account.
5. Take further detailed shots if required. In some scenarios it may be appropriate to photograph individual marks. This would require using lenses such as a 105 mm macro, to allow the operator to get images of sufficient detail. When taking images at close distances it is important to remember to maintain the camera perpendicular to the injury and maintain correct positioning of the scale, as described earlier.
6. Take further images of the person's ID. This helps to demonstrate that the sequence of images is uninterrupted.

Images using photographic filters, or infrared (IR), ultraviolet (UV) or other methods of illumination, may be used to record the injury in addition to unfiltered photographs. When using technologies such as infrared or ultraviolet, such images should be assessed with some prior knowledge and understanding of how to interpret the bite mark outside of the visible spectrum.

10.7 Photographing dentition

The forensic odontologist may require photographs for a visual record of a person's dentition for comparison with the written record and any study models made. The images required for bite mark and identification investigations are essentially the same.

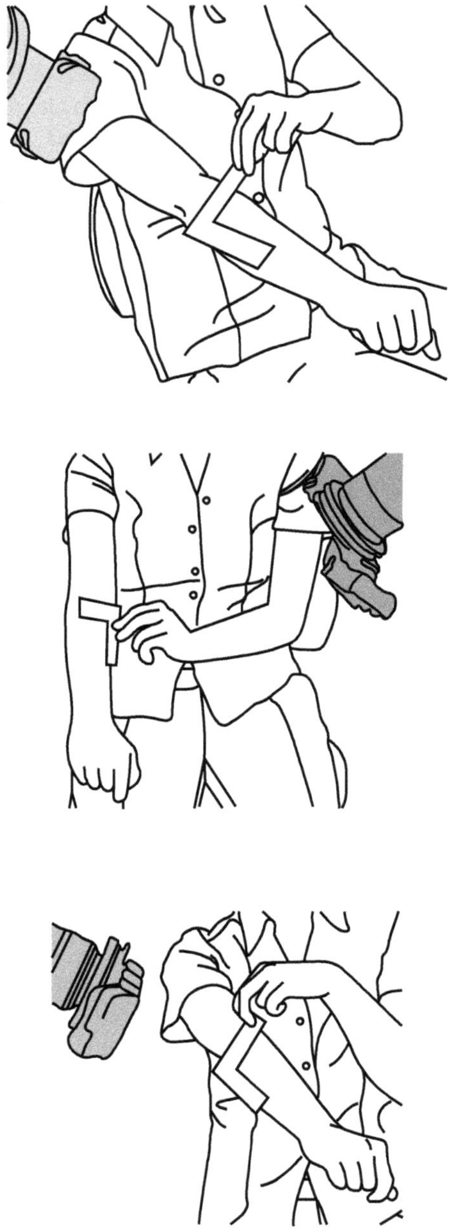

Figure 10.16 Sequence of images for photographing around a curved surface

There are three reasons why a person's dentition may need to be photographed in the context of forensic odontology:

- to make a visual record of the dentition of a suspect in a bite mark investigation
- to make a visual record of the dentition of a victim for identification purposes
- to make a visual record of the dentition for an age estimation investigation.

10.7.1 Equipment

The equipment needed is based on the requirements of standard dental (intra-oral) photography.

Lenses and flash

For a comfortable working distance between the lens and the person's dentition, it is advisable to use a lens with a focal length of around 100 mm. It will be difficult to obtain images of the dentition that have sufficient quality and detail without the use of a DSLR camera and appropriate lens.

It is recommended that a dedicated ring flash be used for intra-oral photography. Flash devices that are positioned on top of the camera or to one side will cause shadows to fall over parts of the dentition and obscure information.

Cheek retractors and mirrors

Often cheek retractors are plastic and are sold as pairs. Plastic retractors can have a limited amount of sterilisation cycles and will change colour, while metal retractors are more expensive but will last longer. Some retractors have a shape that allows the lips to dip over the gingival margin. A more rounded end of the retractor will provide sufficient retraction of the lips and mucosa to avoid the lips obscuring the teeth.

Dental mirrors are commonly coated glass but are available also in stainless steel (Figure 10.17). Glass mirrors provide more reflectance, and so will allow for a smaller aperture giving a greater depth of field. Dental mirrors can be acquired in a wide range of shapes. It is advisable to have mirrors that are suitable for both adults and children. Palatal mirrors are necessary for photographing the upper and lower dental arch views.

Cheek retractors and dental mirrors should be cleaned and sterilised in accordance with current dental infection control procedures.

10.7.2 Sequence of images for the dentition

As when collecting photographic evidence of a bite mark, images of the dentition must conform to the best practice previously stated. Ideally these images will be obtained

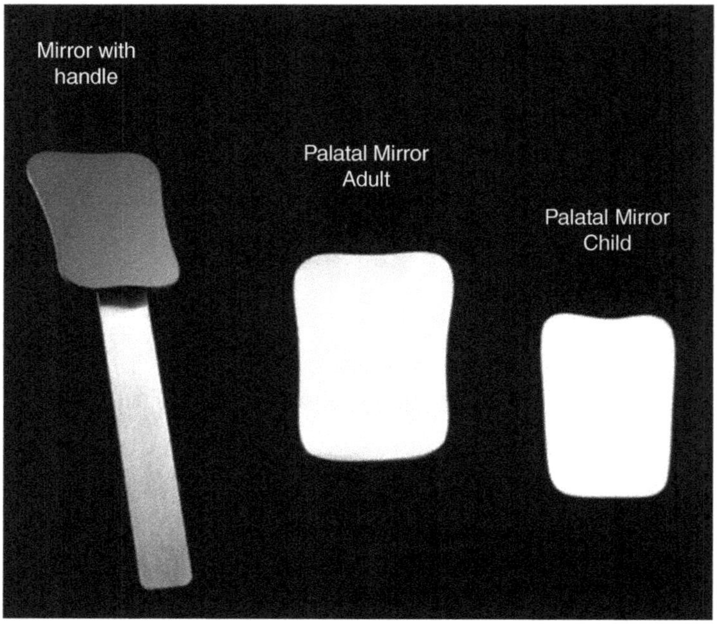

Figure 10.17 Examples of dental mirrors for intra-oral photography

alongside the taking of dental impressions for the dental casts. Unlike photographs of a bite mark, these images are for the purpose of recording the appearance of the teeth and not specifically for forensic analysis. The following is given as an example:

- Image 1 – an image of the person's ID (patient label, consent form etc.). This image is needed to link images of injuries to the person being photographed.
- Images 2 to 4 – anterior and left and right buccal views shot at 1:2 ratio (Figure 10.18).
- Images 5 to 6 – views of anterior teeth with ABFO no. 2 scale (Figure 10.19). The operator must try to ensure that the scale is in the same plane as the incisal edges of the teeth.

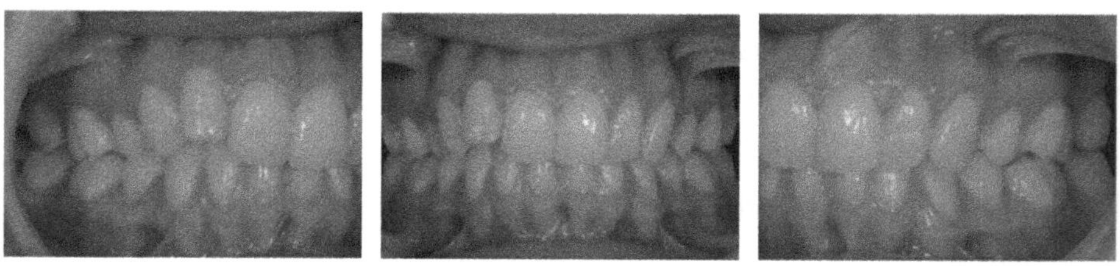

Figure 10.18 Example: views of anterior teeth

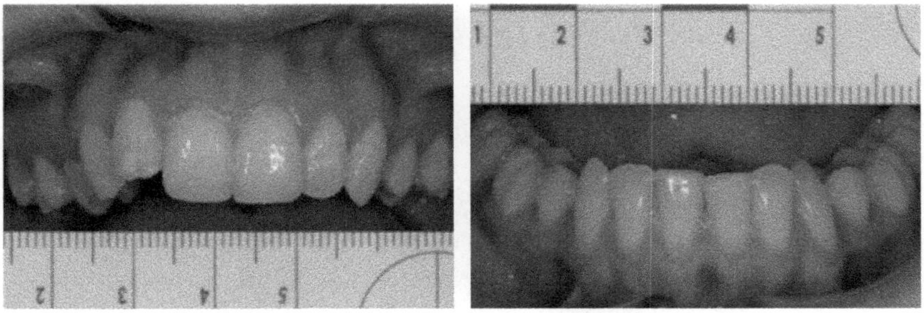

Figure 10.19 Example: views of anterior teeth with scale

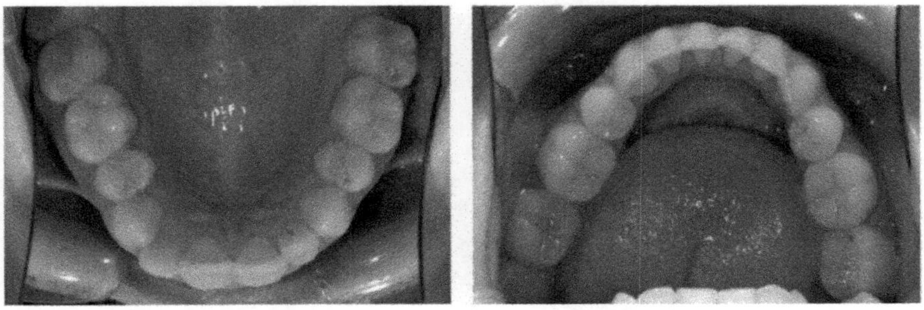

Figure 10.20 Example: incisal and occlusal views

- Images 7 and 8 – The arch views of teeth shot at 1:2.5 ratio (Figure 10.20). The photographer should pay close attention to the anterior teeth; you must be able to clearly see the incisal edges of the teeth.
- Image 9 – again, an image of person's ID (patient label, consent form etc.).

The recording of a person's dentition for the purpose of age estimation is relatively simple. The forensic odontologist may require only a view of the retromolar region of both the maxilla and mandible. This can be achieved by using a palatal mirror or lingual mirror (Figure 10.21).

Images for superimposition

In some cases the forensic odontologist may need to make an identification without the use of ante-mortem radiographs, and so will have to rely on any ante-mortem photographs thought to be of the deceased for comparison. To enable *superimposition* or other methods, the head will need to imaged. This can be done in at least three different ways.

The simplest method (with 2D technology) is to take multiple photographs of the head at various positions – for example, from straight on and then at oblique and

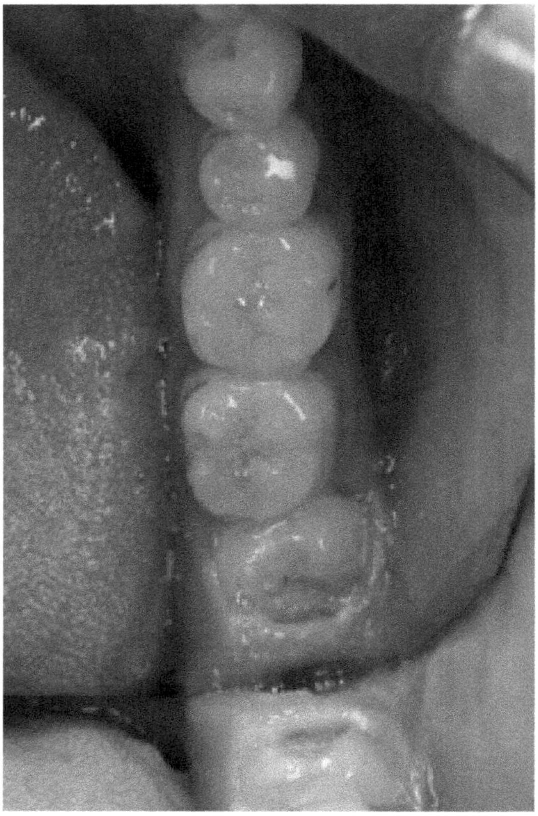

Figure 10.21 View of retromolar region using a mirror

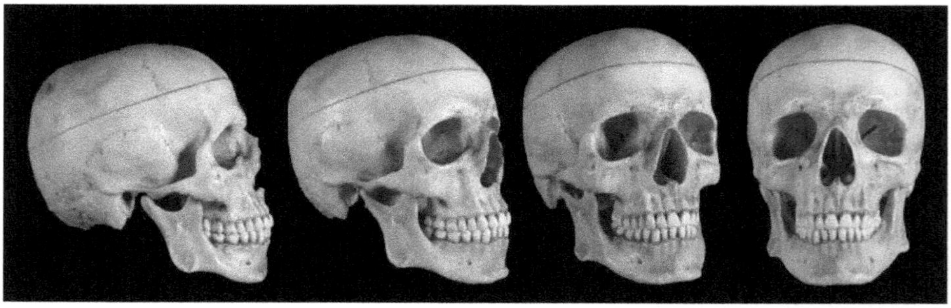

Figure 10.22 Sequence of images for 2D superimposition, post-mortem (for illustrative purposes only)

lateral views of both sides (Figure 10.22). If the investigator is not able to have access to the ante-mortem records, this set of images will allow the investigator to have a photograph that resembles the angle of the face in the ante-mortem photograph (Figure 10.23).

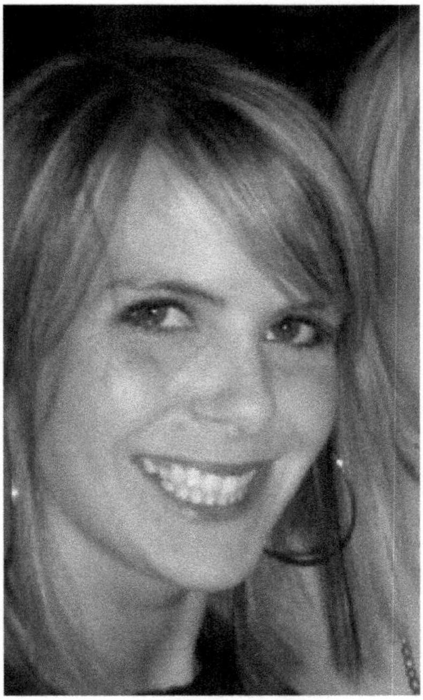

Figure 10.23 Ante-mortem photograph for comparison (this is not from a real case but is intended only for illustrative purposes)

Another method, similar to the one above, is the use of video (a technique developed by Professor D. Whittaker). The method involves rotating the head/skull or the video camera, so as to capture the whole of the head. The video can then be paused at the point that corresponds to the angle of the face in the ante-mortem photograph. (Figure 10.24). The paused video frame can then be exported as an image file to import into image editing software.

A third method is similar to the last. However, this time a 3D capture device is used. This is the most robust and – with the right training – the most useful method. Once a 3-dimensional model of the head/skull has been made, the model can be rotated easily to any position or angle of the face in the ante-mortem photograph. Different 3D devices will work better in different circumstances. A laser scan may produce better images of a skull (Figure 10.25), whereas a stereo photogrammetry device may be better at producing images of a head of the recently deceased.

10.8 Image downloading and storage

Once the images have been taken they need to be transferred to a secure place, such as a hard drive on a computer or on a server. At the very least, the operator needs to ensure that ALL the images for each session are stored in unique folders that relate to each forensic investigation.

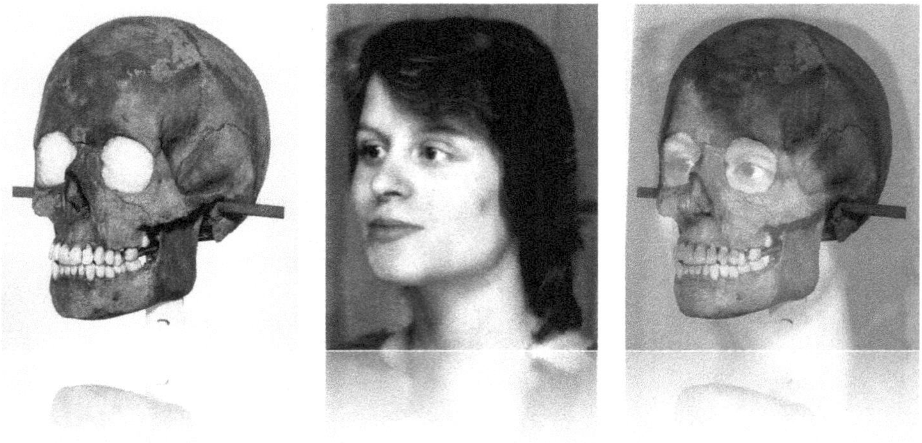

Figure 10.24 Example of video superimposition. Courtesy of Professor D. Whittaker

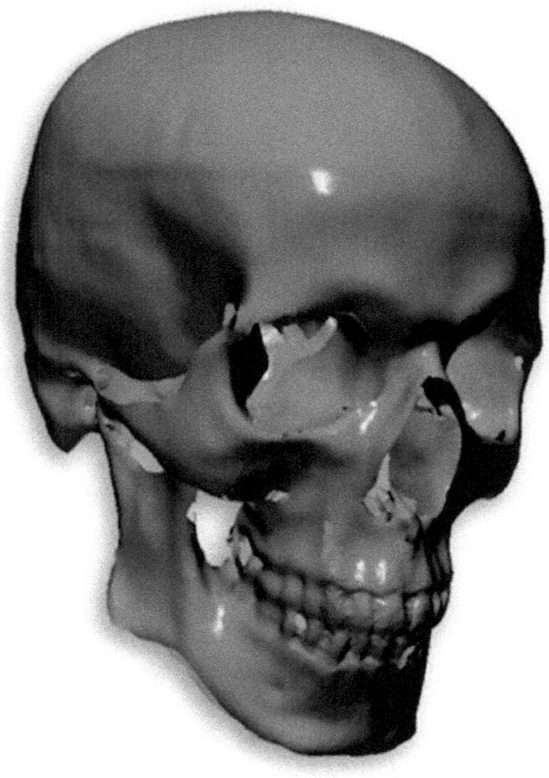

Figure 10.25 Example of a 3-dimensional model of a skull

10.8.1 Guidance on downloading and image workflow

- Download the whole camera card folder from its card(s) to a secure location. Most jurisdictions require individuals and organisations to follow data-protection regulations, so any data storage (computer, server, external disk) needs to have some form of encryption.
- At the secure location, create a new folder named after the case number (e.g. 2012/001).
- Place the camera card folder into a sub-folder called 'RAW' or 'Original'.
- Create a separate sub-folder in the case number folder called 'Tiffs' (for example).
- Open Adobe® Photoshop® and open the RAW files. The files will open up in the RAW file plug-in program (Adobe® Camera Raw converter).
- *Do not perform any alterations to the images* regardless of their quality. Save ALL images to the 'Tiffs' folder you have created. This ensures you have an unedited copy of the images in an open-source file format that will be protected from future legacy issues.
- If it seems necessary to make some enhancements to the images (e.g. levels, curves, or colour removal), save the edited images to a new, separate sub-folder. Name the sub-folder something like 'EditSE' to make it clear that you have edited those images.
- Any alterations to images should be done via the RAW file plug-in program. This will ensure that enhancements will only be done non-destructively and saved as a working copy. All the enhancements done will be saved to the metadata, either directly in the file itself or as a separate file (XMP file).
- Make a copy of the *whole case number folder* on to a DVD or other media. (non-reusable, write-once). This also needs to be secure.

For further guidance, study the documents *Practice Advice on Police Use of Digital Images* (ACPO and NPIA, 2007) and guidelines from the Scientific Working Group on Imaging Technology (2012).

10.8.2 Storage of images

Where to store all your important evidential images is a crucial question. Without proper and safe storage such evidence can be lost. Leaving all your evidence on a laptop at home without the relevant precautions is not acceptable or professional behaviour.

It is extremely important to ensure that all the data are *backed up* (copied to another device) at least twice a day. The most secure and safe approach is to have a dedicated server, which is housed in a separate and appropriate building. This is likely to be out of the reach of most operators who do not work for a large organisation. If a dedicated server is not an option then the minimum requirement is to use an external disk tethered to the computer which has some form of automated software controlling the back-up. Most modern computers and/or the external disk will come 'out of the box' ready for automated back-up.

Running daily back-ups should become routine. All hard disks are vulnerable to some form of system failure (or even virus attack) in which all the data can be lost. Having an automated back-up provides protection against these issues.

Regardless of the amount of gigabytes or terabytes the storage is capable of, the hard disk and the back-up might become filled to capacity with data. At this point space needs to be made available. Methodically the operator should copy images/data to other media (e.g. non-reusable, write-once-only DVD/CD). At least two copies should be made and placed in different locations, as a precaution against loss by fire or theft. This process is referred to as *archiving*.

10.9 Imaging modalities

This section will discuss some imaging modalities available that may help the forensic odontologist, from the use of cameras that are sensitive to different wavelengths of light to the emergence of 3D image capture. Each tool, depending on the circumstances, will demonstrate both benefits and limitations.

10.9.1 Reflected ultraviolet and near-infrared

The light that propagates from the Sun and from electronic devices can be described as an electromagnetic wave (EM), with the light we can perceive and the light we cannot falling within the *electromagnetic spectrum*. The various types of electromagnetic radiation in this spectrum can be classified by their specific *wavelength*, which is measured as the distance between two identical points on the wave (Figure 10.26). Depending on the type of electromagnetic radiation, the wavelength is described at the lower end of the spectrum in kilometres and megametres ('radio waves') to the high end in nanometers ('gamma rays') (Figure 10.27). The components of *visible*

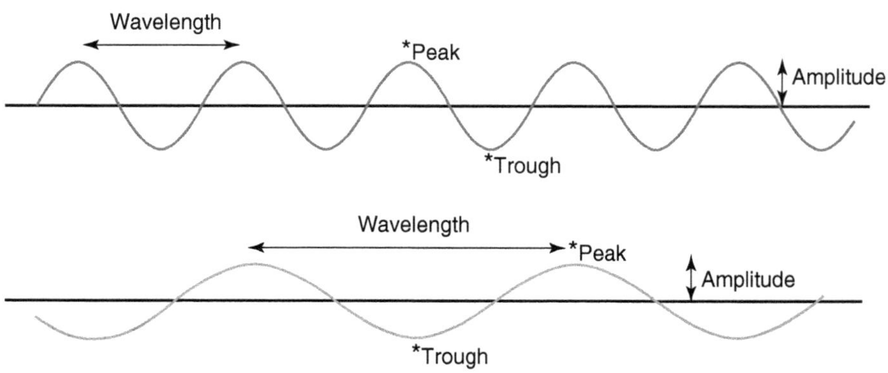

Figure 10.26 An explanation of wavelength. Courtesy of N. Edwards, Cardiff University

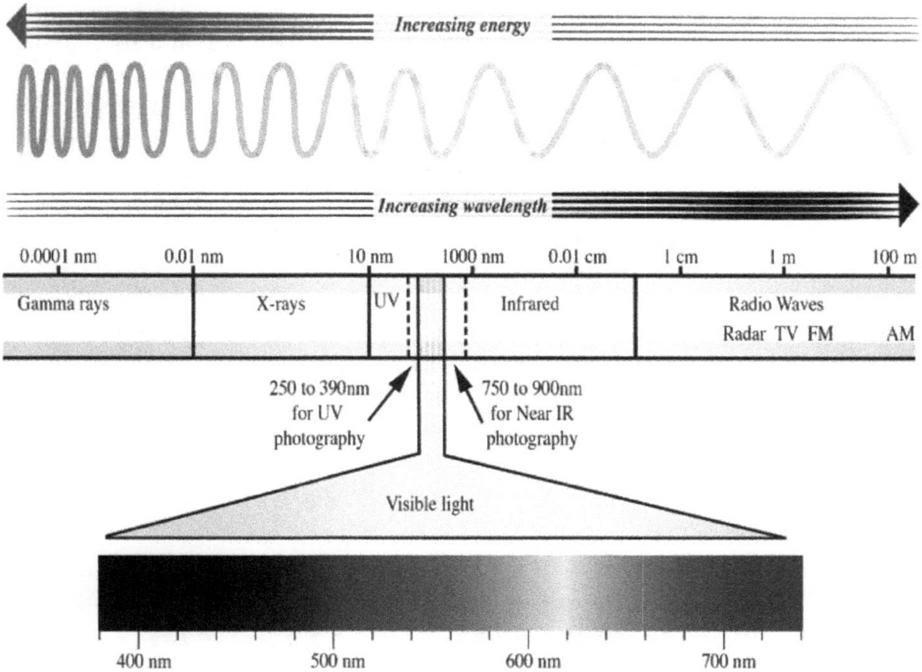

Figure 10.27 The electromagnetic spectrum (For colour details, please see colour plate section.)

light fall within a small portion of the EM spectrum, from violet at a wavelength of approximately 400 nm to red at around 700 nm. For the photography of bruises, some digital cameras can be modified to be sensitive to *ultraviolet radiation* (about 250–390 nm) and *near-infrared radiation* (about 750–900 nm).

For a number of years there has been some discussion on the practical utilisation of reflected ultraviolet (UV) and near-infrared (IR) imaging for the capture of bite marks and other bruises. The belief is that using IR or UV will disclose to the investigator bruises that are not within the visible spectrum, that perhaps a bruise inflicted several months ago will be uncovered for investigation (Wright, 1998a,b, 2010; David, 1990; David and Sobel, 1994; Rowan *et al.*, 2010; Lawson *et al.*, 2010). Whereas some papers have suggested potential benefits of UV and IR for imaging a bruise (Wright, 1998a,b, 2010), other research has suggested that there is a lack of strong evidence to allow for a firm conclusion to be made on the usefulness of such images (Rowan *et al.*, 2010; Lawson *et al.*, 2010; Tetley, 2005).

An issue that can present itself is interpretation. How does the investigator accurately assess the relationship between the information present in the UV or IR image and the suspected injury? There may be several bruises visible in the image, which may have been obtained at different times, as mentioned previously. It is always difficult to confidently state the age of a bruise (Maguire *et al.*, 2005), and this issue can only be compounded when using data obtained from UV or IR imaging.

Without being able to accurately age the bruise, how can the investigator relate the information in the image to the suspected bite mark inflicted on a specific date and not misinterpret it for an injury sustained weeks before? It is understood to what extent both UV and IR light is absorbed by and penetrates the skin. With regard to UV photography, most adapted flash devices emit light within a range of approximately 390 nm and at this wavelength there is very little penetration of the skin (Tetley, 2005). The result of this is it may be rather improbable that UV photography would reveal anything that is not already present to the investigator's own vision. Thus, if the bruise cannot be seen via visible light photography it is unlikely to be apparent in the UV image. However, the development of the bruise over time within the skin can be subject to many variables that may affect how successful the bruise can be imaged. (UV may be useful when imaging an old burn or cut.) Depending on the force of impact or where the impact is – be it over bone or muscle – the bruise may be visible at different stages with the different imaging modalities (Figure 10.28).

Infrared radiation penetrates the skin, and the depth of that penetration depends on the wavelength. Within near-IR photography a wavelength of between 700 and 900 nm

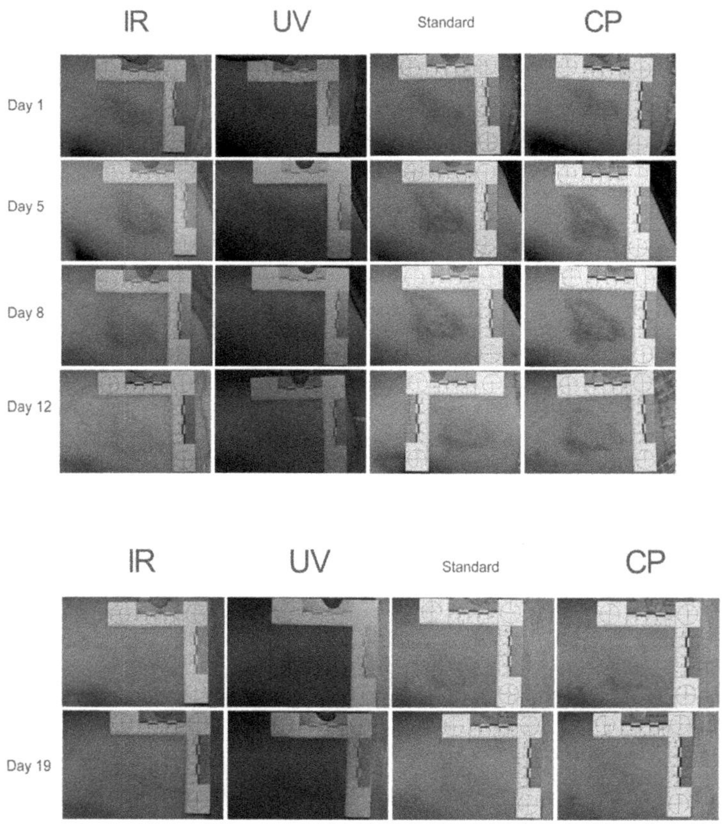

Figure 10.28 Sequence of images over a 19-day period, using IR, UV, CP and standard imaging. Courtesy of child health bruising study, Cardiff University and Medical Research Council (For colour details, please see colour plate section.)

is often used and this has been estimated to penetrate to a depth of approximately 3 mm (Engle, 1968; Zharov *et al.*, 2004). There is limited published research on both IR and UV and specifically to bruises studied longitudinally. Some papers have looked at old bruises (Wright, 1998), but this is restricted to a small case study. Much of the research into bruising employs small sample sizes which reduce the impact of any statistical significance to the data. Currently, there is a lack of research into the interpretation of bruises viewed via these modalities and the use of UV and IR in bite mark investigations. Such techniques cannot be completely disregarded or supported as future research into bruise physiology may reveal some crucial knowledge.

To utilise IR and/or UV digital photography, modified DSLRs and flash units have to be used. There are specialised companies that offer conversion of digital cameras and accompanying flash units. It is worth noting that, when using UV flash units, reference to the Health and Safety Executive's document *The Control of Artificial Optical Radiation at Work Regulations* should be made. Some UV lights are not suitable for prolonged use with people.

10.9.2 Cross-polarised imaging

For many years photographers have used polarising filters to reduce unwanted reflections from water and glass or to increase colour saturation. Polarising filters are also found in LCD screens to reduce glare. In recent years medical and forensic photographers have used the technique of cross-polarisation (CP) to reduce specular highlights reflected off the skin from flash photography. CP photography is demonstrated to great effect when photographing the tongue or buccal mucosa (Figure 10.29; Edwards, 2011).

Cross-polarisation is a simple technique that can have useful results. To understand the process in which the intensity of light is reduced by CP photography, to reduce specular highlights, we again must refer to light as a wave. It is possible to describe in which orientation the light wave is oscillating. Most light sources emit light waves oscillating in multiple orientations, horizontally, vertically or even rotating in orientation while travelling. This kind of light is called *unpolarised* (Figure 10.30). If a linearly polarising filter is placed over such a light source most light waves oscillating

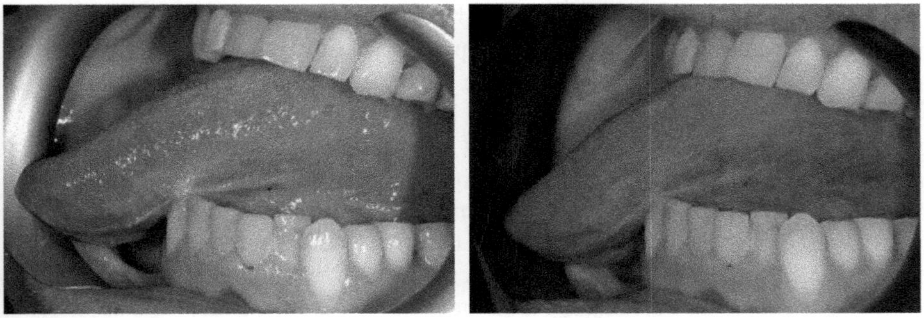

Figure 10.29 Cross-polarised and non-cross-polarised images of the tongue

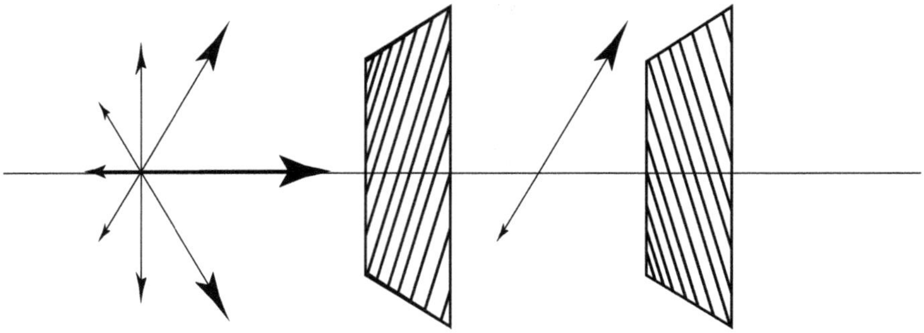

Figure 10.30 Illustration of the cross-polarisation process. Courtesy of N. Edwards

in the various directions can be prevented from passing through the filter, while still allowing, for instance, vertically oscillating waves through. This has the result of reducing the intensity of the light behind the filter by about a quarter.

When the light from an electronic flash with added linear polariser is reflected from an object, some reflected light waves will maintain their oscillation orientation while others will be changed. Specularly reflected light tends to maintain its orientation while diffusely reflected light again contains waves oscillating in all directions, and is therefore unpolarised after reflection. When a mix of specularly and diffusely reflected light enters a camera lens through a second linearly polarising filter located in its front, which is rotated by 90 degrees with respect to the filter in front of the flash, only a proportion of the light can pass through. Thus much of the light will be blocked. The intensity of light that finally reaches the camera's sensor has therefore been reduced. (The absorption and diffusion of light in skin is explained in great detail by Spott *et al.*, 1998.)

An important point to consider when using CP photography is that the filter causes a slight colour shift. This shift is towards the red end of the spectrum and is caused by lengthening of the wavelength of light reaching the camera's sensor, leading to the image having a slightly yellow appearance. Polarising filters used in photography will most likely introduce a yellow tinge, or *bias*; this bias can be expressed as a micro-reciprocal-degree (MIRED) shift. Once the MIRED shift is understood this subtle change in colour can be neutralised by using the shift calculation to change the colour temperature in an image editing application. Correcting colour shift via this calculation is more precise than calibrating the image(s) using the colour balance tool in Photoshop® (If the ABFO no. 2 scale is used in the image, the grey part of the scale can be employed to perform a level of calibration.) It can be argued that any change in distance from the flash to the object will change the colour temperature. Thus you cannot calibrate all images in a series from the colour chart in the first frame. To be consistent you would need to have a colour reference chart in every image, which might be considered impracticable. However, if you use the MIRED shift you can apply the calculation for all the images, if the same filters are used. There is, nonetheless, a slight flaw in this method. It is not always straightforward to obtain the correct MIRED shift for both the filter on the lens and the flash. The manufacturer of the filter should be able to provide its MIRED shift, so once this has been obtained the calculation can be used to convert the MIRED shift into a colour temperature value:

$$\text{MIRED shift} = 10^6/T,$$

where T is the colour temperature in kelvin (K). We can use the known colour temperature of the flash and then calculate the bias caused by the filter. The following is a worked example:

$$\text{Flash unit temperature : 5600 kelvin}$$

$$\text{Filter on flash : +19 mired.}$$

So, $10^6/5600 = 178.6$ mired for the flash. Add to this the filter's +19 mired to obtain 197.6 mired. Then convert this back to its colour temperature: $10^6/197.6 = 5060.7$ K. The value 5060.7 K can now be placed into the 'Temperature' box in the Photoshop® RAW file convertor (Figure 10.31).

Once the filter on the flash has been calculated the bias from the lens filter needs to be neutralised. The light from the flash has a colour temperature of 5600 K. The wavelength of this light is in a range of approximately 500–600 nm. The relationship between the colour temperature and the wavelength is expressed in Wien's law:

$$\lambda_{max} = b/T,$$

where λ is the wavelength in nanometres (nm) and b is Wien's displacement constant (2,897,768). So:

$$\text{For 5600 K, } \lambda_{max} = 517.5\,\text{nm}$$

$$\text{For 5060.7 K, } \lambda_{max} = 572.6\,\text{nm.}$$

There is a limited amount of published research into the use of cross-polarised photography and the imaging of bruises. However, some research carried out has shown

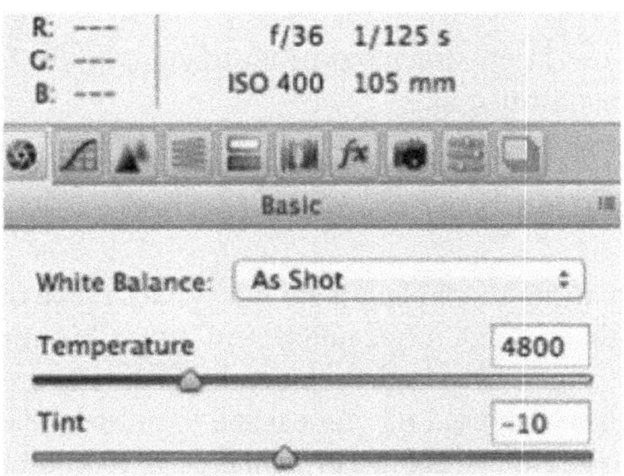

Figure 10.31 Temperature and tint in Adobe® Photoshop® RAW file convertor

that some paediatricians have a preference for CP photography when assessing bruises (Lawson *et al.*, 2010). The benefit of CP photography is greatest when photographing bite marks on oily skin, and especially on curved surfaces such as the forearm. Using a flash device directly in front of the bite mark can cause the specular highlights that cover important information.

When using any modality that is different from the norm, it is vital that the operator takes images of the injury with a standard imaging technique (i.e. without any filters and modifications); those images can then be classed as a reference or control images. This is especially the case when using IR, UV and CP as most people will not be sure how to interpret such images. If these types of modality are not used carefully, the investigator who employs such methods could mislead an investigation or jury.

10.10 Three-dimensional technology

Bruises are often inflicted on to a curved part of the body (Freeman *et al.*, 2005). This requires the photographer to take multiple images around the injury, thus reducing the 3D structure of the human body into a 2D space (using a conventional digital camera). This can cause problems for the accurate representation of depth and the correct placement of the scale. To improve the supportive evidence provided by medical and forensic photographers, the photographic distortion needs to be significantly reduced.

Some short-term fixes have been proposed, such as a device fitted to a camera to keep the camera at 90 degrees to the scale and injury (Smith, 2011). However, for a viable long-term solution it has been proposed that 3D image capture, be it stereo photography or laser scanning, is more precise, accurate and robust than other forms of recording and that it should therefore be explored as an alternative method (Thali *et al.*, 2003; Blackwell *et al.*, 2005; Martin-de-Las-Heras *et al.*, 2007; Evans *et al.*, 2010).

This section examines various types of 3-dimensional capture devices that have been used for various forensic and clinical applications. These scanning devices use two distinctive techniques: passive and active:

- Passive methods include most stereo-photogrammetry devices. The passive method gathers the data via the reflected light already present in the scene.
- Active methods use laser, structured or unstructured light for gathering the data needed for 3D reconstruction.

10.10.1 Triangulation laser scanners (active)

Popular laser scanners using triangulation are the 'Vivid' range of scanners by Konica Minolta. They have been used for a number of years by clinical research teams investigating facial changes (Kau and Richmond, 2008). Pictured in Figure 10.32 is the Vivid 910, which has been used for clinical and forensic applications. Two research studies have demonstrated the scanning of dental casts to good effect with the Vivid 910: examination of the changes in cleft palate patients by Kitagawa *et al.* (2004), and a paper describing the use of such technology for bite mark identification analysis

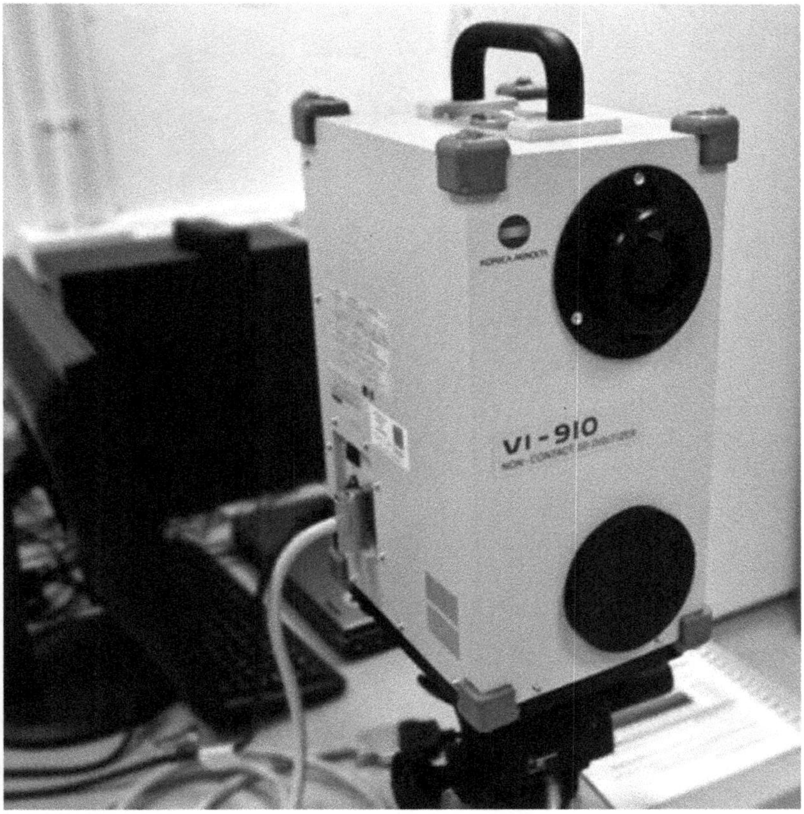

Figure 10.32 The Vivid 910 (approximately 50 cm in height)

by Flora *et al.* (2009). Further applications of the Vivid 910 have been reported in recording whole crime scenes (Cavagnini *et al.*, 2008). Figure 10.33 demonstrates that the Vivid 910 laser scanner produces a very accurate 3D model.

Like other laser scanners, the Vivid 910 uses the stereoscopic principle to generate the 3D model. The scanner directs the light onto the object's surface. The object reflects (scatters) the light back. This light is then collected by a video camera. All the relevant points are located at a known distance from each other. For example, the distance from the scanner to the object and the distance from the laser to the camera are known. Using trigonometry, the 3D (*xyz*) coordinates are then triangulated to create a 3D model of the object.

- Positive factors – superior quality of the data acquired; short scanning times (5 minutes for Figure 10.31) for small objects; quick render time of 3D model; published papers on the use of the Vivid 910 with bite mark analysis; often used for 3D digitization in medical applications.
- Negative factors – tripod-based laser scanners less portable and expensive (the Vivid is priced at up to £30,000).

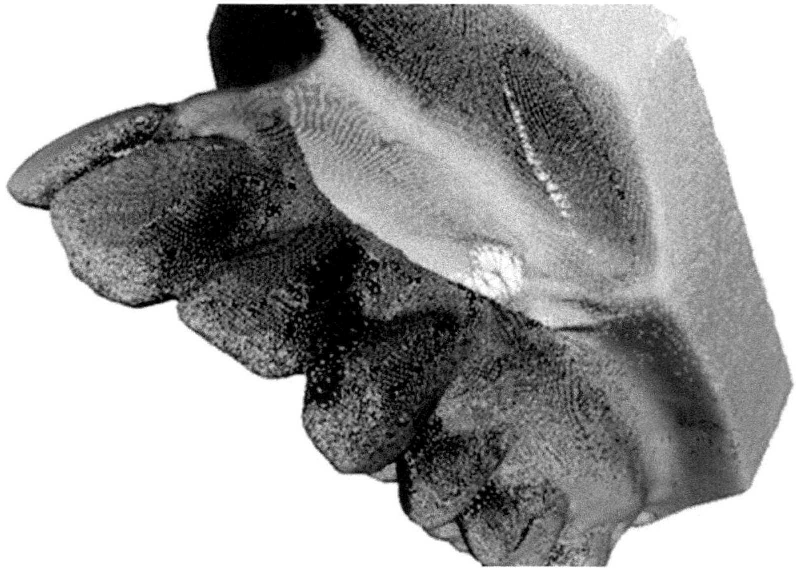

Figure 10.33 Vivid 910 scan of a dental cast

10.10.2 Hand-held laser scanners (active)

Hand-held scanners use the same technological approach to that of the tripod-based Vivid 910. The same triangulation method is used. However, some hand-held scanners can create a live 3-dimensional image. The scanner is often tethered to a computer; the information is collected and the scanner's software generates a 3D model.

The software requires the position of the object in space to be determined. This is done by using reference markers (most commonly adhesive reflective tabs) on the surface of the object that is being scanned. As the scanner scans the object it processes the markers. As long as the previous marker is in sight when the scanner processes the next marker, the software can calculate the coordinates and thus generate a 3D model.

One such scanner on the market is the Handyscan™ from Creaform Ltd. (Figure 10.34). This scanner has been used in forensic applications such as footmark identification (e.g. by Agosto *et al.*, 2008).

- Positive factors – lightweight; easy to use; high-quality colour rendition (VIU colour scanner).
- Negative factors – always tethered to a computer; expensive (approximately £20,000); not extensively tested for forensic odontology.

10.10.3 Structured light scanners (active)

A structured light scanner projects a known pattern of light from a projector housed in the scanner. It uses one sensor (digital cameras) also housed in the scanner, to

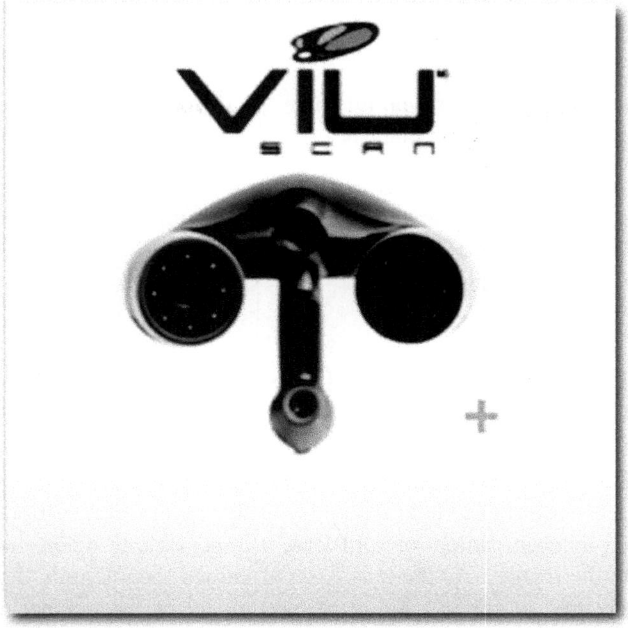

Figure 10.34 The Handyscan™ VIU scanner. Image courtesy of Creaform Ltd

capture images of the object with the patterns projected on it. In order to capture 3-dimensional information, multiple patterns and/or multiple sensors can be used. The stereo cameras/sensors are at a fixed and known distance, enabling triangulation of the coordinates.

One structured light scanner used in forensic applications is a system from Gesellschaft für Optische Messtechnik (GOM). The ATOS II scanner (Figure 10.35) generates a 3D polygon mesh. If a colour render is required then the TRITOP is needed in addition. This instrument uses photogrammetry and reference markers to create a 3D colour render, which is then registered on to the polygon mesh, created

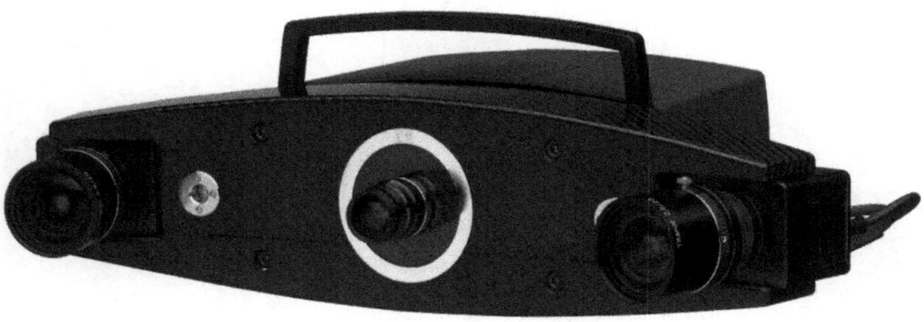

Figure 10.35 The ATOS II scanner. Image courtesy of GOM Ltd

by the ATOS device, in the software. This device has been used extensively in forensic applications (Buck *et al.*, 2006; Thali *et al.*, 2003, 2005).

- Positive factors – superior quality; some use in forensic imaging and some published papers on bite mark analysis.
- Negative factors – expensive (£120,000 plus); the need for two instruments is time-consuming and cumbersome (although the initial ATOS scan is very quick); can take a long time to render final 3D model; length of process depends on the size of the object scanned.

10.10.4 Stereophotogrammetry (passive or active)

Stereoscopic systems employ two methods: using either two or more cameras placed slightly apart from each other; or using a stereo lens with mirrors to collect two images (a pair) on to one sensor (CCD or CMOS). By analysing the slight differences between the images seen by each camera or split lens, it is possible to determine the distance at each point in the images. As the lens is set at known focal length, the principles of triangulation are used to create a 3-dimensional model by the scanner's software.

Some of the most widely used stereoscopic scanner systems are from 3dMD Ltd. (Figure 10.36). They are used mainly for clinical and surgical applications as described by Popat *et al.* (2008). The system needs to be highly accurate in order to satisfy the requirements for surgical planning. The 3dMD systems can record in both still and motion with the 3dMDface system using unstructured infrared light. This is therefore an active method.

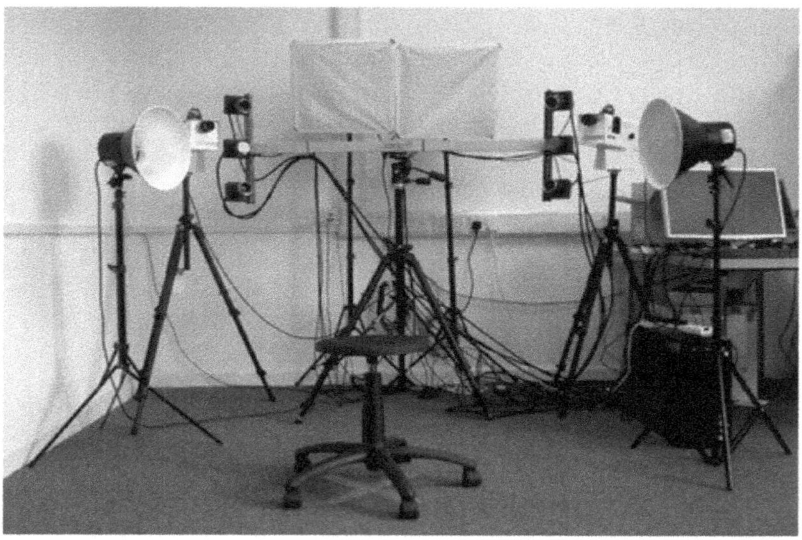

Figure 10.36 The 3dMD system. Courtesy of J. Djordjevic

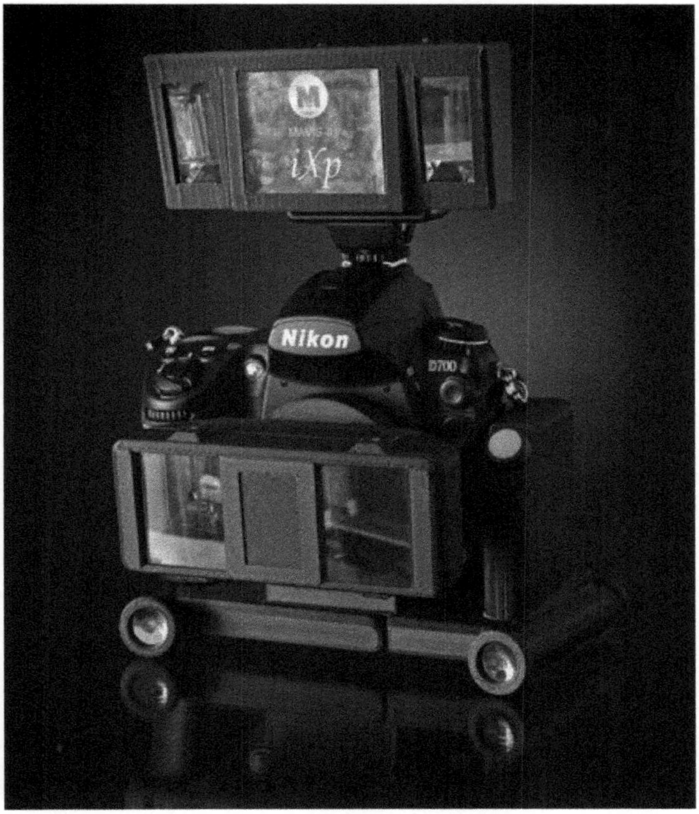

Figure 10.37 The MAVIS camera with Nikon D700 body

- Positive factors – accurate scans; fast scanning time and photo-realistic colour render; widely used within the clinical and surgical community.
- Negative factors – lack of portability as fixed to one room; not tested for forensic application; expensive at £15,000 (cheaper than most 3D scanners); no known tests with dental casts.

The approach of using a stereo lens is employed by the MAVIS stereoscopic camera (Figure 10.37). This was designed initially for the measurement of leg ulcers and diabetic foot ulcers by Plassmann and Peters (2002). The MAVIS II system is constructed from a digital SLR (a Canon 450D) with a stereo lens attached to the lens mount. The device shown is the MAVIS II camera system using a Nikon D700.

- Positive factors – portable and lightweight; easy to use; very fast render of 3D model; inexpensive at approximately £5000; fast capture time.
- Negative factors – confined to scanning small surface areas; poor scanning of dental casts.

10.10.5 Other 3-dimensional devices

Time-of-flight scanners work by emitting a laser at an object and measuring the time it takes for the light to reflect back to the scanner; as the speed of light is a known constant, the exact position of the object in space can be calculated. Time-of-flight scanners have been used in the fields of archeology, building construction and engineering. Such scanners are good at collecting data of very large areas such as the topography of a particular landscape or buildings. Time-of-flight scanners tend to produce less accurate results on small objects with fine details.

An example of a time-of-flight scanner used in forensics is the Lieca ScanStation C10TM (Figure 10.38). It has been used by police forces to demonstrate a reconstruction of a whole crime scene (Buck *et al.*, 2010). Such a device would likely struggle to provide detail results from a bite mark on skin.

Touch probe scanners (coordinate measuring machines, CMM) are used in the engineering and automotive industries. One example is the C3 V bridge CMM manufactured by Nikon (Figure 10.39), which is used in the production of magnesium diecast components for engines. Another example is the PIX 3, which has been used

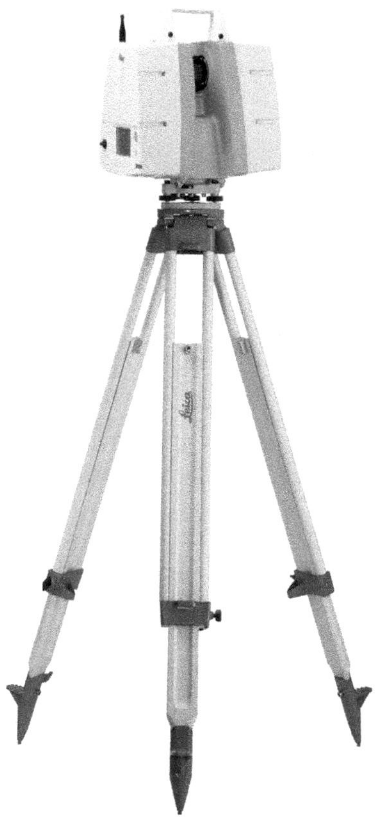

Figure 10.38 The Lieca ScanStation C10^{TM}. Image courtesy of Leica

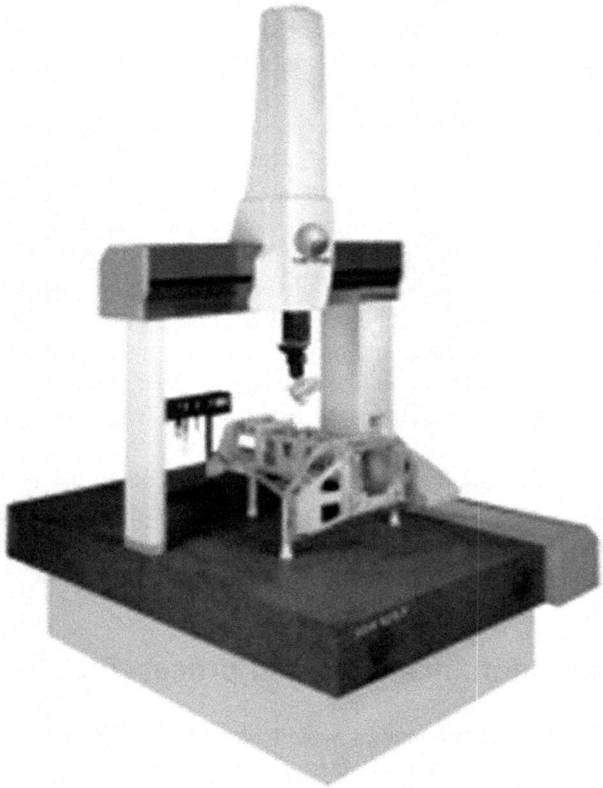

Figure 10.39 The C3 V bridge CMM™. Courtesy of Nikon UK

to scan dental casts in two relevant papers on bite mark analysis (Martin-de-las-Heras *et al.*, 2007, 2009).

Although using such scanners has been demonstrated as a possible solution to collecting 3-dimensional data of a dental cast, the author believes that a touch probe machine would be far too slow in recording sufficient data. A non-contact scanner such as the Vivid 910 described earlier would be better suited for use with a dental cast. A CMM scanner would be an impracticable solution for 3D capture of a bite mark injury, as physical contact on the injury would be required.

10.10.6 3D versus 2D

The precision and accuracy of the image capturing device are of vital forensic importance. However, our current understanding of bruise physiology is not sufficient (limited published data) to allow an accurate record of the true shape and size of a patterned injury. Thus, testing the true accuracy of an image capturing device is difficult to ascertain in the case of a patterned bruise. Research of 2D and 3D methods has shown the apparent limitations of 2D camera capture. When the operator fails to follow gold-standard techniques while using a 2D camera, the distortion introduced reaches unacceptable levels. 3D capture is more precise and reduces perspective and angular distortion (Evans *et al.*, 2012).

At the time of writing, investigators at the University of Bern who are using the GOM system have been the only team to have successfully presented 3-dimensional evidence, from stereo photographic capture to computer-generated modelling, of bite mark evidence to a court of law. However, two issues arise with the GOM device. First, the price (£120 upwards) is prohibitive for most institutions in the UK, especially for forensic purposes. Second, the portability of the device is problematic. In many situations bite mark cases involve photography of living subjects, often children. This necessitates that any 3D system should be practical and consistent if it is to replace the current 2D systems. There are some high-quality lightweight hand-held 3D capturing devices (Agosto *et al.*, 2008), such as the Handyscan^{TM} which has to be tethered to a computer.

It is the opinion of the author that greater improvements in the technology, in the form of portability and the imaging of both the bruise and dental cast need to be made and further research into the robustness of the method needs to be conducted before 3D imaging of bite marks will be commonplace in the courts of the world.

10.11 Image enhancement and processing

At the start of this section the author would like to issue an important caveat. All images, digital or otherwise, that are intended for use as evidence should be treated with great care. Any operator applying enhancement or restoration techniques to images must be mindful of artefacts, and in general creating a false appearance in the images. Artefacts are created when a high level of contrast and/or heavy compression is applied; this may cause some pixels to become blocks of black or white, which, if care is not taken, may introduce false information into the image that is to be analysed.

This section will look at some of the current methods in use. All of these techniques have benefits and limits in the context of admissibility in a court.

10.11.1 Examples of enhancement

Every year companies produce cameras with increasingly advanced technology and capabilities. This development often presents itself with sensors (which transform the light into binary information), with greater amounts of megapixels, and with higher levels of light sensitivity. An increase in quality gives the operator greater tonal range and less noise, thus better images. This development has an impact on photographic forensic evidence. A simple extrapolation could be that, the more information that can be collected by the camera, the greater latitude for image enhancement and thus the possibility for the investigator to examine subtle information in the evidence.

The increasing use and development of digital photography has made it possible to apply digital enhancements. This gives the operator the possibility of achieving a clearer or finer definition in an image. This process can be of help to the forensic odontologist in the analysis of bite mark injuries. Using robust protocols and audit trails, a number of studies have demonstrated the use of computer software to enhance the edge definition of patterns within images in different forensic applications. Some examples include *colour separation*, which uses algorithms within Adobe® Photoshop® for removal of distracting background patterns from fingerprint and handwriting evidence (Berger *et al.*, 2005); and red/green/blue (RGB) *channel extraction*, which removes one or more of the three RGB channels to decrease background interference in a variety of crime scene images (Dalrymple, 2002, 2004). A similar method is used in footmark analysis, whereby details are extracted and the background information is reduced by viewing the image separated into RGB and cyan/magenta/yellow and key (CMYK) colour channels (Smith, 2006).

The layers containing information or distractions can be identified and, following a mixture of blending and removing colour layers, the subject can be made clearer (Blitzer *et al.*, 2008). Each of these methods in essence removes a colour channel (Figure 10.40), making the image 'greyscale'. This can in some instances make the bite mark appear to have better edge definition (Figures 10.41, 10.42 and 10.43).

Further edge definition can be achieved by applying contrast, similar to the method used with radiographs. Caution should be used when applying high levels of contrast, especially if the image has been compressed. If high levels of contrast are applied to a JPEG file, for example, it is likely that artefacts will appear and may even mask parts of the bite mark (Figures 10.44 and 10.45).

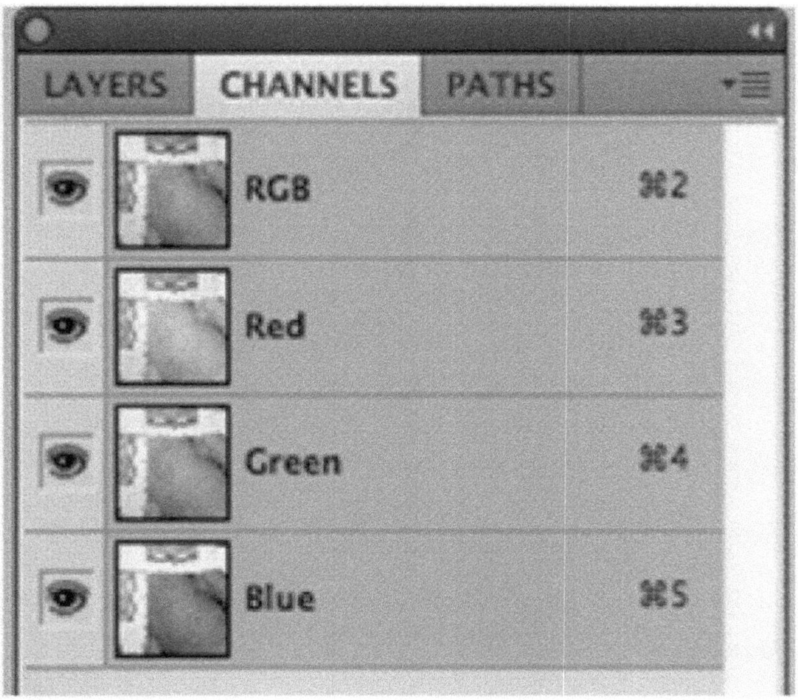

Figure 10.40 RGB channels of an RGB image in Adobe® Photoshop®

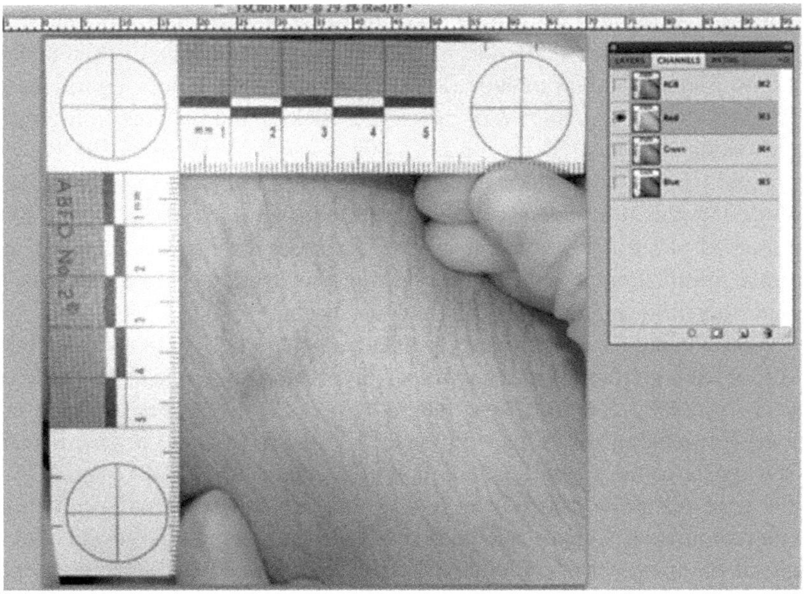

Figure 10.41 Image of bite mark with the red channel selected

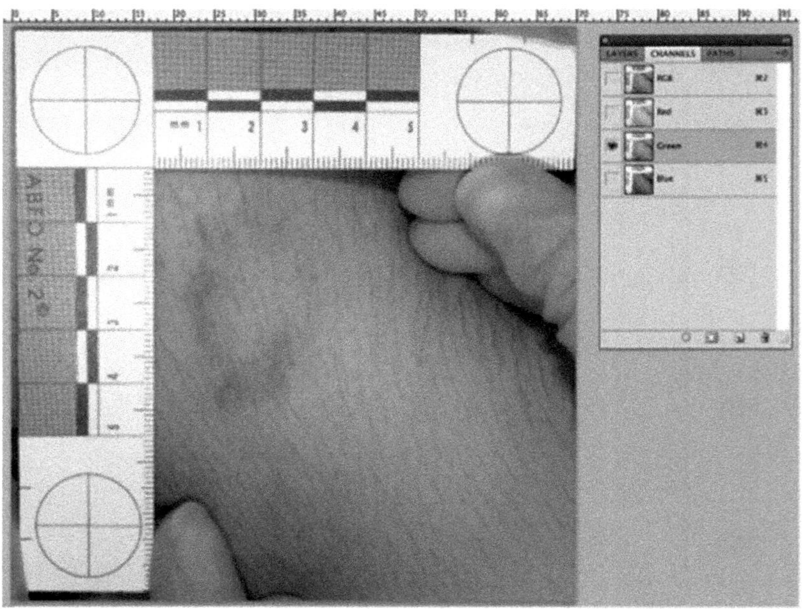

Figure 10.42 Image of bite mark with the green channel selected

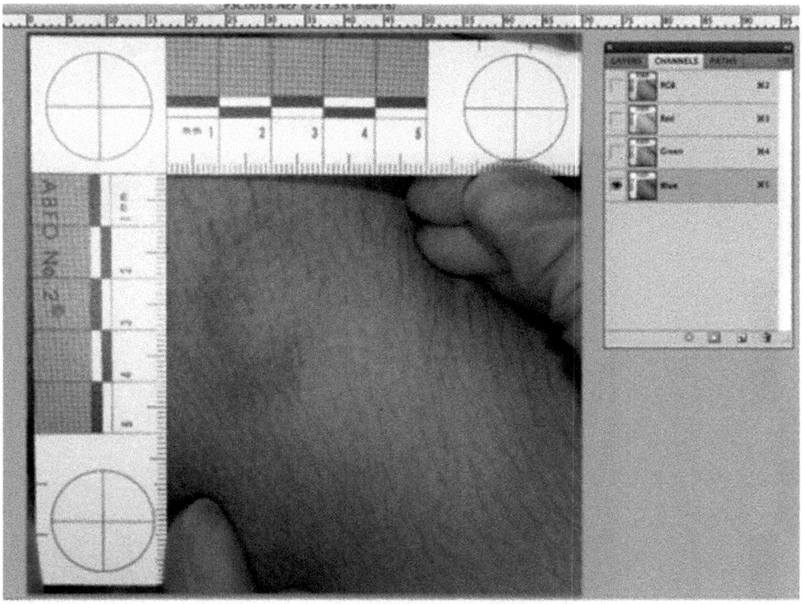

Figure 10.43 Image of bite mark with the blue channel selected

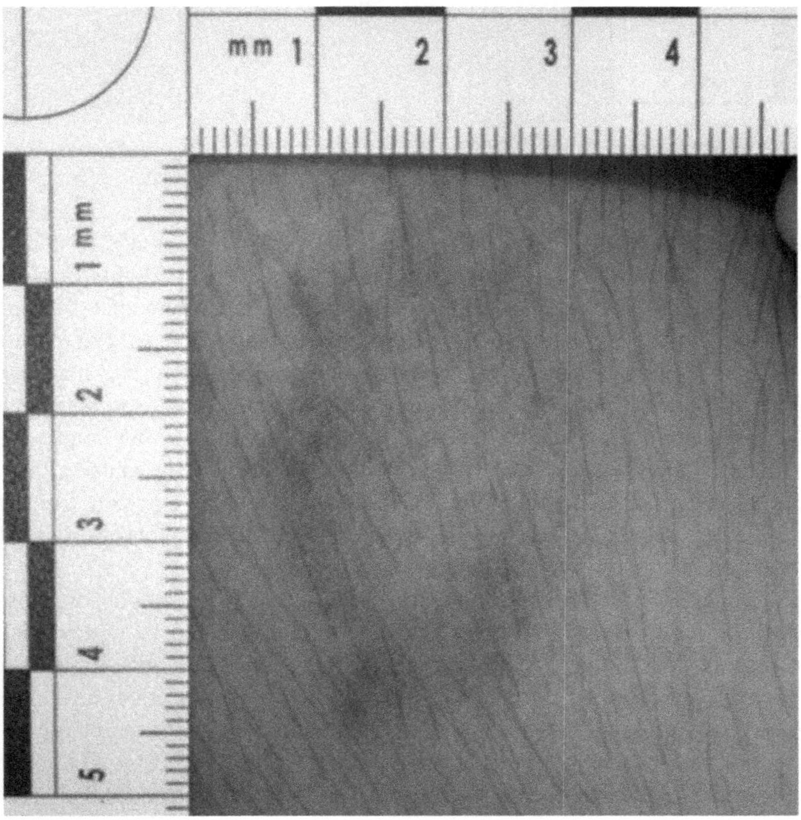

Figure 10.44 Image without contrast adjustment

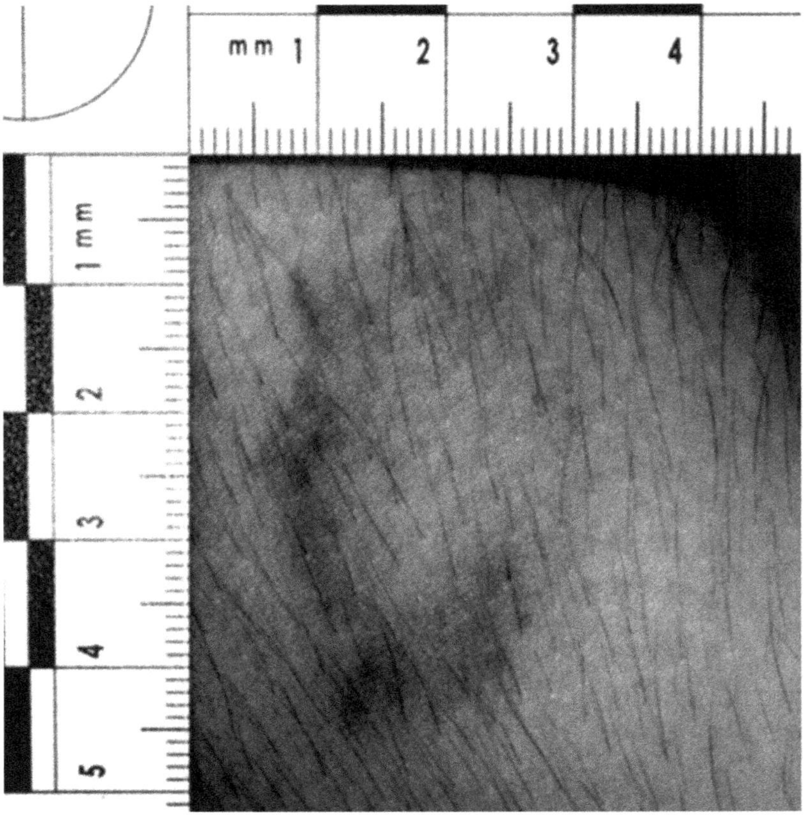

Figure 10.45 Image with heavy contrast adjustment

Note that adjusting the contrast or removing a channel in an image does not bring forth any previously unseen information (Evans *et al.*, 2013). A digital enhancement can only be applied to information that is already visible, albeit faint and diffused. Any enhancement should only be used in conjunction with an unchanged reference image for comparison. Enhanced images can have a potential benefit to bite mark analysis with regard to the definition of bruise edges. However, it should be noted that any forensic assessment made when examining the enhanced image and concluding that there is greater detail in that image is likely to be a subjective conclusion that could vary among experts. All methods of image enhancement will benefit from further research to understand how such images behave when adjusted. Further variability in the process of bite analysis would be an unwelcome addition.

Digital imaging in the forensic community is a relatively recent phenomenon, with perhaps little more than 10–15 years of common use. It could be argued that legal systems need time to properly digest all the issues and implications of how far image enhancement can be pushed. In the UK, several rulings and publications have discussed the way in which digital evidence should be handled – mostly in regard to using an audit trail and following operating procedures. A particular example is the Select Committee on Science and Technology's fifth report (1998). Further to that, in section

60 of the *Youth Justice and Criminal Evidence Act 1999* (which superseded the repealed section 69 of the *Police and Criminal Evidence Act 1984*) there is clear indication that any digital evidence that has been altered or enhanced must be declared and that any work on the image must not affect the accuracy of the record. It is especially important to make sure that all editing is done on a working copy rather than the original; utilising RAW image files will ensure that the original cannot be overwritten.

10.11.2 Published guidelines

Two important publications address the processing of digital imaging in relation to evidence, which are summarised below.

Practice advice on police use of digital images (ACPO and NPIA, 2007)

This document is helpful with regard to good practice and definitions of digital enhancement and processing.

What is considered admissible under the term 'enhancement'?

- *Brightness adjustment.* This is a simple procedure of brightening or darkening all the pixels in the image. This can be achieved in all imaging software. Each pixel in the image is given an RGB value. If each channel (red, green or blue) has a value of 0 then that pixel is black. If the value is 255 then that pixel is white. When the brightness level is changed, ALL the pixels are uniformly moved towards white or back.
- *Contrast adjustment.* This is a simple adjustment to increase or decrease showing how darker areas compare with lighter areas.
- *Colour cast removal* (colour correction is assumed to be routine processing). This can be done either by performing automatic white balancing in the image editing software (which can on occasion produce unexpected results) or calibrating the image by using the dropper tool on a colour/grey chart that is present in the image.
- *Noise removal.* This uses mathematical models to remove noise (which is commonly in the form of graininess). The software will replace each pixel in the image with a pixel that has been made with the average value of its neighbouring pixels. When too much noise removal is performed the image will become blurred.
- *Edge enhancement.* This is an image sharpening tool that attempts to identify sharp edges of an object against a background of a dissimilar colour – exaggerating the differences, thus making the edge more pronounced. However, this process may result in a loss of detail if too much enhancement is made.
- *Histogram stretching.* This has the effect of increasing the contrast of the image. This can lead to the image having an unnatural appearance and extreme contrast.

What is considered admissible under the term 'restoration'?

Any restoration to an image must be validated by mathematical modelling. The investigator should be aware that any restoration applied to the image may need to be justified and described to the court. *Restoration applies only to techniques that do not add information* (interpolation of pixels without proper explanation is inadmissible).

- *Blur removal.* This particular action can be difficult for the non-expert. First the operator will need to identify whether there is motion blur or focus blur. It is essential to have an advanced understanding of this process before this technique is used.
- *Greyscale linearisation.* This is a process whereby the operator can select which areas or objects to brighten, rather than the whole image (global adjustments).
- *Colour balancing.* This is the action of restoring the colour of the image to what is thought to be the original colour. It is important to make sure that there is some form of reference in the image, against which to balance the colour.
- *Warping.* This consists of restoring an image that has been distorted by either image manipulation or optical aberration. Again, this is an area that should be attempted only by advanced practitioners with in-depth knowledge of the software and the mathematical modelling that is being used.
- *Geometric restoration.* This includes the correction of geometric distortion from a wide-angle lens, such as a fisheye type. It must be noted that interpolation is not admissible; any corrections must be justified mathematically. Some research has indicated that angular distortion can be corrected. However, correcting perspective distortion in a bite mark image without prior knowledge of the specific angle may be problematic.

Restoration techniques may in some circumstances be on the edge of what is considered admissible. If the process is not fully understood by the investigator, or has a lack of basic research, then it should be approached in a very careful way. In some instances the edited version may appear to demonstrate forensic significance that is not present in the original, this may need to be explained to the court when presenting the evidence.

The Scientific Working Group Imaging Technology

In the United States, SWGIT has produced a detailed booklet with (at the time of writing) 22 sections on subjects from image handling to image enhancement. According to SWGIT, in the context of imaging technology in the criminal justice system:

> Digital images that have been enhanced are admissible when the enhancement can be explained by qualified personnel. ... All personnel utilizing imaging technologies shall be trained and competent in the operation of the relevant imaging technologies.

The SWGIT document suggests that any enhancements made that follow the traditional darkroom methods and used in the digital sphere are likely to be admissible.

The SWGIT document organises types of enhancement and processing into various categories, in a manner similar to that of the practice advice on police use of digital images considered above. Traditional enhancement techniques include:

- *Brightness adjustment* (same as above).
- *Colour balancing* (same as above).
- *Contrast adjustment* (same as above).
- *Cropping*. This is simply marking off an area of interest (perhaps a close-up of the bite mark) and removing the superfluous information.
- *Dodging and burning*. This comes from techniques performed in the traditional darkroom. In dodging, the operator stops some light for a portion of time over one part of the image, making that part lighter than the rest of the photograph. Burning requires the operator to allow the light more exposure time, thus making the image darker. In the imaging software the operator uses the dodge or burn tool to select a specific area to lighten or darken.

Non-traditional enhancement techniques include:

- *Colour processing*. This consists of transforming the hue of an image and the saturation. This can be done within an image to a particular area/object.
- *Linear filtering*. This can be applied to increase contrast to an area in the image. The type of filtering includes sharpening, deblurring and edge enhancement (as mentioned above).
- *Non-linear contrast adjustments*. This can be used to apply contrast to selected areas in the image.
- *Restoration techniques*. The SWGIT document follows the same categories as above for restoration.

10.11.3 Case law

In terms of admissibility of digital imaging evidence, both the Daubert and Frye tests can be used in the context of enhancements and alterations. There have been some cases in courts around the world that are relevant to digital imaging.

State of Connecticut v Alfred Swinton

This relates to the use of enhanced images in a murder case in which bite mark evidence was included. The images were subjected to enhancement with software called LucisPro (www.lucispro.com). During the appeals process the defendant questioned the admissibility of the evidence from the forensic odontologist, which included both enhanced images and overlays made in Photoshop®. The court found in favour of the enhanced images. It was explained that the expert witness who performed the enhancements was an advanced operator and could express their knowledge to the court. However, in regards to the overlay images, the expert witness who testified on the overlays did not did not actually create the overlays and was thus unable to explain the process to a satisfactory level to the court. The court subsequently decided that the overlays were not admitted properly.

It seems that the court requires that there be not only a reliability of the evidence itself but also the ability of the expert witness to give sufficient explanation. There must be testimony by a person with some degree of computer expertise, who has sufficient knowledge to be examined and cross-examined about the functioning of the computer.

Bryant v State of Florida

This case is interesting as it refers to the need to compare an edited version with that of the original. The defendant in this case argued that enhanced video had been admitted without the defence team being able to examine the original video data for comparison by their own expert witness. The court decided that enhanced video evidence was edited in such a way that disrupted the time sequence of the video; subsequently the case was remanded for a new trial.

Kennedy v State of Florida

Image enhancement on fingerprint evidence was performed to increase the contrast of the print. The defendant questioned the lack of a Frye hearing to determine the robustness of the method. The court concluded that this test was not needed as the experts did not use a novel scientific method and that, due to the experts explanation, no alteration to the evidence took place.

People v Perez

This relates to the enhancement of images of a shoe print. The defendant protested that the image was enhanced using Photoshop® and was subject to a 'new scientific technique' which was then not subjected to a Frye test before the trial and should not have been used. The court declared that using Photoshop® does not constitute using a scientific technique but is rather another way to develop film or pictures. This alludes to the reference that such enhancements that follow traditional darkroom, which methods are admissible. Importantly, is was declared that the method did not alter the image/representation of the shoe print.

Further cases in the US and Canada

These include image enhancement and computer generated evidence:

- *State of Florida v Victor Reyes* (2003)
- *R.v Jamieson* (Ontario Superior Court of Justice)

- *Commonwealth of Virginia v Robert Douglas Knight* (1991)
- *State of WA v Eric Hayden* (1995)
- *State of Washington v Hayden* (1998)
- *University of Regina v Pettick* (Saskatchewan Court of Appeal)
- *United States v. Beeler* (1999).
- *Nooner v State of Arkansas* (1995)
- *State of Ohio v Jones* (2000)
- *State of Ohio v Hartman* (2001).

10.11.4 Comment

Digital imaging enhancement techniques, if used with due care, are not often questioned. It could be argued that it is not necessarily the tools that need to be doubted but the methods and interpretation of the images by the expert witness that need to be carefully controlled. The benefit of digital technology is that any editing that has been done by the operator is recorded in the *image metadata*, and this allows a second expert witness to repeat the method easily – thus ensuring verifiable results. *One cannot overstate the need for comprehensive operating procedures and audit trails when editing images for analysis and presentation to the court.*

10.12 References

ACPO and NPIA (2007) *Practice Advice on Police Use of Digital Images*. Available at www.npia.police.uk/en/6533.htm (accessed: 13 July 2012).

Agosto E. *et al.* (2008) Crime scene reconstruction using a fully geomatic approach. *Sensors* **8**: 6280–6302. Sensors [Online]. Available at www.mdpi.com/journal/sensors (accessed: 13 July 2012).

Berger C. E. H., De Koeijer J. A., Glas W. and Madhuizen H. T. (2005) Color separation in forensic image processing, *Journal of Forensic Science* **51**: 100–102.

Blackwell *et al.* (2005) 3-D imaging and quantitative comparison of human dentitions and simulated bite marks, *International Journal of Legal Medicine* **121**(1).

Blitzer H. L. and Jacobia (2007) Storing and archiving images. In: *Forensic Digital Imaging and Photography*, 2nd edn. New York: Academic Press.

Blitzer H.L., Stein-Ferguson K. and Huang J. (2008) *Understanding Forensic Digital Imaging*. New York: Academic Press.

Bowers C. M. and Johansen R. J. (2000) *Digital Analysis of Bite Mark Evidence Using Adobe Photoshop*. USA: Forensic Imaging Services.

British Association of Forensic Odontology (2002) What is a forensic odontologist and what is the scope of their work? Available at www.bafo.org.uk/guide.php (accessed: 13 July 2012).

Buck *et al.* (2006) 3D documentation of footwear impressions and tyre tracks in snow with high-resolution optical surface scanning, *Forensic Science International* **171**.

Buck *et al.* (2010) 3D bloodstain pattern analysis: ballistic reconstruction of the trajectories of blood drops and determination of the centres of origin of the bloodstains. *Forensic Science International* **206**(1): 22–28.

Cavagnini G. *et al.* (2008) Reverse engineering from 3D optical acquisition: application to crime scene investigation. In: *Virtual and Rapid Manufacturing*. London: Taylor & Francis.

Dalrymple B. (2002) Optimized digital recording of crime scene impressions, *Journal of Forensic Identification* **52**: 750–761.

Dalrymple B. (2004) Background subtraction through exhibit substitution, *Journal of Forensic Identification* **54**: 150–157.

David T. J. (1990) Documentation of a seven-month-old bite mark with ultraviolet photography. Presented to the Annual Meeting of the American Academy of Forensic Sciences, Cincinnati, February.

David T. J. and Sobel M. N. (1994) Recapturing a five-month-old bite mark by means of reflective ultraviolet photography, *Journal of Forensic Science* **39**(6): 1560–1567.

Engle C. (1968) *Photography for the Scientist*, 4th edn. London: Academic Press.

Edwards N. (2011) Cross-polarisation: making it practical, *Journal of Visual Communication in Medicine* **34**(4): 165–172.

Evans S., Jones C. and Plassmann P. (2010) 3D imaging in forensic odontology, *Journal of Visual Communication in Medicine* **33**(2).

Evans S., Jones C. and Plassmann P. (2012) 3D imaging for bite mark analysis, *Imaging Science Journal*. http://dx.doi.org/10.1179/1743131X11Y.0000000054.

Evans S., Noorbhai S., Lawson Z., Stacey-Jones S. and Carabott R (2013) Contrast enhancement of bite mark images using the grayscale mixer in ACR in Photoshop, *Journal of Forensic Science*, **58**(3): 2013.

FBI Laboratory (2005) Digital Imaging Guidelines. Photographic Operations and Imaging Services Unit, Federal Bureau of Investigation.

Flora M. *et al.* (2009) Forensic bite mark identification using image processing methods. In: *Proceedings of the 2009 ACM symposium on Applied Computing*, USA, pp. 903–907.

Freeman *et al.* (2005) Seven hundred seventy eight bite marks: analysis by anatomic location, victim and biter demographics, type of crime, and legal disposition, *Journal of Forensic Science* **50**(6).

House of Lords Select Committee on Science and Technology fifth report (1998) Available at www.parliament.the-stationery-office.co.uk/pa/ld199798/ldselect/ldsctech/064v/st0501.htm (accessed: 13 July 2012).

Kau and Richmond (2008) Three-dimensional analysis of facial morphology surface changes in untreated children from 12 to 14 years of age, *American Journal of Orthodontics and Dentofacial Orthopedics* **134**(6).

Kitagawa *et al.* (2004) Dentoalveolar growth of patients with complete unilateral cleft lip and palate by early two-stage furlow and push-back method: preliminary results. *Cleft Palate–Craniofacial Journal* **41**(5).

Lawson Z., Nuttall D., Young S., Evans S., Maguire S., Dunstan F. and Kemp A. (2010) Which is the preferred image modality for paediatricians when assessing photographs of bruises in children? *International Journal of Legal Medicine*. Doi: 10.1007/s00414-010-0532-7.

Langford M. (1975) *Advanced Photography*, 3rd edn. London: Focal Press.

Martin-de-Las-Heras *et al.* (2007) Effectiveness of comparison overlays generated with DentalPrint software in bite mark analysis, *Journal of Forensic Science* **52**(1):

Martin-de-Las-Heras and Tafur (2009) Comparison of simulated human dermal bitemarks possessing three-dimensional comparison attributes to suspected biters using a proprietary three-dimensional comparison, *Forensic Science International* **190**(1).

Maguire, Mann, Sibert *et al.* (2005) *Archives of Diseases in Children* **90**: 187–189.

Payne-James J. (2012) Rules and scales used in measurement in the forensic setting: measured – and found wanting! *Forensic Science, Medicine, and Pathology*. Doi 10.1007/s12024-012-9320-7.

Plassmann P. and Peters J. M. (2002) Recording wound care effectiveness, *Journal of Tissue Viability* (12): 1.

Police and Criminal Evidence Act (1984) Section 69: Evidence from computer records. [Online]. Available at www.legislation.gov.uk/ukpga/1984/60/contents (accessed: 13 July 2012).

Popat H. *et al.* (2008) Three-dimensional motion analysis: an exploratory study. Part 1: Assessment of facial movement, *Orthodontic Craniofacial Research* **11**.

Rowan P., Hill M., Gresham G. A., Goodall E., Moore T. (2010) The use of infrared-aided photography in identification of sites of bruises after evidence of the bruise is absent to the naked eye, *Journal of Forensic Legal Medicine* **17**(6): 293–297.

Scientific Working Group on Imaging Technologies (SWGIT). Available at www.theiai.org/guidelines/swgit/index.php (accessed: 13 July 2012).

Sheasby and MacDonald (2001) A forensic classification of distortion in human bite marks. *Forensic Science International* **122**(1).

Sheets and Bush (2010) Mathematical matching of a dentition to bitemarks: use and evaluation of affine methods. *Forensic Science International*. Doi:10.1016/j.forsciint.2010.09.013.

Smith E. R. (2011) Device for reduction of angular distortion in photography. USA: US 7,997,808 B1.

Smith J. (2006) Image enhancement and Adobe Photoshop: using calculations to extract image detail. *Journal of Forensic Identification* **57**: 493–505.

Spott *et al.* (1998) Application of optical diffusion theory to transcutaneous bilirubinometry. Proceedings Paper. Doi: 10.1117/12.297907.

Tetley and Tetley (2005) The photography of bruises. *Journal of Visual Communication in Medicine* **28**(2): 72–77.

Thali *et al.* (2003) Bite mark documentation and analysis: the forensic 3D/CAD supported photogrammetry approach, *Forensic Science International* **135**(2).

Thali *et al.* (2005) Virtopsy: scientific documentation, reconstruction and animation in forensics: individual and real 3D data-based geo-metric approach including optical body/object surface and radiological CT/MRI scanning, *Journal of Forensic Science* **50**(2).

Wright F. D. (1998a) Photography in bite mark and patterned injury documentation: Part 1, *Journal of Forensic Science* **43**(4): 877–880.

Wright F. D. (1998b) Photography in bite mark and patterned injury documentation: Part 2, *Journal of Forensic Science* **43**(4): 881–887.

Wright F. D. and Golden G. S. (2010) The use of full-spectrum digital photography for evidence collection and preservation in cases involving forensic odontology, *Forensic Science International*.

Zharov V. *et al.* (2004) Infrared imaging of subcutaneous veins, *Lasers in Surgery and Medicine* **34**: 56–61.

11

Role of the forensic odontologist in the protection of vulnerable people

Barbara Chadwick
School of Dentistry, College of Biomedical and Life Sciences, Cardiff University, UK
Catherine Adams
UKDVI & Powys Teaching Health Board, UK

11.1 Introduction

Somebody may abuse or neglect a child or vulnerable adult by inflicting harm, or by failing to prevent harm. It must be remembered, though, that most injuries are accidental and may be simply explained. Also, it is not possible to diagnose whether an injury is accidental or non-accidental in origin from the appearance alone. CORE INFO is an excellent online source of up-to-date information from systematic reviews of the world literature with regard to child abuse and neglect, and it includes reviews on bites, dental neglect and oral injuries (www.core-info.cardiff.ac.uk).

The mobility of children and vulnerable adults is an important consideration when deciding whether the explanation of an injury from carers is consistent with the physical abilities of the person concerned. For example, a torn upper labial frenum is not uncommon due to accidental falls in children learning to walk, and due to falls from, for example, bicycles in older children. However, a non-ambulant child or adult is not as likely to sustain this type of injury accidentally, so bruising and laceration of the upper labial frenum should arouse suspicion as it can be non-accidentally caused by forcible bottle feeding or gagging, gripping and violent rubbing of the face. Injuries to the palate, vestibule and floor of the mouth can occur during forceful feeding and may be caused by a feeding utensil. Again it must be recognised that these types of injury can also be due to falls with objects in the mouth, and this applies to young children and adults with limited physical ability.

Usually, the issue of main concern to the forensic odontologist is that of bite mark analysis. However, the issue of dental and oral neglect is common to both

Forensic Odontology: An Essential Guide, First Edition.
Edited by Catherine Adams, Romina Carabott and Sam Evans.

children and vulnerable adults. A multi-agency approach to any cases of suspected abuse or neglect is essential in terms of communication and coordination between all the agencies involved.

Physical abuse

This is defined as 'inflicting an injury that is not accidental'. Consideration that the injury is non-accidental in origin should be raised when any (or a combination) of the following are present:

- The explanation is inconsistent with the injury or the developmental stage of the injured.
- There is a history of frequently repeated injury.
- The injuries are of different ages, other than common sites of accidental injury of a child of that age.
- There is facial bruising (other than over bony prominences), particularly around mouth, eyes or ears.
- there are unexplained or inadequately explained burns, bite marks, severe bruising or any combination of these.

Neglect

This may be defined as the 'failure to meet the basic needs of a child or a person in your care'. It includes the following considerations:

- The person has inappropriate or inadequate clothing.
- The person is left unsupervised or with a variety of different carers.
- There is persistent failure to seek or follow medical or dental advice.
- There is persistent failure to ensure appropriate safety.

11.2 Bite marks and vulnerable people

Any person may be the recipient of a human bite mark, but children and vulnerable adults are especially at risk. The interpretation of bite marks in children and adults in the care of others is especially difficult. In common with human bite marks in general, the bites may be defensive, offensive or self-inflicted. In cases where mental disability in the form of mental retardation is an issue, bite marks may often be self-inflicted. Some self-inflicted injury behaviour is a feature of non-specific mental retardation, Lesh–Nyhan syndrome, Rett syndrome, Cornelia de Lange syndrome, Torette syndrome, familial dysautonomia, choreoacanthocytosis, sensory neuropathies and several psychiatric disorders. Of these, individuals with Lesh–Nyhan syndrome,

Cornelia de Lange syndrome, and familial dysautonomia recurrently display loss of tissue as a consequence. From a dental perspective, individuals with Lesh–Nyhan syndrome displays distinctive features of biting the tongue, lips and fingers, which are diagnostic features of this syndrome.

Bite mark analysis is covered comprehensively in other chapters of this book.

11.3 Dental neglect in childhood

11.3.1 Introduction

In the last decade, high-profile deaths of children in the UK as a result of severe child abuse have received massive media attention and led to profound changes in the way child protection is undertaken in the UK. The enquiry into the death of Victoria Climbié drew attention to the failure of multiple agencies (police, social and health services) to intervene or share information and highlighted multiple failures in the systems in place to protect children from harm. Lord Laming concluded that this was not an isolated incident and that most children who die from abuse are known to several agencies (Laming, 2003). Child protection is a shared responsibility and everyone's responsibility, including the dental team (Harris *et al.*, 2006).

It is widely reported that oral and facial injuries are common in physical abuse. However, the inclusion of dental caries as a possible marker of neglect in the National Institute for Health and Clinical Excellence (NICE) commissioned clinical guideline on when to suspect child maltreatment (National Collaborating Centre for Women's and Children's Health, 2009) has emphasised the importance of a dental examination – and therefore the dentist – in protecting children at risk of neglect.

Sadly, child maltreatment is relatively common. For example, as of 31 March 2010 in the UK 46,705 children were on child protection registers or were the subject of child protection plans, and as such were considered at high risk of harm from maltreatment. (National Society for the Prevention of Cruelty to Children, 2012). Neglect is by far the most common reason for a child to be on the register, accounting for 45% of cases, and it follows that dentists are likely to see both neglected children and neglected dentitions. However, dental caries is still common, affecting up to 53.4% of 5-year-olds in some areas of England (NHS DEP, 2008). The question therefore becomes: when is dental caries a sign of neglect, or what is dental neglect?

11.3.2 Defining dental neglect

NICE guidance

Dental neglect may occur in isolation or as part of the wider features of general neglect. The suggested interventions for dental neglect are based on those for general neglect, and it is therefore helpful to consider recent *NICE guidance* on child maltreatment before considering how to recognise and deal with dental neglect specifically.

The aim of the NICE guidance was to summarise the 'alerting clinical features' of maltreatment for healthcare professionals who were not specialists in child protection.

Where evidence was lacking, an expert panel (including four dentists) used a consensus approach. The alerting features were used to define two categories according to the level of concern, with recommendations to either 'consider' or 'suspect' maltreatment. 'Consider' means maltreatment is one possible explanation for the alerting feature or is included in the differential diagnosis. 'Suspect' means you have a serious level of concern about the possibility of child maltreatment but not proof of it.

If an alerting feature prompts you to consider child maltreatment, look for other alerting features of maltreatment now or in the past, and do one or more of the following:

- Discuss your concerns with a more experienced colleague.
- Gather collateral information from other agencies and health disciplines.
- Ensure review of the child or young person.

If an alerting feature prompts you to suspect child maltreatment:

- Refer the child or young person to children's social care, following local procedures.

The guidance suggests that neglect is a failure or provision and/or supervision, summarising it as:

> the persistent failure to meet the child or young person's basic physical or psychological needs that is likely to result in the serious impairment of their health or development. This may or may not be deliberate. There are differences in how parents and carers choose to raise their children, including the choices they make about their children's healthcare. However, failure to recognise and respond to the child or young person's needs may amount to neglect. ... There is no diagnostic gold standard for neglect and therefore decision-making in situations of apparent neglect can be very difficult and thresholds hard to establish. It is essential to place the child or young person at the centre of the assessment.

Oral health

Oral health is specifically considered within the NICE guidance. Although it acknowledges that current evidence is not strong enough to confirm a relationship between poor oral health and child maltreatment, it does include alerting features for poor oral health. It may present as untreated dental caries, gum disease, mouth ulcers or teeth that appear dirty and uncared for. The specific recommendations are as follows:

1. *Consider* neglect if parents or carers have access to, but persistently fail to obtain, National Health Service (NHS) treatment for their child's dental caries (tooth decay).
2. *Suspect* neglect if parents or carers fail to seek medical advice for their child to the extent that the child's health and well-being is compromised, including if the child is in on-going pain.

The increasing acceptance of untreated dental disease as a potential sign of child neglect is reflected in specific guidance in the Department of Health funded educational online resource *Child Protection and the Dental Team* (Harris *et al.*, 2006) and a recent policy document on dental neglect produced by the British Society of Paediatric Dentistry (Harris *et al.*, 2009).

Before trying to specifically define dental neglect, it is first helpful to consider further the concept of oral health which was defined by the Department of Health in 1994 as:

> the standard of health of the oral and related tissues which enables an individual to eat, speak and socialise without active disease, discomfort or embarrassment and which contributes to general well-being.

This definition places oral health and well-being as an integral part of general health. Similarly, when trying to define dental neglect, starting from the more general definition for neglect is helpful. There are many different definitions for neglect, but within the UK neglect is defined officially (HM Government, 2006) as:

> the persistent failure to meet a child's basic physical and emotional needs, which can lead to impairment of the child's health and development.'

In contrast to other forms of child maltreatment, neglect is characterised by failing to do something in the child's best interest rather than by causing specific harm. The British Society of Paediatric Dentistry (BSPD) policy document on dental neglect in children (Harris *et al.*, 2009) used the UK definition of neglect as the basis for their definition of dental neglect:

> the persistent failure to meet a child's basic oral health needs, likely to result in the serious impairment of a child's oral or general health or development. It may occur in isolation or may be an indicator of a wider picture of neglect or abuse.

The parallels between the UK definition of general neglect, the wording of the NICE guidance and the BSPD dental neglect definition are obvious and deliberate, emphasising the same key phrases:

> persistent failure ... basic needs ... impairment of child's health.

Although, as the NICE guidance indicates, there are many different oral issues that might be considered as demonstrating neglect, it is perhaps dental caries that is most commonly encountered. An understanding of the issues surrounding this disease process are therefore important.

11.3.3 When is decay neglect?

The Child Dental Health Survey in 2003 found that 43% of 5-year-olds and 50% of 8-year-olds had obvious caries in their primary teeth (Lader *et al.*, 2004). In other words, dental caries remains common in the UK and while it is preventable its presence, even in high levels, cannot be taken as evidence of dental neglect. Nor is it possible to set a threshold based on the number of carious teeth at which a diagnosis of dental neglect can be made.

Many variables determine levels of dental health in individuals, including well-recognised regional and social inequalities in both disease experience and access to services and treatment. Within the UK there are also clear differences of opinion on the management of dental caries particularly in the primary dentition, with prevention, restoration and extractions all being suggested as appropriate management strategies in some circumstances. For very young children, who cannot easily tolerate treatment while conscious, the management of the disease is often limited to prevention alone in the absence of symptoms.

Diagnosing dental caries is difficult for both lay and indeed many medical professionals. Some disease may be obvious but also be well-controlled or arrested, while active disease may remain undetected (Figures 11.1 and 11.2). However, it is not the presence of disease but the impact of the disease on the individual child and the parental response to the disease that is important when determining dental neglect.

Pain and infection are the most common and well-known sequelae of dental decay. But there is increasing evidence to suggest that children with untreated dental disease have poorer oral-health related quality of life than those with no disease and treated disease, and they may also be under-developed for their age (Sheiham, 2006). Importantly, treating the disease allows children to recover and catch up. Assessing general development in terms of height and weight compared to the average child is therefore important when reviewing the potential impact of dental disease.

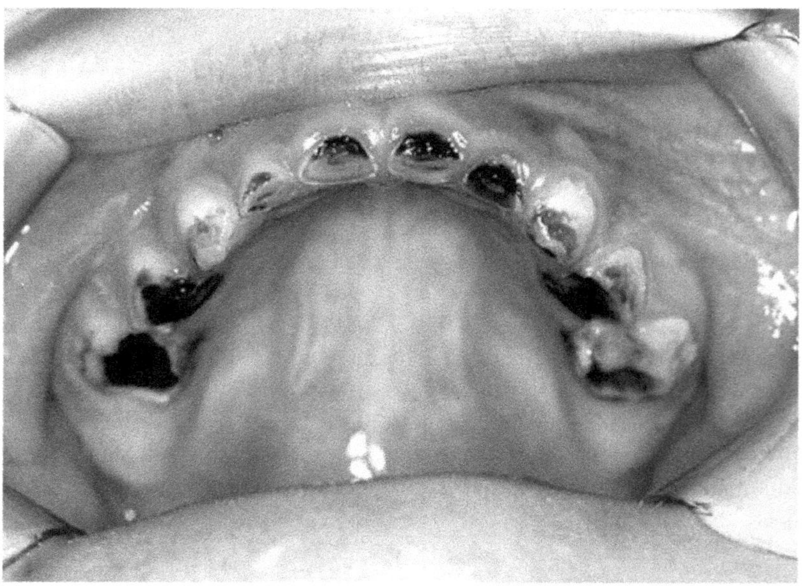

Figure 11.1 Upper arch of a 5-year-old boy. All teeth show obvious decay, but the decay is dark and arrested. The family are attending for regular reviews and no new lesions have appeared over a 2-year period. Dental neglect is not considered at this stage

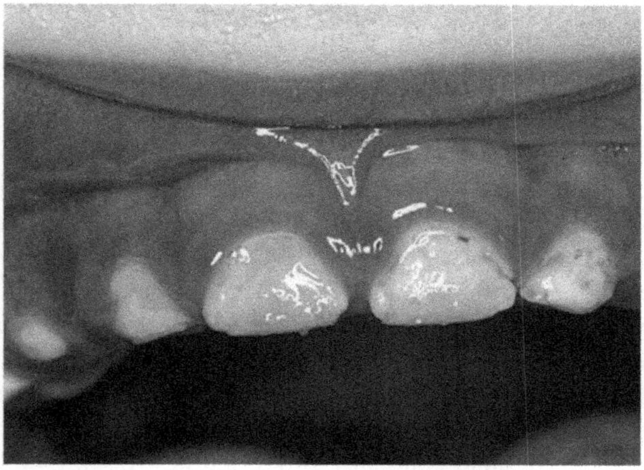

(a)

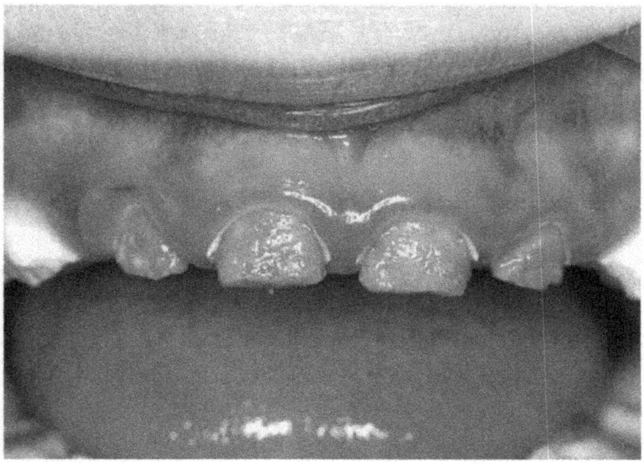

(b)

Figure 11.2 (a) Upper arch of a child aged 17 months. Early enamel changes as a result of decay associated with prolonged bottle feeding are already evident. At this stage, preventive dental team management is appropriate. (b) Upper arch of same child aged 23 months. The child presented in pain, having missed two review appointments. The decay is active, there is no enamel on the incisors and the erupting canines are already showing evidence of decay in enamel. The child was scheduled for extractions under a general anaesthetic. At this stage, preventive multi-agency management should be considered

Questioning children themselves about their oral symptoms is the best way to identify oral problems, but this is difficult in very young children, so parents' and carers' views should also be obtained. There is increasing evidence that children with chronic oral problems may not always report pain but the oral discomfort may affect them in many different ways – altering their eating patterns, disturbing sleep, stopping them playing and even increasing time off school (Slade *et al.*, 1996; Shepherd *et al.*, 1999). Careful questioning is required to identify these effects.

11.3.4 Parental response to dental disease

As we have already stated, dental decay is common in children in the UK – which in itself implies a lack of awareness among parents and carers on both the aetiology and prevention of the disease. Parents may expect children to brush their own teeth when they are in fact far too young to undertake this complex process. If they do not assist with tooth brushing they may not regularly look in their child's mouth and will not see early signs of disease. A lack of knowledge may lead them to believe that tooth decay is normal and that nothing can be done. Parents who are fearful of the dentist themselves may find in difficult to engage with dentists and may also fail to seek care for their children. Family stress, poverty or illness may all contribute.

Once a child has attended for dental assessment and appropriate preventive advice has been received, failure to follow preventive protocols or change harmful behaviours may be of concern if the child continues to develop new disease or symptoms – or indeed if a younger sibling begins to develop signs and symptoms of oral disease. A detailed history from the parent and child may reveal repeated attendance with different services for the same problem. Children or families who present repeatedly when in pain, but who do not respond to offers of appropriate treatment, are a cause of particular concern.

The views of the child are increasingly important and his/her views need to be considered when planning treatment. When assessing dental neglect in older children, their competence to consent to or refuse treatment needs to be considered. Where the child's refusal to accept or even attend for treatment is compounded by dental anxiety, identifying appropriate support mechanisms for both the parent and child are important. Multi-agency management may be required to assist these children to overcome their anxiety and receive appropriate dental care; and the role of the dental team in these instances is to ensure that an appropriate referral, with consent of the family, is considered and made if required.

The BSPD definition of dental neglect includes the words 'persistent failure', and severe untreated dental disease is clearly a persistent failure. Some definitions include the word 'wilful' when defining dental neglect (American Academy of Paediatric Dentistry, 2010), but severe disease can result without intent; however, its consequences are just the same for the child. While severe untreated disease may develop as a result of poor parental knowledge and failure to follow preventive guidelines, failing to take action is not in the best interests of the child. The welfare of the child is the paramount consideration (HM Government, 1989), and putting the needs of the child first and supporting the family to do this is the overarching aim of all safeguarding legislation and the duty of all clinicians.

11.3.5 Identifying neglect in dental practice

When a diagnosis of neglect is being considered a thorough assessment and accurate records are essential. Because dental neglect requires *persistent* failure to respond to a child's needs, it is usually seen over a period of time, so recording relevant detail and concerns for all children at every appointment is essential. For example, a child who attends on a single occasion in clothes that are dirty and do not fit may be explained, but when it is observed at every visit, neglect should be considered. While concerns over dental neglect may be raised by a preschool child presenting with severe untreated dental caries, it is the response of the carer to the suggested management that determines whether the problem can be managed within the dental team or requires multi-agency management.

The history, oral and clinical examination are therefore critical to the diagnosis of dental neglect, but other factors are important too – the attendance history and symptoms, response to preventive strategies, and general appearance of the child are also important (Table 11.1).

The history should be taken from the child and/or carer, depending on the child's age. It should include a full medical, dental and social history. The social history allows details of other siblings' and the family's current tooth brushing and diet habits to be assessed.

Where dental disease is obvious or symptoms are reported, a detailed history of symptoms and adverse events (e.g. previous attendance with toothache, severe infections, repeat use of painkillers and antibiotics, previous general anaesthesia for dental extractions for all children in the family) is required.

A detailed clinical examination should include assessment of soft and hard tissues. Poor oral hygiene, gingival inflammation, dental caries, trauma, ulceration and signs of infection should be recorded. Radiographs should be used as appropriate.

From the information gathered a diagnosis and treatment plan can be made. The relevant clinical and radiographic findings should be shown to the child and carer and treatment options discussed and agreed; this should include management of pain if present, appropriate prevention and ongoing management of disease including follow-up. At this stage the aim is to ensure the child receives appropriate care to safeguard his/her welfare, not to blame the family for the disease.

Clearly the carer's circumstances, understanding and ability to manage the child's oral care are important; but if, despite attempts to assist them, they are unable

Table 11.1 Examples of neglect in the dental setting (based on Balmer *et al*., 2010)

Dental features	General features
• Child presenting with extensive, untreated oral disease • Late presentation of obvious severe oral pathology • Attendance only when in pain with failure to attend for follow-up appointments • Severe dental trauma in the absence of appropriate supervision • History of multiple repeat dental general anaesthesia for extractions • History of multiple missed appointments • Failure to administer antibiotics for acute dental abscess	• Child consistently presents with ingrained dirt on hands, and clothes are smelly • Child consistently dressed inappropriately (e.g. for the weather or the child's size) • Severe and persistent headlice on successive appointments • Diet history reveals inadequate or very limited diet (with no input from other agencies)

or unwilling to provide the necessary support a diagnosis of dental neglect should be considered.

11.3.6 Responding to neglect in dental practice

When dental neglect is recognised, one of three tiered levels of intervention is considered (Harris *et al.*, 2006):

- preventive dental team management
- preventive multi-agency management
- child protection referral.

Preventive dental team management

At this level the emphasis is on supporting families to attend for care and institute rigorous preventive strategies. Missed appointments are flagged and followed up. At this stage, sharing information with other agencies (health visitors, general medical practitioners) is essential. Identifying reasons for non attendance, referral to more local dental facilities or addressing underlying dental anxiety management may resolve the problem.

Preventive multi-agency management

If concerns remain or the situation is deteriorating, help from other agencies may be required to ensure appropriate dental care. Parental consent to involve other professionals (health visitor, school nurse, doctor, social workers, paediatrician) should be sought. A joint action plan can then be agreed to address concerns. Where the reason for referral is for repeated failed appointments, it may not be possible to gain consent – but it may still be appropriate to proceed.

Child protection referral

This may occur if all previous interventions fail but may happen at any point if a child is suffering significant harm from dental neglect. A child protection referral following local child protection procedures should be made. The exact arrangements vary slightly in different countries within the UK but are broadly similar.

Set-by-step guidance on local child protection procedures, case histories and example referral letters to health visitors to assist practitioners can be accessed online for all areas of the UK, and can be accessed from the Child Protection and the Dental Team website (www.cpdt.org.uk).

11.4 Legislative framework for child protection in the UK

The legislative framework for child protection within the UK can appear complex because no single piece of legislation covers it. Over time, a series of laws and guidance have been amended, updated and revoked. Statutory laws are amended by new legislation passed by Westminster, the Welsh Assembly Government, the Northern Ireland Assembly and the Scottish Parliament. Case law, based on interpretation in the courts, may lead to an amendment. But not all laws affect all parts of the UK. Practitioners must therefore ensure that they consult the guidance for their locality.

The Children Act 1989/2004

Within the UK the Children Act is the most pertinent, replacing most other legislation regarding the welfare of children. It details the legal framework for local authority responsibilities for the care and protection of children. The *paramountcy principle* means that a child's welfare is paramount when making any decisions about a child's upbringing. It introduced the notion of parental responsibility, partnership and participation of the child in decision making.

In 2004, following the inquiry into the death of Victoria Climbié, the Act was amended – bringing all local government functions of children's welfare and education under the statutory authority of local Directors of Children's Services. It placed a strong emphasis on 'safeguarding' across all sectors and at all levels. It is the duty of all those working with children to make their safety and well-being paramount (sections 25(2) and (5)).

In both England and Wales, Area Child Protection Committees (ACPC) were replaced by Local Safeguarding Boards, giving them increased influence over strategic decisions and providing them with more senior management commitment.

UN Convention on the Rights of the Child 1989

The UN Convention on the Rights of the Child was ratified by the UK in 1991, with some reservations. Governments of countries that have ratified the Convention are required to report to, and appear before, the UN Committee on the Rights of the Child periodically to be examined on their progress with regard to the advancement of the implementation of the Convention and the status of child rights in their country. For example, Article 19 states specifically that children should be protected from all forms of neglect and negligent treatment. Wales is the first, and so far only, part of the UK to embed the principles of the UN Convention into its own laws. The National Assembly for Wales passed the Rights of Children and Young Persons (Wales) Measure on 18 January 2011.

11.5 Protection of the vulnerable adult

11.5.1 The dentist and the vulnerable adult

In their publication *Child Protection and Vulnerable Adults*, the General Dental Council (GDC; www.gdc-uk.org) considers the term 'vulnerable adult' to mean:

> a person above the age of 18 years who is or may be in need of community care service (including healthcare) by reason of mental or other disability, age or illness; and who is unable to take care of him or herself, or unable to protect him or herself against significant harm or exploitation.

People with learning disabilities or mental health problems, older people and disabled people may fall into this definition, particularly when their situation is complicated by additional factors such as physical frailty or chronic illness, sensory impairment, challenging behaviours, social or emotional problems, poverty or homelessness. Domestic abuse may also be included within the definition of vulnerable adults.

The General Dental Council expects that all registrants are aware of the procedures involved in raising issues about the possible abuse or neglect of children and vulnerable adults. Further, the GDC state that:

> dental professionals have a duty to find out what the local procedures are in their area, whether they work for the NHS or in private practice.

They have a responsibility to raise any concerns they may have about the possible abuse or neglect of vulnerable adults. In common with child protection, the procedures for vulnerable adults may vary between countries in the UK but will be broadly similar. The definitions of abuse, neglect and safeguarding for vulnerable adults apply to children and adults alike.

If a dental professional makes a professional judgment and decides not to share his/her concern with the appropriate authority, then they must be able to justify how they came to this decision.

Suspicions of abuse, neglect or exploitation of vulnerable adults may also be triggered by observations of the patient's presentation or by concerns or comments about the lack of appropriate care at their home or residential placement.

It is important that caregivers realise that the Department of Health has established a consensus that identifies 'neglect and acts of omission' as a form of abuse. This includes ignoring medical, oral and physical care needs, failure to provide access to appropriate health services, and withholding the necessities of life, such as medication, adequate nutrition and comfort.

11.5.2 Confidentiality

Ethical and statutory codes with respect to confidentiality are in place to protect individual patients. However, they are not intended to prevent exchange of information between professionals who have a responsibility to ensure the protection of children and vulnerable adults. Furthermore, where there are safeguarding concerns, there is a duty to share all relevant information with those who need to know. This may be done without the permission of the child or vulnerable adult or the parents or carers when it is believed that the concerns may pose an additional risk to those in their care.

Vulnerable adults and children are entitled to the same duty of confidentiality from professionals provided they have the ability to understand the choices and their consequence in respect of any intervention. Vulnerable adults are assumed to have mental capacity unless proven otherwise (Mental Capacity Act, 2005) as detailed in the next section.

> There is nothing within the Caldicott Report 1997, the Data Protection Act 1998, or the Human Rights Act 1998, which should prevent the justifiable and lawful exchange of information for the protection of children or prevention of serious crime. (Carlile Review, 2002)

11.5.3 The Mental Capacity Act 2005

Principles (section 1)

1. A person must be assumed to have capacity unless it is established that he lacks capacity.
2. A person is not to be treated as unable to make a decision unless all practicable steps to help him to do so have been taken without success.
3. A person is not to be treated as unable to make a decision merely because he makes an unwise decision.
4. An act done, or decision made, under this Act for or on behalf of a person who lacks capacity must be done, or made, in his best interests.
5. Before the act is done, or the decision is made, regard must be had to whether the purpose for which it is needed can be as effectively achieved in a way that is less restrictive of the person's rights and freedom of action.

Adults who lack capacity (section 2)

1. For the purposes of the Act, an adult lacks capacity in relation to a matter if at the material time he is unable to make a decision for himself in relation to the matter because of an impairment of, or a disturbance in the functioning of, the mind or brain.
2. It does not matter whether the impairment or disturbance is permanent or temporary.
3. A lack of capacity cannot be established merely by reference to a person's age or appearance, or a condition of his, or an aspect of his behaviour, which might lead others to make unjustified assumptions about his capacity.
4. In proceedings under this Act, any question whether a person lacks capacity within the meaning of the Act must be decided on the balance of probabilities.

Inability to make decisions (section 3)

1. For the purposes of section 2, a person is unable to make a decision for himself if he is unable:
   - to understand the information relevant to the decision
   - to retain that information
   - to use or weigh that information as part of the process of making the decision, or
   - to communicate his decision (whether by talking, using sign language or any other means).
2. A person is not to be regarded as unable to understand the information relevant to a decision if he is able to understand an explanation of it to him in a way that is appropriate to his circumstances (using simple language, visual aids or any other means).
3. The fact that a person is able to retain the information relevant to a decision for a short period only does not prevent him from being regarded as able to make the decision.
4. The information relevant to a decision includes information about the reasonably foreseeable consequences of (a) deciding one way or another, or (b) failing to make the decision.

11.6 Record keeping

Accurate, contemporaneous record keeping is a fundamental recommendation for healthcare professionals and forms an essential component of the accountability for child protection and the protection of vulnerable adults. It is these records that will be used in any multi-agency functioning.

It is essential that the following are accurately documented:

- Date, time and location of presentation.
- Name and professional details of any referring party if relevant.
- Name and relationship status of any accompanying person.
- History from child or vulnerable person and their carers (if appropriate).
- Description of the location of the injury, including diagrams. Figures 11.3, 11.4 and 11.5 show examples of useful body diagrams that may be used by dental professionals.
- Size and shape of the injury. Photographs with appropriate scales included (ABFO no. 2 rigid right-angled scale) will be especially important, but these are normally professionally taken once the child or vulnerable person has been referred to

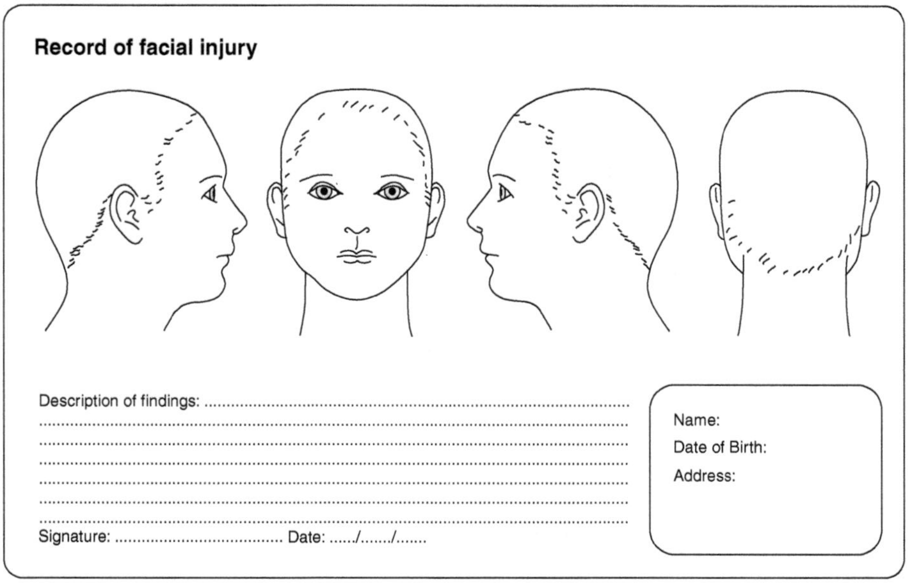

Figure 11.3 Recording facial injury. Courtesy of Ruth Bowen, Medical Illustrator, Cardiff University

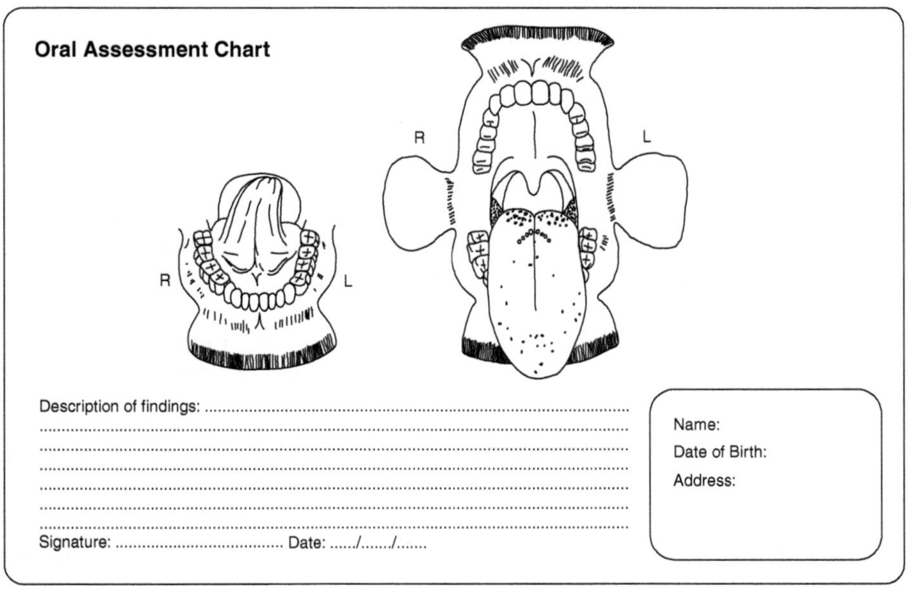

Figure 11.4 An oral assessment chart. Courtesy of Ruth Bowen, Medical Illustrator, Cardiff University

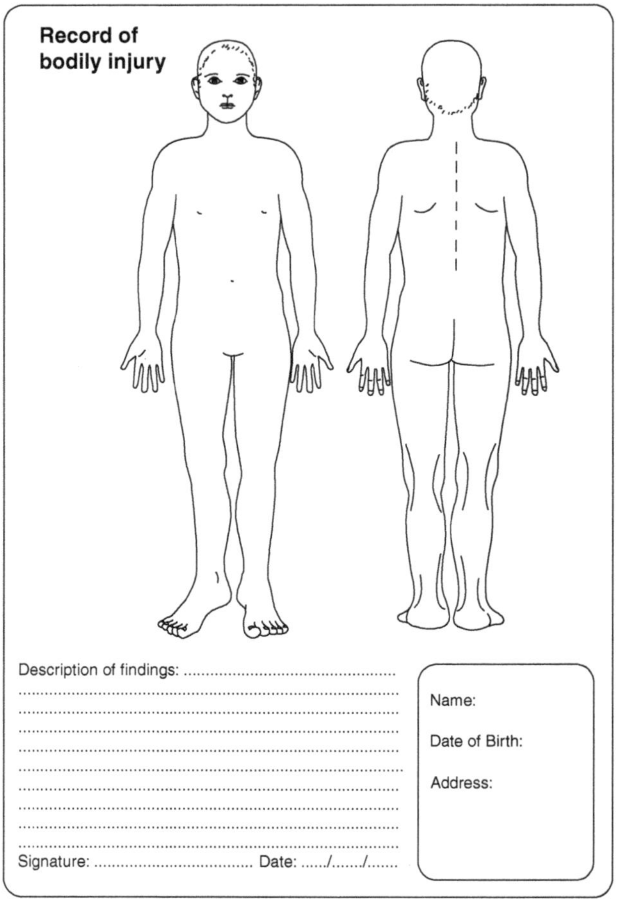

Record of bodily injury

Description of findings: ....

Signature: .... Date: ....../......./.......

Name:

Date of Birth:

Address:

Figure 11.5 Recording bodily injury. Courtesy of Ruth Bowen, Medical Illustrator, Cardiff University

the appropriate safeguarding team. It must be remembered that dental, oral and bite mark injuries should be photographed by experienced, appropriately trained clinical photographers.

- Observations relating to the behaviour, presentation and comments made by the accompanying person(s).

Further information will be taken by the forensic dentist and these are detailed elsewhere.

11.7 Summary chart

A summary of the actions to be taken when suspecting abuse or neglect in children and vulnerable adults may be seen in Figure 11.6.

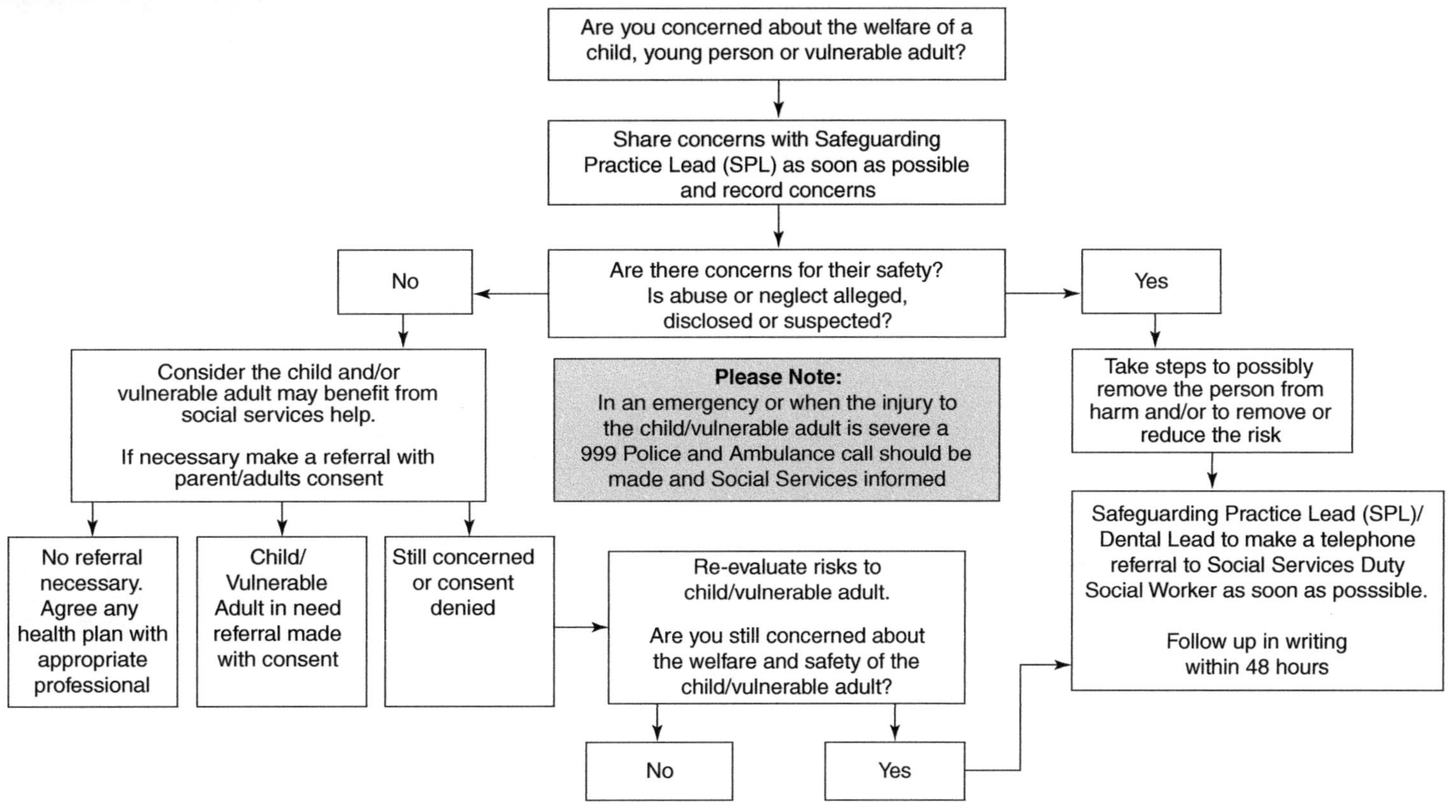

Figure 11.6 Safeguarding vulnerable groups flowchart. Courtesy of Ruth Bowen, Medical Illustrator, Cardiff University

11.8 Further reading

United kingdom

- Child protection and the dental team (www.cpdt.org.uk/index.htm)
- When to suspect child maltreatment – NICE clinical guideline 89, 2009 (www.nice.org.uk/CG89)

Scotland

- Child protection (www.scotland.gov.uk/Topics/People/Young-People/children-families/17834

Wales

- Safeguarding in dental practice – adults and children (www.wales.nhs.uk /sitesplus/888/page/54347)
- Child protection (www.core-info.cardiff.ac.uk)

Northern Ireland

- Child protection (www.dhsspsni.gov.uk/child_protection)

11.9 References

American Academy of Paediatric Dentistry (AAPD). *Definition of Dental Neglect.* Available at www.aapd.org/media/Policies_Guidelines/D_DentalNeglect.pdf (accessed: 14 March 2012).

Balmer R. C., Gibson E. and Harris J. (2010) Understanding child neglect, *Current Perspectives in Dentistry: Primary Dental Care* **17**: 105–109.

Carlile Review (2002) *Review of Safeguards for Children and Young people Treated and Cared for by the NHS in Wales.* Available at www.wales.nhs.uk/publications/ English_text.pdf.

Department of Health (1994) *An Oral Health Strategy for England*. London: DH.

Harris J., Sidebottom P., Welbury R. *et al.* (2006) *Child Protection and the Dental Team: An Introduction to Safeguarding Children in Dental Practice*. Sheffield: Committee of Postgraduate Dental Deans and Directors. Available at www.cpdt.org.uk.

Harris J., Balmer R. C. and Sidebotham P. D. (2009) British Society of Paediatric Dentistry: a policy document on dental neglect in children. *International Journal of Paediatric Dentistry* 14 May 14. [Online]. Doi: 10.1111/j.1365-263X.2009.00996.x.

HM Government. The Children's Act 1989. London: The Stationary Office 1989.

HM Government (2006) *Working Together to Safeguard Children: A Guide to Inter-Agency Working to Safeguard and Promote the Welfare of Children*. London: The Stationery Office. Available at www.everychildmatters.gov.uk (accessed: 15 December 2011).

Lader D., Chadwick B., Chestnutt I. *et al.* (2004) *Children's Dental Health in the United Kingdom, 2003: Summary Report*. London: Office of National Statistics.

Laming L. (2003) *The Victoria Climbié Inquiry: Report of an Inquiry by Lord Laming*. London: The Stationery Office.

National Collaborating Centre for Women's and Children's Health (2009) *When to Suspect Child Maltreatment*. London: RCOG Press.

National Society for the Prevention of Cruelty to Children (2012) *Prevalence and Incidence of Child Abuse and Neglect.* Available at www.nspcc.org.uk/Inform/research/statistics/prevalence_and_incidence_of_child_abuse_and_neglect_wda48740.html (accessed: 5 January 2012).

NHS Dental Epidemiology Programme for England – Oral Health Survey of 5 year old Children 2007 / 2008. Accessed 5 January 2012. URL: http://www.nwph.net/dentalhealth/reports/NHS_DEP_for_England_OH_Survey_5yr_2007-08_Report.pdf

Sheiham A. (2006) Dental caries affects body weight, growth and quality of life in preschool children, *British Dental Journal* **201**: 625–626.

Shepherd M. A., Nadanovsky P. and Sheiham A. (1999) The prevalence and impact of dental pain in 8-year-old school children in Harrow, England, *British Dental Journal* **187**: 38–41.

Slade G. D., Spencer J., Davies M. J. *et al.* (1996) Intra-oral distribution and impact of caries experience among South Australian schoolchildren, *Australian Dental Journal* **41**: 343–350.

United Nations High Commissioner for Human Rights. United Nations Convention on the Rights of the Child. Geneva, Switzerland: Office of the United Nations High Commissioner for Human Rights, 1989 [WWW document]. (accessed 15 December 2011). URL: http://www2.ohchr.org/english/law/crc.htm

Index

References to images are given in *italic* type, references to tables are given in **bold** type.

A London Borough Council v K, 46
abrasion
  skin, 173
  teeth, 102–3
abuse
  neglect, *see* neglect
  physical, 278
  see also children; vulnerable adults
Adobe Photoshop, 217, 265
adolescents, 146–8, 150–151
age assessment, 2–3, 68, 102
  accuracy, 141–5
  adults, 151
  apical translucent zone, 152
  biomarkers, 153
  children and adolescents, 146–8, 150–151
  chronological age, 138–9
  dental age, 139–40
  disaster victims, 131
  importance of, 137–8
  infants, 69–70, 149–50
    neonatal, 148–9
  invasive, 141
  non-invasive, 140–141
  post-mortem comparative identification, 72–3
  pulp ratio, 15, 25
  report writing, 153–5
amelodentinal junction (ADJ), 19
amelogenesis, 19–20
amelogenins, 19
American Board of Forensic Odontology, 84–5, 204
Anatomical Pathology Technologists, 49, 54–6
  responsibilities, 55–6
  training and qualifications, 55
ante-mortem data collection, 78–80
  disaster identification, 130
  radiography, 88–9
appliances, dental *see* dental appliances
archiving, 250
Association of Anatomical Pathology Technology (AAPT), 54
asylum seekers, 137
Atlas of the Mouth, 145
ATOS II scanner, 259
Auld, Lord Justice Robin, 26

babies *see* infants
Bengston's stages, *144*
biomarkers, 153
bite mark analysis, 167
  anatomical location, 170–171, 174
  assessment, 212–14
  biological comparison, 188
  bite mark incidence, 174
  class characteristics, 192–3, 212–13
  dentition and mouth parts, 167–9

Forensic Odontology: An Essential Guide, First Edition.
Edited by Catherine Adams, Romina Carabott and Sam Evans.

bite mark analysis (*continued*)
dentition prediction, 196–8
evidence collection, 211–2
feature-based analysis, 194–201, 214
causal dentition prediction, 196–7
comparative, 198–200
dental casts, 198–9
for identification, reliability, 1–2
individual characteristics, 192
limitations, 204–7
mark distortion, 174–8
primary, 175–6
secondary, 177–8
see also photography, distortion
nature of injury, 172–3
open and closed populations, 218–19
photography, 185–8, 185–90, 195–6, 223–6, *304*
images for superimposition, 245–7
magnification ratios, 240
physical comparison, 191–4, 214–17
metric and non metric, 192–3
reliability, 204–5
reporting, 202–3, 220–221
self-biting, 174, 278–9
severity, 171, 2
skin, 169–71
suspect exclusion, 201, 217–18
suspect inclusion, 201–2
tissue damage, 173
transparent overlays, 191–2, 216–17
uniqueness of dentition, 179–84
interpretation, 182–4
representation, 180–182
vulnerable people, 278–9
wax casting, 216
bleaching trays, 99
blur removal, 270
bone morphogenic proteins (BMP), 13
Bosnian war, 137
Boxing Day tsunami, 1, 3, 3–4, 120
DVI process, 120–121
brassières, 176
breasts, 176, *177*, *304*
brightness adjustment, 269
British Association for Forensic Odontology, 125
British and Irish Legal Information Institute, 41
Brown, Simon Dennis, Baron Brown, 46
bruising, 170, 173
Bryant v State of Florida, 272

calcined material, 77
calcium, 21
cameras, 224
maintenance, 234
stereoscopic, 261
canine teeth, 73
distance between, 168, 198–9, 212–13
tooth marks, 168
Canon, 224
caries, 279, 282
catenary curve, 168
Cell Rests of Mallassez, 17
cementoblasts, 17
cementocytes, 17
cementum formation, 17
cervical loop, 12
charting systems, 85–7
cheek retractors, 243
chemical, biological, radiological and nuclear (CBRN) threats, 2
Child Dental Health Survey, 281–2
Child Protection and the Dental Team website, 286
children, 170
abuse by carers, 277–8, 279
age assessment, 147–8
Demirjian's method, 150–151
bite marks, 174, 198
court rules, 27
neglect, 281–3
identification, 284–6
response, 286
parental response, 284
record-keeping, 291–2
Children Act, 1989/2004, 287
chronological age, 138–9
circuit judge, **41**

civil court proceedings, 26–7
  contempt, 47
Clarke, Anthony, Baron Clarke, 120
cleaning, 60–61
clinical examination, 285
  age assessment, 154
  bite mark suspects, 187–8
clinical waste, 61
closed disasters, 117
clothing, 59–62
colour charts, 230–231, 254, *306*
computed tomography, 93, 132, *133*
cone-beam computed tomography (CBCT), 93
conflict (of interest) statement, 36
contempt of court, 47
contrast adjustment, 269
Control of Substances Hazardous to Health Regulations (COSHH), 57, 60
Cornelia de Lange syndrome, 278–9
Coroners, 68, 130
  tooth extraction, 109
Court of Appeal, 47
court proceedings
  criminal, 26–7
  evidence presentation, 36–41
    cross-examination, 37–8
  forms of address, 40–41, **41**
  perjury, 47
  rules of, 26
craniofacial superimposition, 107
criminal court proceedings, 27
  perjury, 47
criminal responsibility, 138
cross-examination, 37–8
cross-polarised photography, 253–6
crown stage, 13–14

date of birth, 137
Daubert v Merrell Dow Pharmaceuticals, 205
deciduous teeth, 104, 131, 140
declaration of awareness, 35–6
declaration of compliance, 35
decontamination, 60–61
degree courses, 5–6
Demirjian's age assessment, 150–151
dental age, 139–40
dental appliances, 93–7
  bleaching trays, 99
  denture marking, 97–9
  fixed prostheses, 99–100
dental arches, 168
dental basement membrane, 13
dental casts, 94–5
  bite mark analysis, 198–9
dental development *see* tooth development
dental follicle, 11
dental identification, 2–3
  age estimation, 68
  ante-mortem data collection, 78–80
    radiography, 88–9
  comparative
    post-mortem examination, 70–76
    problems, 85–7
    reconciliation, 80–5, 130–132
  craniofacial superimposition, 107
  dental appliances, 94–7
  incinerated remains, 77
  radiography, 87–9
  without presumptive identification, 67–8
Dental Identification Manager (DIM), 121
dental lamina, 9, 9–10
dental materials, 77
  see also fillings
dental models, 94–5
dental papilla, 110
dental profiling
  dental restorations, 106
  ethnicity, 101–2
  facial reconstruction, 106–7
  gender, 101
  habits, 102–3
  isotope and trace element analysis, 105–6
dental radiography, 2
dental records, 2, 78–9, **79**, 125–7
  digital, 87
  reconciliation, 130–131

dental restorations, 106, 168–9
dentine
 intertubular, 16
 intratubular, 16
 mantle, 15–16
 primary, 16
dentinogenesis, 14–16
dentures, 97–9
Department for Work and Pensions, 57
dermis, 170
development of teeth *see* tooth development
developmental tooth anomalies, 103
Diplomates Reference Manual, 56
disaster management, 118–19
Disaster Victim Identification, 117
 documentation, 122–5
  dental records, 125–7
 equipment, 132–4
 planning, 119–20
 post-mortem examination, 127–9
 team morale, 135
 team structure, 121
disinfectants, 60, **61**
dissection techniques, 57
district judge, **41**
DNA analysis, bite marks, 188
DNA tests, 72, 107–10
documentation
 Disaster Victim Identification, 122–5
 see also dental records
dynamic (bite mark) distortion, 175

ectomesenchyme, 9
edentulous individuals, 97–9
edge enhancement, 269
elderly people, 170
electromagnetic spectrum, 250–251, *309*
emergency mortuaries, 49–50
ENAM gene, 19–20
enamel, 107–8
 aprismatic, 20
 biomineralisation, 20–21
 interprismatic, 20
enamel epithelia, 12
enamel formation, 14
enamel knot, 13
enamelin, 19–20
epidermis, 169
epithelial band, primary *see* primary epithelial band
epithelium, 18
equipment, Disaster Victim Identification Team, 132–4
eruption, 131, 140, *144*, 150
ethnicity, 101–2
 dental age and, 139
evidence, 23–4
 collection, 211–12
 documentary, 24
 oral testimony, 24
 real, 24
 see also expert evidence and witnesses
evidence-in-chief, 37
excision, 91
expert evidence and witnesses, 24–5, 25
 acting as a single joint expert, 43–4
 addressing the court, 40–41
 admissibility of evidence, 206
 bite mark analysis, 204–7, 220–221
 contempt and perjury, 47
 evidence at court, 36–41
  cross-examination, 37–8
  evidence-in-chief, 37
  questioning, 38–40
  re-examination, 38
 expert's duties, 28–30
  overriding, 29
  report writing, 30–31
 experts' meetings, 42–3
 feedback, 44–5
 misconduct, 46–7
 negligence, 45–6
 report writing, 30–36
 role in court proceedings, 25–6
 rules of court and, 26
 wasted-costs orders, 47
 written questions, 42
extraction forceps, 72

facial dissection, 57
facial reconstruction, 106–7, 130
facial trauma, 66

familial dysautonomia, 279
family court proceedings, 26, 28
Family Law Week, 41
Family Procedure Rules, 2010, 27, 31–2
feedback, 44–5
fetal material, 69–70
fibroblast growth factors, 13, 15, 18
fillings, 74, *75*, *300*
  see also dental materials
fixed prostheses, 99–100
flash devices, 228–9, 243
fluorosis, 103–4
forceful feeding, 277
forms of address, 40–41

gender, 101
geometric restoration, 270
greyscale linearisation, 270
Guide for Good Practice in Bite Mark Investigation and Analysis, 223

hand-washing, 59
Handyscan VIU, 259
health and safety, 57–61
  personal protective equipment, 60
Health and Safety Executive, 57
hearsay rules, 25
Hedgehog (Hh) signals, 13
Hertwig's Epithelial Root Sheath (HERS), 16–17
high court judges, **41**
histo-differentiation, 11
histogram stretching, 269
hot tubbing, 42–3
Human Tissue Act, 50–51, 71, 73
  licence issue requirements, 51–2
hydroxyapatite (HAp), 20
hygiene, 59
hypodermis, 170

identification
  bite mark, *see* bite mark analysis
  dental, *see* dental identification
  methods, 66–7
  necessity of, 65–6, 117–18
Ikarian Reefer, 28–9
image enhancement, 264–9
  case law, 271–3
  guidelines, 269–71
image files
  downloading, 247–9
  formats, 231–5, *313*
  restoration, 270
  storage, 249–50
imaging, 125, 134
  three-dimensional *see* three-dimensional imaging
  see also photography
immunisation, 62
incinerated remains, 68–9, 77
  dental materials, 77
incisor teeth, 73, 212
  tooth marks, 168
infants, 69–70
  neonatal, 148–9
  skin bruising, 170
infection hazards, 58–9, **58**
infectious agents, 54
infrared photography, 252–3, *314*
inner enamel epithelium, 12
Innocence Project, 1
instruments, 60–61
inter-canine distance, 168, 198–9, 212–13
International Organisation of Forensic Odonto-Stomatology, 4–5
Interpol Forms, 74, 84, 122–5, *302*
intratubular dentine, 16
isotope and trace element analysis, 105–6

jaw resection, 56–7, 57
Jones v Kaney, 45–6
JPEG file format, 232
Judiciary of England and Wales, 41

Kennedy v State of Florida, 272

laceration, 173
Lactobacillus, **58**
laser scanners, 256–7
  handheld, 258
Lassa fever, **58**
lenses 225–8, *227*, 243

Lesh-Nyhan syndrome, 278–9
Lieca ScanStation, 262–3
Lollia Paulina, 1
London Mass Fatality Plan, 49–50
love bites, 171
LucisPro, 271–2

magistrates, **41**
Management of Health and Safety at Work Regulations, 57
mandibular arch, 194
Manning v King's College Hospital NHS Trust, 40
mantle dentine, 15
Marchioness disaster, 120–121
mass fatalities, 1
  see also Disaster Victim Identification
matrix proteins, 20–21
MAVIS camera, 261
maxillary arch, 168, 194
memory cards, 235
Mental Capacity Act, 2005, 289–90
mental status, 172
Merton Age Compliance Guidelines, 138
micro-reciprocal-degree (MIRED) shift, 254
mirrors, 243, *244*
misconduct, 46–7
mitochondrial DNA, 108
mobile phones, 226
molar teeth, 72, 107
  for DNA analysis, 108
Moorees' stages
  double-rooted teeth, *143*
  root resorption, *144*
  single-rooted teeth, *142*
morpho-differentiation, 11
mortuaries
  disaster areas, 117, 118–19
  equipment, 54
  health and safety, 57–8
    cleaning and decontamination, 60–61
    immunisation, 62
  layout, 52–4, *53*, *99*
    clean areas, 53
    dirty areas, 53–4
  permanent, 49
  safe working practices, 58–9
  specimen transport, 54
  see also Anatomical Pathology Technologists
multi-detector computed tomography (MDCT), 132, *133*
multi-slice computed tomography (MSCT), 4, 93
multiple-fatality incidents, 117–18
Mycobacterium tuberculosis, **58**

National Institute for Health and Clinical Excellence (NICE), 279
neglect, 279–86, 282
  identification, 284–6
  response, 286
negligence, 45–6
Neilsen, Keiser, 1
New Zealand Disaster Victim Identification team, 3
Nikon, 224
noise removal, 269
non-amelogenins, 19–20

occupational tooth abrasion, 102–3
odontoblasts, 14
  differentiation, 14, *16*
  matrix secretion, 16
odontogenesis *see* tooth development
Odontogenic Homeobox Code, 19
odontogenic keratocysts, 14
odontoscopy, 191–2
old age, 170
open disasters, 117
oral assessment chart, 290, *291*
oral health, 280
oral testimony, 24
orthodontics, 126
outer enamel epithelium, 12
overlays, 191–2, 216–17
overriding duties, 29

pain, 282
palatal rugae, 95–6
particular duties, 29–30
Pearce v Ove Arup, 29

People v Perez, 272
perjury, 47
permanent mortuary, 49
permanent teeth, 140
photography
  bite marks, 185–8, 195–6, 223–6
    distortion, correction, 239–40
    photographic filters, 241
    sequences of images, 240–241, *242*
  case law, 271–3
  colour charts, 230–231, 254, *306*
  colour reproduction, 224
  cross-polarised, 253–6
  dentition, 241–3
  depth of field, *312*
  distortion
    correction, 176–8, 196, 239–40
    minimisation, 235–9
  equipment, 243
    cameras, 224
    flash devices, 228–9
    lenses, 225–8, *227*
    mobile phones, 226
    preparation, 234–5
  image files
    downloading, 247–9
    enhancement, 264–9
    formats, 231–5
    guidelines, 269–71
    restoration, 270
    storage, 249–50
  imaging modalities, 250–253
  magnification ratios, 240
  post-mortem dental identification, 71, 74
  scales, 229–30
  superimposition, 245–7, *248*
  three-dimensional, 256–64
    see also three-dimensional imaging
  ultraviolet and infrared, 250–253
  see also images
polarised photography, 253–5
polymerase chain reaction (PCR), 108
post-mortem examination
  dental identification, 70–6
    equipment, 72–3
    photographs, 71, 74
    quality assurance, 74
    radiography, 74–6, 89–91
    tooth cleaning, 71
    tooth removal, 73
  Disaster Victim Identification, 127–9
  Human Tissue Act, 50–51
post-traumatic stress disorder (PTSD), 135
posture distortion, 176
pre-dentine, 14
primary dentine, 16
primary epithelial band, 9, *10*
prime lenses, 225
profiling, *see* dental profiling
Public Prosecutor v Torgerson, 205
pulp ratio, 15, 25

questioning, 38–40

radio-frequency ID (RFID) tags, 98–9
radiography, 87–9, 146
  age assessment, 138, 151–2
  ante-mortem, 87–9
  Disaster Victim Identification, 127–9
  neonatal infants, 148–9
  post-mortem, 89–91
Raja Chandra, 98
RAW image format, 232–3
Re F (Children: DNA Evidence), 32–3
Re M (Adoption: Leave to Oppose), 39
re-examination, 38
reconciliation process, 80–85, 130–132
reconstructive identification *see* dental profiling
record keeping
  child and vulnerable adult protection, 290–291
  see also dental records
refugees, 137
reliability of evidence, 205–6
removable dental appliances, 96–7
report writing, 30–36, 217–18
  age assessments, 153–5
  bite mark analysis, 202–3
  conflict statement, 36

report writing (*continued*)
contents of a report, 31–2
drafting suggestions, 32–4
errors, 33
factual disputes, 33
procedural requirements, 34–6, **34**
declaration of compliance, 35
scope and source of instructions, 36
statements of truth, 34–5
reasoning, 33–4
report length, 33
resection techniques, 56–7
risk assessments, 58–9
root formation, 16–17
root resorption, *144*
Royal Society of Public Health, 54
RP v Nottingham City Council and the Official Solicitor (Mental Capacity of Parent), 25
rules of court, 26–8
Ruxton, Isabella, 107

safe working, 58–9
scales, 237–9
Scientific Working Group Imaging Technology, 270–271
Select Committee on Science and Technology, 232
self-biting, 174, 278–9
sharps, 61
short tandem repeats (STR), 108
signalling events, 18
single joint experts, 43–4
skeletonised remains, 91, 150
skin, 169–71
hypodermis, 170
skull bones, 102
State of Connecticut v Alfred Swinton, 271–2
statements of truth, 35–6
stellate reticulum, 13
stereophotogrammetry, 260–261
stomatodeum, 9, *10*
stratum intermedium, 132
Straumann company, 100
Strengthening Forensic Science in the United States: A Path Forward, 1–2, 206
structured light scanners, 258–9
sucking/suckling, 169
Supreme Court, 45–6
suspect exclusion, 201

technical explanations, 39
tetracycline staining, 105, *301*
three-dimensional imaging, 4, 256–63
computed tomography, 93
TIF image format, 232
time-of-flight scanners, 262
time-related tissue distortion, 176
tissue (bite mark) distortion, 175
Tome's Process, 20
tongue, 169
tooth anomalies, 103
tooth decay, 279, 281–3
parental response, 284
tooth development, 140, *303*
amelogenesis, 19–20
dentinogenesis, 14–16
early life, 9–13
bud stage, 9–10
early bell stage, 13
epithelial/mesenchymal interactions, 17–18
later life, 13–14
crown stage, 13–14
late bell stage, 13–14
Moorees' stages, *142–4*
morpho- and histo- differentiation, 11–12
schemas, 145–6
tooth placement, 19
tooth root formation, 16–17
tooth eruption, 131, 140, *144*, 150
tooth extraction, 108
tooth germs, 9
tooth marks, 168–9
tooth preservation, 152
touch probe scanners, 262
training, 4–6
transcription factors, 18

transforming growth factor beta (TGFβ), 18
Trauma Risk Management (TRiM), 135
triangulation laser scanners, 256–7
twins, 179

ultraviolet (UV) photography, 252–3, *300*, *314*
uniqueness of dentition, 179–84
United Kingdom Border Agency, 146
United Nations Convention on the Rights of the Child, 146, 287–8

vestibular lamina, 9
Vivid 910 laser scanner, 257
Voluntary Registration Council, 54–5
vulnerable people, 288–90
  bite mark analysis, 278–9
  confidentiality, 289–90
  decision-making capacity, 290

Wall, Sir Nicholas, 30
warping, 270
waste disposal, 61
wasted-costs orders, 47
Woolf, Harry, Baron Woolf, 26
written questions, 42

X-ray fluorescence spectroscopy, 77
X-ray units, 3–4, 76, 91, 134

yes/no answers, 39

zoom lenses, 225

www.ingramcontent.com/pod-product-compliance
Ingram Content Group UK Ltd.
Pitfield, Milton Keynes, MK11 3LW, UK
UKHW051035091026
15624UKWH00011B/438

9 781119 9